PSYCHOTHERAPY OF ADDICTED PERSONS

Psychotherapy of Addicted Persons

EDWARD KAUFMAN

Foreword by
Edward J. Khantzian

THE GUILFORD PRESS
New York   London

© 1994 The Guilford Press
A Division of Guilford Publications, Inc.
72 Spring Street, New York, NY 10012

Printed in the United States of America

This book is printed on acid-free paper.

Last digit is print number: 9 8 7 6 5 4 3 2 1

Library of Congress Cataloging-in-Publication Data
Kaufman, Edward.
    Psychotherapy of addicted persons / Edward Kaufman.
       p.   cm.
    Includes bibliographical references and index.
    ISBN 0-89862-116-X
    1. Substance abuse—Treatment.   2. Psychodynamic
psychotherapy.   I. Title.
    [DNLM: 1. Substance Dependence—psychology.
    2. Psychotherapy—methods. WM 270 K21p 1994]
    RC564.K379 1994
    616.86′ 0651—dc20
    DNLM/DLC
    for Library of Congress   94-8644
                                        CIP

Foreword

Addiction develops in context—in the context of a biologic–genetic matrix that leaves individuals at risk before they know or feel their feelings, have their first thoughts, or initiate their first impulse or independent act or action; in the context of families who already are in part or whole enmeshed in addictive substances or addictive behaviors and dysfunction; and in the context of cultures and social settings, in some more so than others. But ultimately alcoholism or addiction occurs predominantly in a personal context; that is, it is a person who is or has become disordered, who uses, abuses, and becomes dependent on substances. Thus, this book is most appropriately titled, *Psychotherapy of Addicted Persons*.

In this volume, Edward Kaufman exhaustively reviews and discusses these contexts that are the underpinnings for the development of addictive disorders, but it is the last context, namely, that of the person or personality factor, that he explores in greatest depth in order to arrive at the main thrust of this book—how to treat addicted individuals in psychotherapy. As Kaufman indicates, there is considerable overlap and co-occurrence of different personality disorders in individuals with substance abuse, and it is more likely that the personality disorder(s) is (are) more indicative of significant dysfunction than any distinct personality type in individuals who suffer with these disorders. Although Kaufman indicates there are individual, social class, and gender differences that we must appreciate, ultimately his review convincingly documents the existence of a more or less disordered, dysfunctional person involved in substance abuse, and suggests that this person (man or woman, socially privileged or underprivileged, over-defended or vulnerable) suffers and is in need of understanding, and benefits from psychotherapeutic treatment. I share with Kaufman the notion that appreciating the nature of the personality disorder or dys-regulated person is critical for understanding the treatment needs of substance abusers, and the modification we must make in techniques (or our treatment approach with our patients) to successfully access and modify what ails and compels them.

Like all good clinician-therapists, Kaufman appreciates the importance of a careful assessment, especially at the outset of treatment. He advocates proceeding on a flexible but appropriately informed basis in order to fine tune and respond to the patient's needs. Kaufman cuts through the negative and counterproductive stereotype of addicts as unengageable and unmotivated. Instead, he matter-of-factly demonstrates that substance abuse patients will commit to the task of therapeutic work, that a bond is formed, and that a therapeutic alliance can be initiated and maintained. Kaufman demonstrates how much of this is accomplished in the nitty-gritty aspects of exploring the patterns of drug/alcohol use, and carefully exploring the severity of psychological and physical dependence. Furthermore, the specifics of the hows and whys of approaching detoxification and achieving abstinence, including appropriate choice of setting, become crucial to building the foundation for subsequent phases of treatment. The reader will also be provided with helpful guidelines in helping patients to work concurrently with Twelve-Step programs and other treatments aimed at achieving and maintaining abstinence.

One of the main strengths of this book is that it offers an integrated approach to the treatment of addicted individuals, an objective that Kaufman is explicit about at the outset. It avoids the pitfalls of previous reports and texts that either focus too narrowly on the disease concept—chemical dependency literature on the one hand—or draw too narrowly on a psychodynamic or psychiatric perspective of addiction as symptom on the other. This is evident in the way he uses descriptive findings (including his own observations from work with his patients) and psychodiagnostic and psychodynamic studies. He describes their relevance to social class and genetic factors, family of origin issues, and personality characteristics; and then helps us to make sense of how all of the above pertains to and is consistent with the chemical dependency literature and the utility, if not necessity, of integrating our clinical paradigms with the practical "step-by-step" benefit and wisdom of Twelve-Step approaches. This is no mean achievement. Others have tried it with mixed results, but Kaufman embraces the task in a more systematic and comprehensive way, this being most evident in his review of how concepts from the Twelve Steps can be used differentially and discriminately in successive phases of therapy to achieve abstinence, human connectedness (or interdependence), and an understanding (i.e., insight) of the self-defeating defenses and character flaws associated with addictive illness. Kaufman also describes explicitly how he integrates cognitive-behavioral concepts used in relapse prevention with a contemporary psychodynamic approach. The latter is based on an appreciation of developmental handicaps and structural deficits that predispose to reliance on substances, and relapse once abstinence has been achieved. Most importantly, Kaufman clearly advocates empathy, timing, patience, and support as mainstays to the psychotherapeutic work, and the techniques employed must allow for the work to take place interchangeably in the contexts of the psychotherapy and Twelve-Step programs. This will depend on patients' needs, their progression, and what recovery expectations can be best sustained and met in which context at what phase of treatment.

Kaufman's openness about his interactions with his patients in the useful case vignettes he provides, and his reflections about what to work on or leave alone in the therapy, and if or when to use the patient's Twelve-Step program, are refreshing, germane, and helpful in demonstrating technique and how the work of psychotherpay and recovery unfolds. Some of the richest, most practical, and most helpful aspects of this book are covered in the chapters on countertransference, interactive issues, and integrating individual therapy with group and family therapy. Again, the author is frank and open about his experiences and preferences, and succeeds in covering complex theoretical and technical issues in clear and comprehensible terms. Kaufman is consistent here, as he is throughout the book, in his commitment to integrating approaches, espousing flexibility that tailors specific combinations to meet each individual's needs. Thus any combination of individual therapy, Twelve-Step work, group therapy, and family treatment might be employed. In some instances, two or more, if not all, might be necessary over time. To quote a former associate (C. Treece), in the case of substance abusers, "more [often] is better," and Kaufman appreciates this well.

Kaufman's book is meritorious in a number of respects, but especially in that it introduces the novice to basic concepts without the burden of jargon or psychobabble; for the more advanced clinician seeking an understanding of theory and practice, it exhaustively reviews the more complex aspects of the theory of substance abuse, and its application for practice, in deceptively clear and useful ways. This book

is scholarly, balanced, and practical. Its integration of multiple perspectives and approaches should serve students and practitioners
very well, and it promises to be an important mainstay as a scholarly reference and practical guide to the treatment of the addicted person.

EDWARD J. KHANTZIAN, M.D.
President, American Academy of Psychiatrists
in Alcoholism and Addictions

Associate Clinical Professor of Psychiatry,
Harvard Medical School at the Cambridge Hospital

Associate Chief of Psychiatry,
Tewksbury Hospital, MA

Preface

My purpose in writing this book is to present a workable, successful, pragmatic method of psychodynamic psychotherapy for persons addicted to drugs and/or alcohol. This method can be utilized by a broad audience of therapists at varying levels of training in psychotherapy and/or substance abuse. I believe that the reason so many practitioners hesitate to treat substance abusers is their failure to utilize such a method.

This therapeutic approach has evolved from my work with substance abusers in a wide variety of settings, dating back to my clinical years in medical school in the late 1950s. The settings that followed included Los Angeles County General Hospital (where I served a rotating internship); Columbia-Presbyterian Medical Center/New York State Psychiatric Institute (where I spent a broad clinical residency, including research in diagnosis and the effects of drugs and detoxification on the sleep-dream cycle); Columbia Psychoanalytic Clinic (where I was taught by Sandor Rado, one of the first theorists in the addictions, and Nathan Ackerman, the father of family therapy); Lewisburg Federal Penitentiary, Pennsylvania (where I served as chief psychiatrist, with about 200 of the 1,000 inmates incarcerated for drug-related offenses); Reality House (where I worked in a full-day program for addicts in New York City's Harlem); St. Luke's Hospital, New York City (where I was director of psychiatric emergency services, with many addicts and alcoholics among the patients); the New York City Prison System (where I was director of prison mental health services — about 80% of the 13,000 inmates had substantial substance abuse problems); the Lower East Side Service Center (where I served as medical director of a program with over 1,000 methadone maintenance patients, a therapeutic community, and seven outpatient programs); the University of California at Irvine (where I was direc-

tor of psychiatric education and a professor of psychiatry, with a focus on teaching and research on addiction and the family); and, lastly
and presently, Capistrano by the Sea Hospital in Dana Point, California (where I am associate medical director for chemical dependency).
In addition to these institutional positions, I have always maintained
a private practice, with a substantial number of my patients having
substance abuse as a primary problem.

The model I am proposing has evolved out of more than 30 years
of trial and error, during which I used the techniques that I learned
in the settings noted above. Thus my major influences include adaptational psychoanalysis; object relations; cognitive-behavioral therapy; methodological research in the psychosocial, psychotherapy and
biomedical areas; structural family therapy; pharmacotherapy; psychodynamic group therapy; the techniques of ex-addicts in the therapeutic community; and the Twelve-Step movement (Alcoholics Anonymous
[AA], Cocaine Anonymous [CA], Narcotics Anonymous [NA], Al-
Anon, etc). I prefer to view my use of these varied therapeutic systems
as a pragmatic, individualized integration, and dislike a label of "eclec-
tic," which does not convey the systematization of my approach. I feel
that I have taken what is most applicable to the treatment of substance
abuse from each of these varying methods of therapy.

The word "pragmatic" has many interesting meanings (*Webster's
Third New International Dictionary,* 1981). These include "skilled in
law or business," "practical," "matter of fact," "dealing with events
in such a manner as to show their interconnections," and "prescribing
the means necessary to the attainment of happiness" (p. 178). I hope
that by the end of this book, the reader will agree that pragmatic psychodynamic psychotherapy for addicted persons meets all of these defi-
nitions.

I have chosen to use the term "addicted persons" in the title because of the recent return to popularity of the word "addicition," as
used in addiction medicine and addiction psychiatry. In this book the
term "addictive disorder" is synonymous with "addiction," "substance
dependence," "psychoactive substance dependence," and "chemical dependence." Severe substance abuse that falls short of addiction is essentially handled in the same manner, as it is so often a final step before
full substance dependence. In the text the acronym SA is used for "substance abuser." It may be used to denote a drug addict, an alcoholic,
or a serious abuser of psychoactive substances.

My discussion of addictive disorders is limited to disorders involving psychoactive substances. I do not deal separately with other com-
pulsions that have been termed "addictions," such as inordinate cravings
for gambling, sex, food, love, relationships, work and exercise. These

compulsive or, if you will, addictive behaviors play a critical role in every SA's problems, from the onset of the illness to addiction and recovery. Thus, they are discussed as an integral part of every SA's treatment, but not as addictive disorders per se.

I hope to reach a wide audience, including alcoholism counselors, recovering addict therapists, social workers, psychologists, addiction medicine practitioners, psychiatrists, and psychoanalysts. Some readers may find a section too elementary or another too complex to understand. Other readers may take the reverse view of the complexity and relevance of the same two sections. My hope, however, is that all readers will be stimulated by the systematic integration of several methods of therapy, as well as by the illustrative case histories. Thus, perhaps, addiction therapists will learn how to utilize psychodynamic constructs more effectively in understanding and treating SAs, and psychoanalysts will learn how to incorporate the Twelve Steps and the tools of sobriety into their treatment.

The chapters that follow provide the details necessary for understanding and treating SAs with pragmatic psychodynamic psychotherapy.

Chapter 1 focuses on the personality, psychopathology, and psychodynamics of SAs in general and male SAs in particular. This knowledge is one of the cornerstones of my method of psychotherapy. The others are defense mechanisms; the therapist's knowledge of self (countertransference); a three-stage method of psychotherapy; and an integration with Twelve-Step groups, group therapy, and family therapy. Even this chapter on psychodynamics draws from a broad-based literature and observational viewpoints. Thus, a topic such as drug of choice is examined from the perspectives of family systems, gender, social pressures, and substance availability as well as psychodynamics. I have chosen to write a separate chapter on female SAs (Chapter 2) because of the specific gender-related psychological issues and needs for treatment of women. For all too long, female SAs were lumped together with males.

Fortunately, over the past 20 years, rapidly emerging research findings have focused on the special needs and issues of female SAs. These issues are perhaps more important in women than in men, because their use of substances is much more closely related to such psychodynamic issues as incest, abuse, illness, and loss.

The need for an entire chapter on defense mechanisms (Chapter 3) could be questioned. My decision to enter the field of psychiatry was influenced greatly by my fascination with Anna Freud's (1966) *The Ego and the Mechanisms of Defense,* which I read as a medical student. I also found the concept that recovering persons require con-

solidation and support of certain aspects of defenses—even denial—
in the early phases of therapy a very helpful one (Wallace, 1985). In
Chapter 3, various defense mechanisms are discussed from several
different frameworks. In addition to Anna Freud's classic defense
mechanisms, newer concepts of defenses, such as splitting and projective identification, are extremely helpful in the therapy of SAs. These
defenses are peeled away during the latter phases of therapy—a process
that is facilitated by AA and other Twelve-Step groups. The first of
four major case histories is introduced here as illustrative of the
relevance of defense mechanisms, as well as of personality disorders
in (see Chapter 4).

A separate chapter on personality disorders (Chapter 4) is included,
because these account for very critical aspects of the behavior attributed
to SAs. The three major personality disorders most commonly seen
in SAs are examined: antisocial, narcissistic, and borderline. Passive
aggressive personality disorder, and other personality disorders and
traits, are also briefly discussed. The literature on the psychodynamics and treatment of personality disorders is reviewed and specifically
applied to SA's.

Chapters 5, 6, and 7 describe the method of psychotherapy in three
phases, which in the chemical dependence field would be labeled: (1)
achieving abstinence, (2) early recovery (sobriety), and (3) advanced
recovery. More psychodynamically, they would be termed (1) the therapeutic contract, (2) cognitive-behavioral skills training, and (3) work
on autonomy and intimacy (learning to work and to love). In each
of these three chapters, the role of psychodynamic aspects in assessment and in phase-appropriate treatment is delineated. The role of AA
and similar groups is also discussed, as well as the steps that are specifically focused on in each phase. One specific case is followed in detail as his therapy is traced throughout the three phases.

Thus Chapter 5 describes evaluation, motivation, detoxification,
involvement of the family and social network, developing a method
for abstinence, and delineating a workable treatment contract. In this
phase, the therapist is at first a confronter (to motivate the patient to
enter treatment), then a supporter and educator. Phase 1 ends when
the patient has been discharged from the hospital or other intensive
treatment setting, and the treatment contract has been developed and
mutually agreed upon.

Chapter 6, which covers Phase 2, focuses on methods for maintaining a drug- and alcohol-free state. The term "sobriety" not only
includes abstinence from all abusable substances, but implies a dedi-
cation to growth and self-awareness. Here the primary approach is
cognitive-behavioral, supportive, and psychoeducational. Relapse

prevention strategies are taught and practiced, so that the patient can develop a variety of coping techniques. Part of the educational process is the recognition of affects—the situations that provoke them, their relationship to relapse, their psychodynamic significance, and their appropriate expression. Other psychodynamic issues are explored, but the need for the patient to maintain a sober core is always kept in mind. Thus any issues that severely threaten sobriety are labeled as such and postponed until sobriety is more stable (Phase 3). Phase 2 generally requires from 6 months to several years.

Chapter 7 describes Phase 3, which includes the achievement of more standard analytic goals: the ability to love in an intimate way, self-sufficiency in work and creativity, and the achievement of relaxing, pleasurable leisure skills. With continued emphasis on the sober core, any method of deep insight-oriented psychotherapy can be used in this phase. Several major themes are worked on in this phase; these include grief, childhood trauma, transference-countertransference resolutions, relinquishing narcissistic entitlement (and other characterological issues), healthy self-care and achieving intimacy. Here the case history described in Chapters 5–7 is brought to termination of therapy.

Chapter 8 develops the concept of countertransference, from the early psychoanalytic view through object relations and interpersonal approaches. Thus there is a focus on the therapist's role in transference and countertransference, as well as on the substantial value of interactional methods to create change, particularly in personality-disordered SAs. Specific types or aspects of countertransference that are discussed include objective versus subjective countertransference; positive and negative countertransference; empathy; idealization; gender-related issues; and projective counteridentification. Related phenomena are also described, such as parallel process; therapist codependence, denial, enabling, and burnout; and therapist family-of-origin issues. These generally disparate concepts are synthesized into a phase-related utilization of countertransference in order to enhance understanding and facilitate change. A third case history is presented here; this one demonstrates the patient's splitting and projective identification, as well as the therapist's projective counteridentification and utilization of countertransference.

Chapters 9 and 10 focus on the integration of group and family therapy with the proposed individual therapy model. Prior to the utilization of the type of integrated model that I am proposing, group therapy was considered the treatment of choice for SAs. In the present book, it is viewed as one among several essential modalities in providing a comprehensive approach. A phase-related model of group therapy for SAs is presented in Chapter 9; multiple-family and couples group treat-

ment are also described here. The final chapter, on the integration of
individual and family therapy, uses a fourth case history, but in this
case (unlike the preceding ones) the patient describes her own view
of the treatment process. My previously described method of family
therapy is summarized here, as is the integration of family therapy into
the overall method. A synthesis of several family therapy approaches,
with an emphasis on structural and psychodynamic family techniques,
is presented.

Contents

Personality, Psychopathology, and Psychodynamics of Addicted Persons

A clearer dichotomy exists in the field of substance abuse treatment than in the treatment of any other major diagnostic category. On one side are chemical dependence counselors, physicians recovering from drug and alcohol abuse, and dedicated members of Alcoholics Anonymous (AA) and other Twelve-Step groups. On the other extreme are psychoanalytically trained therapists who regard substance abuse essentially as a symptom of underlying psychological conflict. Many if not most members of the former group have had misfired attempts at psychotherapy with the latter group, and hence are prejudiced against it. Years later, sober as a result of Twelve-Step work, they are quite critical of therapists who let them drink or use drugs and deteriorate for years before they became sober. More recently, many substance abusers (SAs) have been helped to achieve sobriety and happiness by increasing numbers of psychodynamic therapists. These therapists have learned to integrate a variety of psychotherapeutic approaches with the Twelve Steps, while maintaining the importance of an understanding of the unique psychodynamics of each patient. This chapter summarizes the wide variety of schools of thought that are helpful in achieving a full understanding of the psychology of SAs.

Early psychodynamic studies of SAs viewed them as a homogeneous group, with little if any understanding of the many different types of individuals involved. Early studies in this century focused mainly on males who abused or were dependent on alcohol. Later studies in the 1950s focused on male heroin addicts. Until the 1980s, few distinctions were made between many different types of SAs. Even obvious distinctions, such as those between drug addicts and alcoholics, men and women, older SAs and teenagers, those who abused and those who were addicted, and those who chose stimulants and those who preferred sedatives, were not made. In the last decade, much work has been done to recognize and refine the differences and similarities between the many types of SAs.

SAs have many different behavioral and personality characteristics, some of which are relative to the variables described above and some of which are derived from other factors. Yet there are also aspects of personality that seem relevant to the vast majority of SAs, whether they abuse alcohol only, drugs only, or both. We must keep in mind that factors such as age, gender, social class, culture, ethnicity, stage of chemical dependence, and employment level are often more powerful elements in the shaping of personality than the factors governing the choice of a particular substance. Moreover, many of the behavioral differences between alcoholics and drug abusers develop secondarily after the substance-abusing pattern sets in. These differences are attributable in part to the life style factors resulting from the legality of alcohol, as opposed to the illegality, expense, and criminal activities often necessary to obtain drugs such as heroin, cocaine, and amphetamines.

One powerful argument for viewing alcoholics and drug abusers as one group is the widespread use of combinations of the two by SAs. Abuse of multiple substances has been separated into four major groupings (Kaufman, 1977): (1) the abuse of drugs by primary alcoholics and problem drinkers; (2) the abuse of alcohol by primary drug abusers; (3) "polydrug abuse," which is the simultaneous or sequential abuse of alcohol and drugs; and (4) progressive, or "gateway," abuse (see DuPont, 1984). Thus, the usage of drugs by alcoholics and of alcohol by drug abusers is common. The present widespread nature of inextricably woven drug and alcohol abuse compels us to look at both problems together, as well as to attempt to tease them apart.

There is no characteristic personality style that can be called "the addictive personality." However, there are common personality traits, symptoms, and psychodynamic factors that occur in clusters in addicted persons. Interestingly, there are "addictive *personalities*" who can become addicted to almost any substance, from food and caffeinated beverages through over-the-counter drugs to illicit drugs. These individuals also demonstrate addictive propensities to other risk-taking activities (e.g., gambling, motorcycling, skydiving), as well as to exercise, work, relationships, and sex. Although this book deals with the psychotherapy of addicted persons, the major focus, as noted in the Preface, is on those who are addicted to drugs and alcohol. I do not specifically discuss other compulsive behaviors, nor do I deal with the current controversy as to whether these are addictions per se. However, these compulsive behaviors have extremely high comorbidity with substance dependence and often complicate the picture, as many patients shift from drugs to equally destructive behaviors. These behaviors may also lead to conditioned relapse, because they often have been powerfully associated with drugs and alcohol or can lead to stressors such as loss of jobs or relationships, which in turn leave individuals relapse-prone.

Substance abuse and dependence are seen in many different types of individuals with varied personalities and psychiatric diagnoses. The chapters that follow on defense mechanisms (Chapter 3) and personality disorders (Chapter 4) will also help in understanding the psychology of SAs. Finally, similarities and differences between males and females require us to view them both jointly and separately. At intervals throughout this chapter, and in a separate section of this chapter, I discuss specific personality and psychodynamic issues in male SAs. I do the same for female SAs in Chapter 2.

Figure 1.1 provides an overview of the etiological factors that in my opinion, interact to predispose both male and female SAs to substance abuse; Figure 1.2 illustrates various models of how SAs utilize and become addicted to substances of abuse as adults. Figure 1.1 begins with genetics, which can lead to substance abuse directly when parents or other family members are themselves SAs, as well as indirectly through inheritance of temperament, antisocial personality, or depression and/or anxiety. Nine significant childhood experiences and eight adolescent experiences that can lead to substance abuse are then listed. In Figure 1.2, six models of the psychodynamics of substance abuse in adulthood are depicted. In all cases, when substance use grants temporary resolution of psychological wounds or pain, this maladaptive pattern becomes reinforced and addiction results. An integrated psychodynamic model has also been recently proposed by Goldsmith (1993).

PSYCHODYNAMIC THEORIES OF SUBSTANCE DEPENDENCE IN BOTH MALES AND FEMALES

Early theories of substance dependence focused on instincts, drives, the unconscious effects of drugs, and the seeking of drugs for pleasure or self-destruction. In addition, early theories, though purportedly ap-

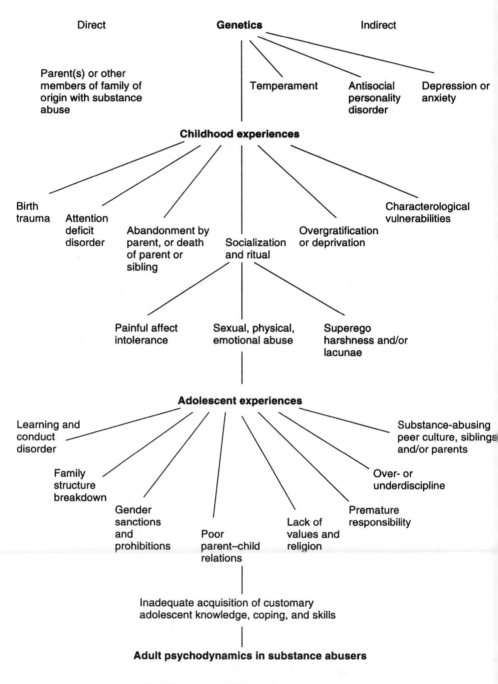

FIGURE 1.1. Childhood antecedents.

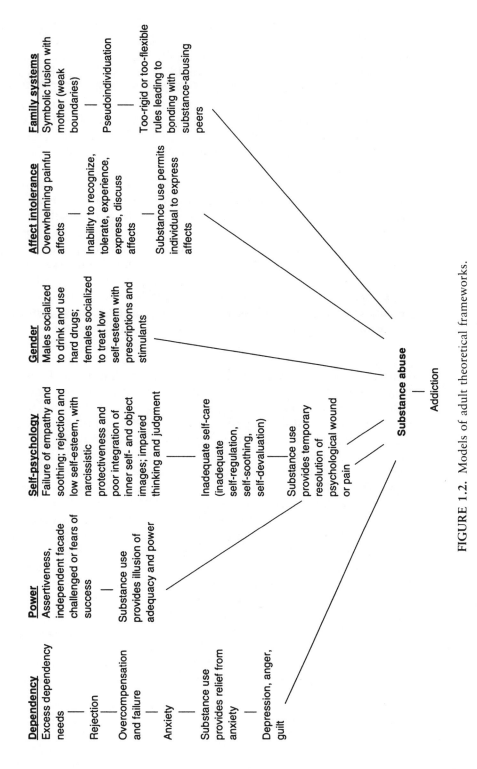

FIGURE 1.2. Models of adult theoretical frameworks.

plicable to both men and women, were in fact based on a male model. Sigmund Freud (1954) in an early letter to Wilhelm Fliess, wrote that masturbation is a primary addiction and that addictions to drugs such as alcohol and morphine are mainly replacements for that primary addiction. Continuing the analogy, Freud stated that masturbation/drug use leads to guilt, anxiety, and diminished self-esteem. Freud postulated that repeated masturbation/drug use occurs to relieve these feelings, and the cycle continues. Addiction has more recently been related to the desire to master the loss of self-esteem resulting from masturbation (Levin, 1987).

A more helpful Freudian concept is that of "repetition compulsion" (1920/1955). This is replayed in SAs' need to use drugs and alcohol repeatedly, to prove they can control their use of these substances. Freud also apparently used cocaine for some time himself in order to augment his own self-esteem, sexual activity, and energy for work, until he encountered difficulty with the drug. Finally, Freud (1928/1961) described addictive gambling as a means of self-punishment for the forbidden wish to masturbate. This may have been the theoretical beginning of the understanding of self-punitive behavior in substance abuse, which is of value today, even though the concept is rooted in Freud's own sexually prohibitive Victorian upbringing.

Rado (1926/1960) was the first psychoanalyst to unite all addictions into one psychodynamic theme, which he termed "pharmacothymia." He stated that chemically dependent persons have an underlying depression that leaves them vulnerable to the rebounding depressant effects of drugs and alcohol, which inevitably follow the initial elation. The compensatory depression leaves SAs even lower in mood than they were before the intoxication. This leads to repeated cycles of milder elation and deepening depression. Rado also equated the power of the early elation to that of a "pharmacogenic orgasm."

Other libidinal theorists (Abraham, 1908/1979; Chein et al., 1964) characterized substance abuse as pleasurable oral regression. Abraham (1908/1979) emphasized a homoerotic component. Fenichel (1945) maintained that men predisposed to becoming addicts or alcoholics react to substances in a specific way: They use the effects of these drugs to satisfy archaic oral longings, which encompass the needs for sex, security, and self-esteem. He hypothesized further that individuals who obtain satisfaction of these needs primarily from drugs cannot have achieved a high level of object relations and are therefore narcissistically fixated. Moreover, he theorized that drugs and alcohol are used to relieve a primitive type of amorphous tension that existed prior to any psychic organization (e.g., the early oral or symbiotic phase).

Of these early libidinal theorists, only Chein et al. (1964) had extensive experience with SAs. Thus, the others applied their existing theories to SAs, rather than developing theories from actual clinical experience with a broad base of substance-abusing patients. Another problem with libidinal theories is their emphasis on the seeking of ecstatic pleasure through drug use; this was representative of a society whose moral condemnation of addicts was based in part on an image of them as pleasure seekers (Khantzian, 1979). Much of the present-day discrimination against SAs in terms of adequate insurance reimbursement is based on anger at them for allegedly self-inflicting their disease in the pursuit of pleasure.

Later theorists, like the earlier ones, emphasized the importance of orality in substance abuse. In the case of heroin ingested by an intravenous route, the rapidity of the onset of action could be considered preoral (Savitt, 1963); smokable substances of abuse enter the body even more rapidly, and in this sense may also be considered preoral. The drug experience has also been linked to an "oral" or "alimentary" orgasm (Chessick, 1960). Fantasies that my own patients have reported experiencing during euphoria have frequently included oral satiation and symbiotic fusion with a breast. In addition, later theorists emphasized a pleasurable state described as a blissful internal homeostasis, which provides relief from anxiety and internal distress. Savitt (1963) and Wieder and Kaplan (1969) stated that the use of drugs compensates for lack of self-esteem and deficiency in self-integration. The work of Chein et al. (1964) marked a shift toward understanding the use of narcotics (or alcohol and other sedatives) as an attempt to cope with painful feelings and overwhelming responsibilities in the outside world. Glover (1932), Khantzian (1979), and I (Kaufman, 1974) have noted the use of sedative and narcotic drugs to dampen overwhelming hostility.

Khantzian (1982; Khantzian et al., 1990), who has worked extensively with SAs, was one of the first psychoanalysts to apply the concepts of self and ego psychology to our understanding of their psychodynamics. He has described ego deficits in SAs including an inability to handle emotions, and/or behavior characterized by swings from over- to undercontrol. Feelings are often vague, ill defined, and confusing when expressed. They are poorly regulated; they are tolerated and expressed mainly through action or somatization. These individuals also tend to overestimate or underestimate their worth, and are unable to maintain an inner sense of cohesiveness, self-comfort, or well-being. The severely dependent adaptation in SAs therefore, may be attributed to ego deficits and vulnerability rather than to oral cravings.

Contemporary psychodynamic theories recognize that much of the psychological dysfunction observed by therapists who treat SAs is the result of drug and alcohol abuse rather than the cause. However, many observers still relate drug taking to the underlying personality organization of the user, albeit in a more contemporary view. They focus on developmental and adaptive factors that influence relationships, self-esteem, judgment, and behavior as well as the capacity to manage stress. My own current view is that personality organization is a function of the integration of pre- and postaddictive experience.

Treece and Khantzian (1986) list the underlying characterological vulnerabilities to substance abuse as (1) inability to experience gradations of feelings, anticipate distress or use affective signals to activate defenses; (2) low self-esteem, with narcissistic protectiveness and poor integration of inner self- and object images; and (3) impaired thinking and judgment relating to immature, rigid defenses and poor adaptive coping mechanisms. These three vulnerabilities lead to deficiencies in the capacity for self-care, characterized by impaired self-regulation, self-soothing, and self-evaluation (Treece & Khantzian, 1986). It is difficult to determine developmentally when these deficiencies in self-care may have evolved. Some vulnerabilities are established through genes and intrauterine environment. Some occur in the first years of life through significant interactions with parent figures. Impaired judgment and inability to distinguish feelings often result when future SAs spend most of their teenage waking hours "stoned" on drugs or alcohol and cannot acquire the basic skills and knowledge of adolescence.

Substance use is generally initiated during a severe crisis in which an individual's usual adaptive capacities are impaired and narcissistic vulnerability is increased. If the user experiences adaptive benefit, continued use and dependence may result. Dependence may develop either from regression to a needy, immature state, or through a misdirected attempt at repair when the drug provides a semblance of normal functioning (Treece & Khantzian, 1986). Dependence may result even when the drug damages ego functioning and self-concept, as when the individual continues to use drugs or alcohol in an attempt to fix the hurt, remembering the moment of euphoria rather than the subsequent crash.

Krystal and Wurmser, along with Khantzian, are the theorists who have made the most outstanding contributions to a contemporary psychoanalytic view of SAs. Krystal (1978, 1985) describes the use of drugs to deal with primitive, overwhelming, preverbal, undifferentiated affects. Wurmser (1987) emphasizes that drugs may be used to deny or "overthrow" a "particularly burdensome and chafing inner authority figure" (p. 170). However, he does not assume the existence of superego lacunae (intermittent punitive and weak areas of conscience), which have been thought to be quite common in SAs. Rather, he emphasizes an excessively brash, punitive superego, which is occasionally overthrown by acting out when the user ingests drugs, but which in turn leads to harsh self-punishment. If Wurmser's theories are correct, they have important implications for treatment. The therapist who provides a great deal of structure, teaches self-preservation, and provides reality testing may be experienced as overly punitive or guilt-inducing. Wurmser (1987) also notes a phobic core within many addicts, with fears of commitment, pressure, or success. Levin (1987), utilizing the self-psychological format of Kohut, sees SAs as having so tenuous a sense of self that they live constantly on the edge of psychic annihilation, with the fear that their barely cohesive selves may fragment at any time. Levin (1987) states that SAs suffer from at least four kinds of self pathology: (1) self-destructiveness, (2) a lack of parts of the self that mediate self-care and maintain self-esteem, (3) excessive self-involvement, and (4) a basic sense of self that is fragile and constantly threatened.

Stanton et al.'s (1982) findings about symptom function in families of drug addicts have also been very helpful in my specific psychodynamic formulations regarding male SAs (see next section). These findings are as follows:

1. The regressive heroin euphoria, which is characterized by infantile fusion with the mother, permits the addict a symbolic reunification with the mother and family of childhood. The drug's blunting effects permit the addict to feel distant from overwhelming fears of incorporation while maintaining an illusory intimacy. This is true of other depressant drugs as well.

2. Heroin produces a sense of power and omnipotence that may unleash aggression toward family members, especially parents. This rage enables the addict to feel temporarily individuated, autonomous, and freed from family bonds. The addict's chosen life style is also a defiant "quantum leap" from that of the family. This combination of temporary assertiveness with family members and a different, drug-oriented life style with frequent failures, which cause the addict to return to the family for protection and nurturance, is known as "pseudoindividuation." True individuation is difficult because of the addict's inability to leave the enmeshed, symbiotic relationship with the family (especially the mother).

3. The regressive, sexually equivalent heroin high, and the resultant "ripping and running" life style, prevent the male addict from developing lasting and intimate relationships, particularly with women. In the latter stages of addiction, drug use eradicates the sex drive, thus

reinforcing the lack of need for women. Drug intoxication provides a pseudosexual experience that, unlike a lasting, sexualized relationship, poses no threat to family loyalty.

4. As a result of the first three factors, as well as an underlying narcissistic personality, addicts form only pseudofamilies of procreation. Thus, in psychotherapy, the most important family work should be that done with the families of origin. In these families, sibling issues are often overlooked but are of critical importance (Stanton et al., 1982).

The psychodynamic concepts of Khantzian, Wurmser, Krystal, Stanton et al., and others described above are, in my experience, always helpful in the treatment of SAs. Their usefulness depends on keeping them in context — not considering them as the sole causes of the substance abuse, not allowing them to be used as excuses for substance abuse, not equating psychodynamic material with psychopathology, and, most importantly, knowing when and how to utilize this material. Indeed, the issue of timing is the essence of psychotherapy with SAs and is discussed in several of the following chapters.

PERSONALITY CHARACTERISTICS AND PSYCHODYNAMICS OF MALE SUBSTANCE ABUSERS

A specific personality typology does not exist among male SAs, but there are some characteristics that help us understand their behavior: (1) Certain clusters of characteristics are frequently seen in male alcoholics; (2) certain personality structures are generally seen in male drug abusers; and (3) some gender issues and underlying psychodynamic conflicts are common to many male alcoholics and drug abusers. These three groupings are discussed separately here.

Male Alcoholics

Again, no specific "alcoholic personality" exists, but there are gender issues and underlying psychodynamic conflicts that are common to many male alcoholics.

Gender-Related Issues

Western society has condoned male drinking for centuries. Despite increasing consumption of alcohol by women in recent years, men still consume 75% of the alcohol drunk in the United States; drink twice as often and become intoxicated twice as often as women (Lemle & Mishkind, 1989); and constitute three-quarters of the alcoholics. Alcohol is considered a symbol of masculinity, in that drinking confirms acceptance from other men. Fifty-six percent of men attend bars without their wives, but only 6% of women do so without their husbands (Lemle & Mishkind, 1989). The more men drink in "masculine" settings, such as in bars and at athletic events, the more likely they are to be problem drinkers.

In order to "drink like a man," one must "take it straight, not sweeten the taste, prefer beer and hard liquor, drink without hesitation and hold his liquor" (Lemle & Mishkind, 1989, p. 213). Tolerance is considered masculine; reactivity or dependence is considered feminine. It fact, it has long been considered a test of adult masculinity to be able to "hold your liquor." The Lord of Dunvegan, a castle on the Isle of Skye in western Scotland, can only assume his title if at the age of 18 he can consume a bottle and a half of claret without falling down. (This custom, which equates the ability to govern a castle with "manly" tolerance to alcohol, may help us understand the high prevalence of male alcoholism in Scotland. However, getting drunk is an almost universal male adolescent rite of passage.)

Men also drink together in clubs as "good old boys," and in bars to feel as if they are "one of the guys." Drinking enhances identification, companionship, and closeness with other males. It is difficult for many men to communicate deeply and at length without getting drunk together, or at least having a few drinks to lower their anxiety. Drinking can also bond men together in hostile and inappropriate sexual advances to women (Bepko & Krestan, 1985).

Men are raised to believe that they must be self-sufficient and independent. Yet they also believe that their emotional and physical well-being is the responsibility of women. They feel entitled to being taken care of and nurtured by women without having to ask for it (Bepko & Krestan, 1985). Furthermore, they deny that they need this care or that they are greatly dependent on being cared for. Men are taught that being dependent or having warm or needy feelings shows weakness; therefore, such feelings are to be denied and avoided at all times. Drinking permits a man to express feelings and to act dependent, yet the alcoholic man will deny these feelings through acting masculine and independent. The drinker is able to express forbidden traits because they are stereotypically female. Thus, he can be irrational, extremely emotional, and hypersensitive, and can shift from the role of emotional distancer to pursuer. However, this behavior ultimately provides reinforcing punishment through guilt and remorse "the day after" (Bepko & Krestan, 1985).

The mass media certainly portray alcohol as masculine. Men who drink are cast in stereotypic roles, such as athletes, working men, and buddies. Men in beer ads vastly outnumber women. Beer commercials are replete with masculine symbols, particularly ritualistic initiation (e.g. the transformation of father–son into man-to-man relationships, male bonding, and advancement in male organizations. In a 1984 study, 74% of all beverages consumed on prime-time television were alcoholic, with men drinking twice as often as women (Lemle & Mishkind, 1989). In popular novels, alcohol is frequently mentioned, usually being consumed by males. The media's pairing of maleness and alcohol exploits and perpetuates this myth. Alcohol is also linked to three other key aspects of the male role: unconventionality, risk taking and aggressiveness.

Though alcohol use is considered male, physiological dependence and its psychological sequelae are not (Lemle & Mishkind, 1989). Feelings of dependence are a very important issue in male drinking and alcoholism. Overt dependence is extremely threatening and intolerable to male alcoholics. Drinking permits them to experience their deep underlying need to be helpless and cared for as they were when they were children (Bepko & Krestan, 1985). It permits them to be undressed and tucked into bed; to sleep late; and to be coddled and protected in other ways from the demands of the world, in which they feel inadequate and in which they are expected to perform as if they were more than adequate. Many male alcoholics deal with their needs for dependence by denying them and trying very hard to never appear dependent. They may overcompensate under the influence of alcohol, and act bossy, aggressive, hostile, and violent. In particular, they may become furious with their spouses when their needs for dependence are not gratified; the taboo against violence towards the "weaker sex" may be broken, and they may become physically violent toward their wives. Another common solution is for male alcoholics to turn to their daughters for gratification of their wishes for dependence. They may also break the incest taboo when intoxicated and seduce or force their daughters to meet their sexual needs.

Under their bravado, most alcoholic men have a pervading sense of low self-esteem and poor self-image. For some, their low self-esteem and lack of confidence are limited to selected facets of their life (e.g., they may feel inadequate at work but not at home, or vice versa). Their drinking is triggered by stresses affecting those areas where they feel most inadequate. Their dependence and low self-esteem often cause them to form heavily dependent transferences rapidly, or to flee from therapy when these and other feelings are overwhelming. They will also seek a fast way out when they are challenged prematurely or when narcissistic needs for admiration are not gratified.

Psychodynamic Issues

In psychodynamic theories, three key male identity issues have been linked to male alcoholism: (1) repressed homosexuality, (2) dependence, and (3) power (Zimberg, 1985). According to Zimberg, alcoholics have latent unexpressable unconscious homosexual cravings and feminine identifications. These men seek close contact with other men, which they can only achieve when intoxicated. The dependence theory is based on reports (Zimberg, 1985) that mothers of alcoholics responded inconsistently to their sons' dependence, and that fathers were rejecting, punitive, and poor as role models. The resulting poor identification with fathers and increased needs for dependence, it is thought, make the sons of such parents feel ungratified and unmasculine. Thus they seek alcohol to provide the substitutive gratification of warmth and comfort while permitting them to act manly. The power theory asserts that heavy drinking occurs in men who are obsessed with manly virtues, yet have real doubts about their masculinity; that is, they feel basically powerless, and alcohol helps them have the illusion of power.

Brown (1985) emphasizes that alcohol itself becomes the prime object of intense dependence. Alcohol serves as the principal means of support and consolation, and the alcoholic comes to rely on it as if it were a faithful friend, lover, or mother. Alcoholic beverages often have soothing brand names (e.g., Southern Comfort, Sutter Home) or gently anthropomorphized ones (Old Grand-Dad, Bud, and Johnnie Walker). Alcoholics feel that, unlike human beings, a bottle will never betray or desert them. Alcoholics may talk to their bottles and even take them to bed. Letting go of such a precious object without a replacement is inconceivable to them. This is a very important concept in therapy with alcoholics, and it is applicable also to some drug addicts (especially those who abuse sedatives). This is why replacements—the fellowship of AA, a nourishing spousal relationship, or even cigarettes—are so important to them.

In comparison with nonalcoholics or heroin addicts, alcoholics show more depression, guilt, anxiety, authority conflicts, and other neurotic traits. They are more emotionally labile and less independent than drug users (Craig, 1982). Fox (1975) stated that in alcoholic men there is often a strong, archaic superego, which tends toward harsh condemnation, a sense of unworthiness and guilt, and masochistic, self-punitive behavior. Fox (1975) also described psychological impotence, ego fragility, sexual immaturity, and excessive homosexual conflicts; however, later research efforts have tended to disprove these last two as common characteristics. Another major dynamic often cited in male alcoholics is drinking to experience a false sense of power over others (Sandmaier, 1980).

The MacAndrew Alcoholism scale has identified Minnesota Multiphasic Personality Inventory (MMPI) characteristics of alcoholics that do not change with drinking and sober cycles (MacAndrew, 1965). Studies of alcoholics using the MMPI have consistently shown two clear subgroups—one characterized by anxiety and depression, the other by antisocial traits (Khantzian, 1982). The former has also been termed the "female" or "reactive" pattern of alcoholism, and the latter has been called the "male" or "essential" type. These two subtypes of alcoholics have been described consistently by a variety of observers, although with different nomenclature.

"Type A" alcoholics are characterized by later onset, fewer childhood risk factors, less severe dependence, fewer alcohol-related problems, and less psychopathology. This group has also been termed "reactive," "delta," "nonfamilial," "affiliative," "milieu-limited," "female," and "Type I." "Type B" alcoholics show earlier onset, more childhood risk factors, familial alcoholism, greater severity of alcohol problems and dependence, polydrug use, chronic treatment history, greater psychopathology, and more life stress. Type B resembles other subtypes labeled "essential," "symptomatic," "gamma," "binge," "familial," "secondary," "antisocial," "male," and "Type II" (Babor et al., 1992).

These typologies have important implications for treatment matching. Litt et al. (1992) found that Type A alcoholics had better outcomes with interactional group treatment, whereas Type B alcoholics did better with coping skills training. The model of interactional group treatment used was that developed by Brown and Yalom (1977) and focused on exploring the participants' relationships with one another, while concentrating on issues and feelings within the group.

Male Drug Abusers

Although, again, there is no specific personality profile for male "hardcore" drug users, a high incidence of antisocial personality traits distinguishes many if not most such individuals from normals and from (nonantisocial) alcoholics. Hard-core drug abusers also exhibit behaviors very different from those of abusers of prescription drugs, marijuana, and the hallucinogens, whose patterns are often similar to those of alcoholics. The term hard-core refers to heroin addicts, heavy cocaine users (particularly regular smokers of "crack" and intravenous users), heavy users of amphetamines (also regular smokers and intravenous users), and abusers of any drugs that are repeatedly obtained through criminal acts other than conning doctors for prescriptions.

However, many criminal addicts are very skilled at these conning behaviors and use them when other sources are exhausted (Kaufman, 1985).

The more individuals resort to illegal behavior to support a drug habit, the more they will acquire antisocial personality traits. When these personality patterns are established, drugs and obtaining them become much more important than people. In order to get drugs and the money to pay for them, hard-core drug users will lie to, cheat, intimidate, steal from, and in extreme desperation attack family members and friends.

Hard-core drug abusers involve themselves in relationships only for what they can get, while giving as little as possible. They often have a history of antisocial behavior before the age of 15, multiple skirmishes with the law, and very unstable relationships; these behaviors are described in detail in Chapter 4. Male drug abusers are more violent than male alcoholics, particularly when they are compared when not under the influence of their substances of choice. The illegal activities necessary to support most drug use forces them into antisocial acts, and resultant repeated incarcerations reinforce their antisocial behavior (Kaufman, 1974). Though they form dependent relationships, they shift their dependence readily from one person to another (e.g., from mother to wife or lover or from therapist to therapist).

A Heroin scale has been developed for the MMPI (the original purpose was to identify addicts in a prison population). The Heroin scale measures depression, ambivalent religious attitudes, resentment of authority, confused psychological development, denial, cunning, and grandiosity (Craig, 1982). Heroin addicts have higher mean scores on this scale than alcoholics, but polydrug abusers score higher than either (Lachar et al., 1979). Heroin addicts are more independent and aggressive than alcoholics, and reportedly have greater ego strength (Craig, 1982).

Khantzian (1980) notes the lifelong preoccupation of heroin addicts with aggression. He also believes that heroin is used specifically as an antidepressant. Wurmser (1987) calls drug use a pharmacologically reinforced denial, as it attempts to blunt the emotional impingement of painful inner and outer reality. He describes the ways in which addicts defend against their phobic core by using an external object (heroin) as protector and by using the defense of turning passive into active. In 1974 I conducted a study consisting of psychodynamic interviews of heroin addicts, and in 1981 I studied multiple-drug abusers and their families of origin. The psychological aspects observed at those times are presented here, and the relevance of these observations to contemporary psychodynamic theory is discussed.

Reasons Given for Initial and Continued Drug Use

Heroin is frequently used initially because it diminishes anxiety about sexual and assertive performance and communication. I found (Kaufman, 1974) that many male patients of all social classes experienced inadequate sexual performances or serious fears about their sexual capacity before their first use of heroin. When they discovered that heroin aided sexual performance through relaxation, elimination of fears and anxieties, or physiological retardation of ejaculation, they gravitated to the drug and became habituated to it.

One patient who had been drug-free for several months reported to me that he had been told by a woman that his sexual performance was inadequate. He left her to purchase and inject heroin, and returned a few hours later; this time his performance was satisfactory. Another patient described heroin as providing "pontoons," which enabled him to sustain his sexual functioning. This particular patient was also totally preoccupied with his violent impulses and found that heroin controlled them. When he was not using heroin, riding a motorcycle offered an alternative expression for his aggression, as did working as a bouncer at a nightclub. The masculinity, exhilaration, autonomy, and potential self-destructiveness involved in motorcycling, compulsive gambling, skydiving, and other risky sports, as well as in buying stocks and commodities on margin, can temporarily substitute for drug abuse. However, those who remain dependent on risk-taking behavior very frequently return to substance abuse, because these behaviors may be powerful paired conditioning stimuli for drug use and/or may produce a euphoria similar to the effects of drugs and alcohol. This "high" may occur through neuropharmacologically triggered cravings involving stimulation of similar neuroreceptors.

I found (Kaufman, 1974) that when assertion-phobic heroin-abusing men were in early recovery and found themselves in situations where they had to be aggressive, they went back to heroin or withdrew. Those who worked in jobs involving public contact (ranging from sales to prostitution) found that they could only function when high on heroin. Many used heroin before psychiatric interviews, when verbal confrontations were anticipated, or prior to any situations where they would have to communicate. Addicts high on heroin found that it totally obliterated concerns with sex, aggression, assertion, or communication. One patient, who said that he felt at first like a sexual "Superfly" on heroin, added that once he was addicted, sex became "number 101" on his list of 100 needs. This observation continues to be valid and is equally applicable to all abusable drugs. In the early phases of its use, cocaine causes an intense degree of sexual stimulation, which leads to regressive, polymorphous, perverse, and often sadistic sexual activities. After long-term use, or even after several hours of continued use (particularly of smokable crack), the sexual drive is rapidly obliterated.

Behaviors Secondary to a Drug-Using Life Style

Many of the "oral" behaviors of heroin addicts are secondary to the life style necessary to obtain drug supplies. Low frustration tolerance, seeing others only as suppliers, manipulativeness, extractiveness, self-destructiveness, and impaired reality testing have all been taken as evidence of addicts' oral character structure (Kaufman, 1974). These traits occur in all opiate addicts, regardless of social class. However, most of those characteristics are secondary, especially in ghetto addicts; they invariably develop once an individual is addicted.

Addicts do not give human relationships priority above their need to find money and drugs to maintain their habits. They are unable to make any personal commitment (except briefly if such a commitment facilitates obtaining drugs), and are virtually untreatable while still on drugs. Many ex-addicts rapidly lose the characteristics listed above when their "street" addiction is removed by detoxification, methadone maintenance, or residential treatment, although some recovering addicts continue to exhibit these traits. Primitive behaviors continue in recovering addicts who are not working to change their behavior (e.g., in methadone maintenance patients who continue to abuse other drugs or alcohol). This hypothesis is not valid for those addicts in whom an accurate history reveals an antisocial or narcissistic personality disorder preceding the onset of drug abuse. These individuals would by definition have demonstrated these oral and other primitive characteristics prior to using drugs.

The untreatability of opiate addicts was formerly taken as further evidence of oral character (Kaufman, 1974); however, opiate addiction has become treatable over the past two decades. Most individuals who remain in treatment lose these primitive personality traits, as do those on methadone maintenance who do not abuse drugs or alcohol and become socially rehabilitated. Giving up these behaviors is the *sine qua non* of successful treatment of the narcotic addict. The orally oriented fantasies and dreams that the heroin addicts I interviewed (Kaufman, 1974) experienced in the early phases of treatment were not necessarily indicative of primitive oral psychopathology. The nature and content of the fantasies could be attributed in part to the pharmacological effects of their drugs of choice, as well as to underlying issues.

Several of my patients (Kaufman, 1974), particularly those from the middle class, described an oral orgasm similar to that mentioned by Chessick (1960). One college student told me that while high on heroin he felt "a rush, a warmth coming from the inside out. It's a visceral warmth [as] opposed to a peripheral. It's different from anything else, even from the warmth you get from the fetal position. Even that does not progress from the center outwards." However, this same patient had another major fantasy when euphoric on heroin — "hot in the sense of sexual sensation. After you heat it, it's warm. It's almost like warm sperm." This patient had a primitive borderline personality, but the multitude and variety of the fantasies that preoccupied him were more indicative of this state than of an oral quality to any primary fantasy. Another student (who was the sickest patient in the college group, having had a series of psychiatric hospitalizations) had no oral fantasies on heroin. He said that without drugs he felt "confused, afraid, and hostile." Heroin relieved his anxiety and depression and helped him sort out his disordered thoughts. Individuals like him, who used heroin to help organize severely disintegrated behavior, tended to be the most seriously mentally ill of the subjects studied. However, the confusion these men experienced was more indicative of their primitive regressed state than was the specific content of their fantasies. In several patients, their primary fantasies when high on heroin involved allowing the expression of aggression or obliterating concern with the destructiveness of their anger. Although such fantasies are generally considered to be at a higher level of psychosexual integration than oral dependent fantasies (i.e., oral aggressive or anal), these subjects did not tend to have more highly integrated character structures than those with oral sucking fantasies. Those subjects who experienced heroin as curative of feelings of disintegration tended to be the most regressed psychologically.

Presently, after working with many recovering addicts longitudinally for 7 or more years who appear to function at a rather high level of adaptation, I have become impressed with their deep and devastating developmental wounds; these cause them to regress rapidly to a primitive, vulnerable state when stressed. However, this regression only occurs if they return to substance abuse. The maintenance of a sober core provides a homeostatic stabilization that permits them to maintain a high level of ego function and not to regress permanently.

Social Class and Psychopathology

The higher the social class of a given male opiate addict, the more likely he is to be suffering from severe psychopathology. For sicker individuals, opiates provide a basic psychological and physical homeostasis. Wieder and Kaplan (1969) noted this phenomenon in middle-class addicts. They theorized that this organizing effect comes from the power of opiates to create, in symbolic terms, a symbiotic fusion with a medicating mother. Psychotic addicts of all social classes tend to use heroin as their tranquilizer of choice, and to experience a sense of homeostatic organization on heroin. In seriously depressed addicts, methadone functions as an antidepressant, though it is perhaps not as effective in that capacity as heroin. This difference may be pharmacological, or it may be a result of the substantial change in life style that usually accompanies an addict's switch from heroin to methadone. This inverse relationship between psychopathology and social class has held up well in my subsequent clinical experience, as my observations about middle-class subjects in the 1974 study (see above) indicate.

Family-of-Origin Issues

Parents: My Own Observations. The most consistent finding in the families of male drug abusers in my own studies (Kaufman, 1976b, 1981), as well as those of other researchers (Stanton et al., 1982), is that an alcoholic father is present in about 50% of cases. With younger drug abusers, there are more fathers who are themselves drug abusers. A father who died or abandoned the family when a drug abuser was young is also quite common. However, I have found that in certain ethnic groups, such as Italians and Jews, fathers neither abandon their families nor are SAs. In Jewish and Italian families, fathers are often emotionally overinvolved with and overreactive to their drug-abusing sons. Almost every Jewish and Italian male drug abuser in my 1981 research was so close to his family of origin that issues of loyalty to spouse versus family were consistently critical. Most of the Italian and Jewish fathers of heroin addicts with whom I have worked with were very hard workers and set very high performance standards for their sons—standards that were not met or even approached. Many Italian sons worked directly for their fathers, and thus were frequently protected from having to meet the usual demands of employment. Perhaps coincidentally, several fathers suffered disabling physical injuries after the onset of their sons' drug dependence, which prevented them from continuing to perform physical aspects of their work (Kaufman, 1981). These disabled fathers' sense of self-esteem was apparently devastated by their injuries and inability to work as they did before their accidents. This led them to be overinvolved with their addicted sons—rescuing the sons to save themselves.

Although many adult male drug abusers frequently appear to be uninvolved with their parents, a closer examination of their contacts reveals that they are actually quite involved, despite their many futile attempts at individuation. Mothers are particularly close to their adult drug-dependent sons; this is the case in every ethnic group with which I have worked. Mothers in these families go through stages of overinvolvement ranging from denial to overprotectiveness to total preoccupation to withdrawal. Enmeshed mothers think, act, and feel for their drug-abusing sons. Several mothers I have worked with regularly took prescription tranquilizers or narcotics, which they overtly shared with their sons. Many mothers suffered an agitated depression whenever their children acted out in destructive ways. Those women who took prescription tranquilizers or abused alcohol frequently increased their intake whenever the addicts experienced difficulty or acted out. Symbiotically relating mothers would do anything for their addicted sons except leave them alone (Kaufman, 1981). Many mothers experienced alcohol abuse, suicide attempts, and severe psychosomatic symptoms, which they blamed on the addicts, thereby reinforcing the pattern of guilt and mutual manipulation. These ethnic- and family-determined psychodynamic patterns have been consistently observed for more than a decade since the original study.

Siblings: My Own Observations. I have found that siblings tend to fall equally into two basic categories of behavior: "very good" and "very bad." The "bad" group consists of fellow drug abusers whose drug use is interwoven with that of the identified patients. The "good" group includes children who assume the role of authoritarian parents when the fathers are absent or disengaged. These children are often highly successful in their own careers; they may individuate from the family, but many remain enmeshed (Kaufman, 1981). A small subgroup of "good" siblings I have encountered in my own work are quite passive and not involved with substance abuse. Some of these develop disorders such as depression, tics, and headaches, which are often related to holding in anger (Kaufman, 1981). The "good" children in these families obey family rules and work hard at school, attempting to meet their parents' high expectations. They bear the burden of the identified patients and of their "incompetent" parents as well. They feel if they can only be good enough, they will erase the effect of the identified patients and make their parents look good. "Good" children are generally rigid and lonely, and may suffer guilt and remorse, often for the rest of their lives.

Enmeshed drug-abusing siblings may provide drugs for each other, inject drugs into each other, set each other up to be arrested, or even pimp for each other. At times, a large family may show both types of sibling relationships. Several drug abusers I interviewed functioned as parental surrogates in their own families of origin and had no way of asking for relief from responsibility except through drugs. More commonly, they were the youngest children in their families, and their drug abuse maintained their "baby" role. They were also frequently the children who got the most attention, and drug abuse kept them from ever having to abandon the parental nest (Kaufman, 1981).

Observations from Other Research. Some of my own findings about male addicts' families, particularly about overinvolved fathers, are at variance with findings from other studies, in part because of the high proportions of Jewish and Italian families in my 1981 project. All studies have emphasized the overinvolved mothers of addicts, but many have described the fathers as detached, weak, absent, or uninvolved (Stanton et al., 1982). Another finding about the fathers in Stanton et al.'s study—one that *is* compatible with my own findings—is that the fathers disciplined inconsistently and often harshly or physically.

Spotts and Shontz (1980) have described the family histories of different types of SAs. They state that chronic amphetamine users grow up in homes with strong, manipulative mothers and passive, ineffectual fathers. As adults, these individuals fear women and deal with them by attempting to conquer, overcome, use, and exploit them. Narcotic addicts come from homes where the fathers were absent or were overpowering tyrants. As adults, they are seriously disabled with poor egos; they are quiet, lonely, and unambitious. Cocaine users describe their mothers as warm and their fathers as strong and encouraging. As adults, they develop an intense need for complete self-sufficiency in order to compensate for their strongly denied need for dependence. Barbiturate users describe neglecting, uninterested fathers and dependent, ineffectual mothers. As adults, they tend to alternate between extreme under- and over-evaluation of relationships, with consequent enthrallment and rapid detachment.

Stanton et al.'s (1982) intensive family studies of heroin addicts have revealed many important psychodynamic factors corresponding to those I have found in my own psychodynamic treatment and interviewing. These factors may be summarized as follows:

1. Fear of success and separation is common in these families; it results from an interdependent process characterized by the families' fear of letting go of the addicts and the addicts' fear of autonomy. The addicts fail whenever they are on the verge of success in treatment, vocational activities, or academic pursuits. Their success is un-

dermined by either their own interpersonal anxiety or the families' re-entrance into crisis or chaos. The addicts' failure then restores the families' homeostasis or resolves their own anxiety.

2. There is multigenerational alcohol dependence, with drug abuse in progeny.

3. Conspicuously "unschizophrenic" conflict is expressed more directly and primitively, but it is relatively free of double binds. Following periods of family conflict, addicts can escape the family by retreating to peer relationships, although many of these peers may themselves be SAs.

4. Alliances between family members, though excessively close and highly conflicted, are clear and readily acknowledged.

5. Mothers are extremely overinvolved with preaddict sons, particularly when the sons are between the ages of 11 and 16.

6. Premature and unexpected deaths occur frequently in these families. Stanton et al. (1982) found not only a high incidence of early parental death, but also a very high rate of early death among paternal grandfathers. In my own studies of these types of families, the premature death of an older sibling was a traumatic factor related directly or indirectly to sibling substance abuse and dependence (Kaufman, 1985). Thus addiction is part of a multigenerational "continuum of self-destruction" often related to cycles of un-worked-through grief.

7. Cultural disparity between parents and children plays an important role in family conflict and addiction, particularly in the case of immigrant and other parents with Old World values who have first- or second-generation American sons.

Male Alcoholics and Drug Abusers

Four key personality traits common to male drug abusers and male alcoholics have been consistently described in the scientific literature: (1) impulsivity (inability to tolerate frustration, and a need to act quickly); (2) repetition of self-defeating behaviors; (3) an overemphasis on immediate euphoria and relief of tension and pain over long-term relief and future problem resolution; and (4) denial of dependence (Kaufman, 1985). They rely excessively on such classical pathological defenses as regression, denial, introjection, obsession, projection, and rationalization (Kaufman, 1985). They also utilize defenses that are more common in SAs, such as pseudocompliance, need for emotional control, omnipotence, avoidance of intimacy, and externalization responsibility (Levinson, 1985). In addition, they may use "all-or-nothing" thinking, conflict minimization and avoidance, passivity and assimilative projection (Wallace, 1985b); repression of grief is also commonly seen (Goldberg, 1985). Several of these defenses are so critical that they are described at greater length in Chapter 3. Lying is also quite common and often so fused with denial that reality and memory become blurred.

As noted separately above in regard to alcoholics and drug abusers, men often use drugs and alcohol to diminish anxiety about self-assertion and conflict in work and social contacts. They use sedating drugs and alcohol initially to obliterate anger and hostility, but these feelings are often released during intoxication. Male drug abusers and alcoholics have difficulty enduring anxiety and tension. Their moods may cycle rapidly from elation to depression, particularly as substance use lowers their emotional thresholds. These mood swings are not necessarily indicative of bipolar disorder or some other mood disorder. Male SAs experience a constant inner battle between feeling weak, dependent, and passive on the one hand, and trying to be aggressive and totally deny their needs for dependence on the other. These strong needs are inevitably frustrated, leading either to depression and despair or to hostility, rages, and fantasies of revenge (Fox, 1975).

Male drug and alcohol abusers have repressed or conscious feelings of omnipotence and grandiosity, together with little ability to persevere and follow through on tasks and goals. Marked narcissism is commonly seen, either overtly manifested or quite close to the surface. Not only do these individuals use both drugs and alcohol, but they often demonstrate other compulsive, self-destructive behaviors that have an addictive quality.

"CODEPENDENT" PATTERNS
IN SUBSTANCE ABUSERS

The word "codependent" has recently achieved broad popular use, but has been criticized in psychoanalytic and other psychodynamically oriented circles as trendy and overgeneralized. Certain primitive dependent and symbiotic characteristics of SAs may nonetheless be understood under the rubric of "codependence." Codependent individuals are ones who have let other persons' behavior affect them to the point of becoming obsessed with controlling those persons' behavior, and/or whose own sense of well-being is totally dependent on the other persons' welfare or attention to them (Kaufman, 1991).

Many addicts' and alcoholics' relationships with significant others are characterized by codependent patterns. Thus the SAs become more concerned with their significant others than with their own development, blaming the significant others for all of their difficulties. The

SAs need to control the others' behavior, particularly to meet their needs, and they have no sense of boundaries between themselves and the others (when a significant other hurts, an SA hurts). When a male addict is trying to earn his way back into his family's good graces, he will temporarily hold back his feelings out of a fear of rejection, which is another behavioral pattern attributable to codependents. Thus SAs may have dysfunctional codependent relationship patterns with sober spouses, parents, and other individuals; they may also be involved codependently with substance-abusing spouses, parents, and others. These relationships may cause difficulties not only because of the inherent exposure to abusable substances, but also because an identified patient may be deeply damaged in the same way a non-SA codependent is (e.g., eventually dragged down to the depths of despair through overconcern about another dysfunctional person). This issue of addict codependence is one of the major stressors leading to relapse, particularly in early abstinence. In later therapy, other typical codependent issues (e.g., fear of intimacy and closeness) are dealt with.

RISK FACTORS PREDISPOSING INDIVIDUALS TO SUBSTANCE ABUSE

Familial and Personality Factors

Over the past decade, child development researchers have addressed the many interacting variables that predispose individuals to substance abuse (see Figure 1.1 for a summary). Their findings have made a substantial contribution to prevention efforts, as well as to attempts to understand the causes of substance abuse. Judith S. Brook, who has followed a large cohort of children and their families since 1975, has made a number of contributions of her own and has synthesized those of others. Brook et al. (1986) have focused on the interrelationship of family patterns, adolescent personality, peer associates, and drug (marijuana) use. They have found that parental adherence to traditional societal values is related to a warm and conflict-free parent–adolescent relationship, as well as to greater identification of adolescents with their parents. The adolescents then introject the parents' conventional values and behavior, and this leads to a drug-free adjustment.

Childhood personality factors found by Brook et al. (1986) to be associated with later substance abuse include rebelliousness, lack of social skills, and aggression. A nonintact family structure, including single parenting, is also associated with substance abuse, whereas religion and regular church attendance are sparing factors. Moreover, in the last decade the reciprocal effects of parent–child interaction have been noted. Brook et al. (1986) term these "bidirectional," in that a parent affects a child at the same time the child affects the parent. (In addition, the child's relationship with each parent is affected by his/her relationship with each of the other family members.)

Parents influence their children through the structure of child-rearing practices and by modeling and subsequent incorporation. Parental substance use (including use of alcohol, tobacco, and tranquilizers) is consistently associated with adolescent marijuana use (Penning & Barnes, 1982). Important positive child-rearing practices include the transmission of warmth; nonpunitive, consistent controls; appropriate closeness; and lack of overpermissiveness (Brook et al., 1986). Through long-term follow-up, Brook and her colleagues have been able to demonstrate that personality risk traits in childhood form the foundations, through personality continuity, for adolescent risk factors and subsequently for drug abuse.

A survey of over 2,000 alcoholics compared with a nonalcoholic group from the general population revealed that alcoholics tend to be only children or last-borns from large sibships (Conley, 1980). This finding echoes one from our (Kaufman & Kaufmann, 1979) study of heroin addicts, which showed a majority of youngest and only children. This phenomenon may be explained by the permissiveness with which youngest and only children are raised (Conley, 1980), or by a family's need to have an infantilized child to take care of or to deflect marital issues when there are no other children present.

Factors Predisposing Individuals to Choose Particular Substances of Abuse

My general premise is that it is difficult to relate a specific personality type to the choice of a specific drug of abuse. This is in agreement with Rado (1926/1960), who, as noted earlier, stated that all types of drug craving are varieties of a single disease called "pharmacothymia." However, a distinction can be made between those who clearly choose either stimulants *or* depressants.

A major difficulty with determining specificity is that many individuals do not have a specific drug of choice or even a pharmacological category of choice. They will use anything that changes their mood, makes them feel whole, clouds their thoughts, obliterates their pain, or places a filter between themselves and the outside world. There are also many drug users who claim that they only abuse or are addicted to certain types of drugs (e.g., "uppers" only or "downers" exclusively). One patient of mine claimed that the only drug he cared for or could become addicted to was Quaalude. Yet when cocaine was readily available he rapidly became addicted, seriously damaging his nasal septum while still claiming that he disliked cocaine. Over the last few years, many allegedly "pure" cocaine addicts have become dependent on alcohol as a result of drinking to come down, to ease the cocaine "crash," or to prolong their euphoria. For these SAs, even a single shot of alcohol or a beer can rekindle the desire for cocaine. More recently, the combination of alcohol and cocaine has been found to form cocaethylene, which prolongs and intensifies the effects of cocaine.

Studies that emphasize specific intrapsychic bases for the use of different drugs overlook many important social factors. This overgeneralization occurs when sampling is restricted to one social class or to limited ethnic groups. Social determinants lead to drug abuse when there is a paucity of alternatives to a meaningful life, as in urban ghettos. In addition, cycles of limited and excessive availability of specific drugs have encouraged the use of other drugs or drug–alcohol combinations (Kaufman, 1977). Nevertheless, there do seem to be some psychodynamic factors governing the substance of choice or at least the chosen pharmacological category for many individuals.

Milkman and Frosch (1973) found a difference between heroin addicts and amphetamine abusers who had experienced both drugs and expressed a specific preference for one of the two. They demonstrated that individuals for whom heroin was the drug of choice suffer from depression and despair, and relieve anxiety by withdrawal from others and repression of conflict through satiation by the drug. In a later work, Milkman and Frosch (1980) emphasized the heroin addicts' need to relieve sporadic rages with opiates. Khantzian (1979) noted the specific muting and stabilizing effects of narcotics on rage and aggression. In a study of over 200 heroin addicts, he found developmental deficiencies that led to outbursts of rage, poor impulse control, and general dysphoria. Heroin then moderated the threat their violent feelings posed to themselves and others. On opiates, they experienced a sensation of total physical relief, which they described as "mellow" and "calm."

As mentioned earlier, heroin retards sexual ejaculation, which some teenage boys find helpful in their initial sexual efforts. Once addiction to heroin sets in, however, their need for sexual contact is often totally obliterated. Heroin and other narcotic addicts need to dampen their sexual and aggressive drives and to reduce the stress of external stimuli. They use narcotics to achieve tranquility. This tendency may also be true of individuals who are dependent on such prescription drugs as codeine, Darvon, Vicodin, and Percodan.

Few differences exist between individuals who choose amphetamines and those who choose cocaine. Stimulant abusers use these drugs to feel active when they are depressed and competent when they are frightened (Milkman & Frosch, 1973). Wurmser (1987) noted that stimulants induce feelings of control and mastery over aggression, which can progress to feelings of grandiosity and invincibility. Khantzian (1979) has remarked that these drugs become compelling for some individuals when they find themselves performing tasks they felt incapable of mastering before taking drugs. Others may use cocaine and amphetamines to relieve a hyperactive, restless life style. Some of the latter individuals may have adult attention deficit disorder, but this diagnosis should be made with caution in drug-abusing adults. Wieder and Kaplan (1969), like Wurmser and Khantzian, noted that use of amphetamines initially enhances feelings of mastery, leading to greater frustration tolerance, feelings of competence, and self-esteem. However, they also noted that as stimulant use progresses, this feeling of power reverses as the user feels increasingly threatened in relatively harmless circumstances. Cocaine users are often intensely competitive men who take risks to be successful; they find that cocaine helps drive them to this success. This feeling of competence may backfire as violent fantasies and acts are triggered by stimulants.

Stimulants initially enhance sexual fantasy and performance, but later eradicate sexual desire. One unique effect of cocaine on sexuality is that cocaine is associated with the release and acting out of polymorphous perverse sexual fantasies. Many male cocaine addicts whom I have treated had relatively mundane sexual lives until they went on cocaine binges. On such binges they might devote themselves exclusively to achieving their wildest sexual fantasies, often with younger women who were also using cocaine. Of course, sexual desire evaporates after repeated use of cocaine or stimulants, and severe impotence and lack of desire become common.

Until recently, psychodynamic patterns in alcoholics have been considered separately; however, current researchers have observed patterns similar to those of alcoholics in sedative, hypnotic, and minor-tranquilizer abusers. Khantzian (1979) has found that sedative abusers have rigid personality structures, with unstable defenses against primitive narcissistic and aggressive impulses. The sedatives overcome rigid defenses, so that affection and aggression can be expressed in the absence of ego structures that modulate such drives (Khantzian, 1979). Sedative abusers repeatedly engage in behavior that seems to tempt fate to destroy them (Spotts & Shontz, 1980). These drugs provide their users with a passport to oblivion in which they can deny failure and release inhibitions. They experience a memory loss for fights and accidents, which lets them disavow guilt. Alcohol and the sedatives relax sexual fears and allow the user to overcome sexual inhibitions, which are often unconscious. Methaqualone (Quaalude) was widely believed to have an aphrodisiac effect, which is probably mythical. Once abuse sets in, the calming effects of sedatives backfire and often lead to violence, as inhibitions are lost or rebound excitability occurs.

Hallucinogens are used by sensation seekers to counteract boredom; marijuana also lets the user relax or withdraw from competitive pressure (Hendin, 1980). Users of stimulants and sedatives, as noted above, take these drugs to alleviate depression, anxiety and helplessness. Carrol and Zuckerman (1977), comparing users of these different drug types on the MMPI and the Sensation Seeking Scale, found that stimulant use was associated with high scores on the MMPI Hypochondriasis, Hysteria, Paranoia, Schizophrenia, and Hypomania scales. Hallucinogen use was correlated with high scores on the first four of these, along with high Depression and Social Introversion scores.

The effects of all substances depend on expectations and setting. For example, if sleeping pills are taken with the expectation that they will help the user sleep, then they produce somnolence. If they are taken at a party to release inhibitions, then they lead to initial activation.

Recently specific receptors in the brain have been discovered for opiates, amphetamines, methylphenidate (Ritalin), benzodiazepines, and possibly a host of other psychoactive drugs. This research may lead to the discovery of a strong neurochemical basis for drug preference, related to receptor sensitivity or deficits in endogenous psychoactive substances, but unrelated to personality or psychopathology. Further research in the next decade on the biological aspects of drug abuse may reveal a great deal about specific organic etiologies for or abuse of various drugs, and may substantially contribute to effective treatment.

Genetic Factors

These social and psychological explanations for the etiology of alcoholism and drug abuse are in no way meant to minimize the importance of genetic factors, which have repeatedly been demonstrated in scientific studies. For example, male children of alcoholics are four times more likely than normals to become alcoholics, even if they are adopted and raised in homes without an alcoholic parent (Goodwin, 1981). McKenna and Perkins (1981) studied male and female alcoholics with varying combinations of alcoholic parents; twice as many female as male alcoholics had two alcoholic parents. (Alcoholics with two alcoholic parents have a much more severe and rapidly progressive alcoholic disease course.)

Genetic studies of drug abusers are just beginning. The incidence of parental alcoholism in drug abusers has been repeatedly noted in this chapter. Cadoret et al. (1986), in a study of adoptees, noted that drug abuse was highly related to three factors: antisocial personality in a biological parent, alcoholism in a biological parent, and divorce or psychiatric disturbances in the adoptive family. The finding in regard to antisocial personality disorder suggests that a predisposition to substance abuse may be not only directly transmitted, but indirectly linked with various familial factors. Other such factors that have been investigated include temperament and major mental illness (particularly depression and anxiety).

CONCLUDING COMMENT

The contemporary psychodynamic view I have set forth on this chapter draws from the chemical dependence literature as well as the psychological, psychiatric, and psychoanalytic literatures. I find this type of integrative understanding critical to the psychotherapy of SAs as developed in the following chapters.

CHAPTER 2

Personality, Psychopathology, and Psychodynamics of Addicted Women

I have chosen to write a separate chapter on female SAs because so many of their issues are quite different from those of male SAs. (Although women are viewed here as a group, there are obviously also differences among individual women, and the chapter takes at least some of these into account as well.) The issues unique to female SAs were not appreciated until the past 20 years, as they were generally not delineated by earlier researchers, clinicians, or the self-help movement. Today there is a rapidly expanding base of knowledge involving female drug and alcohol abuse.

Women differ significantly from men in patterns of usage, as well as in many aspects of personality, psychodynamics, and psychopathology. Men use more alcohol, marijuana, heroin, cocaine, hallucinogens, and inhalants. Women use more legal drugs, most of which are prescribed by male physicians to keep them calm (passive and depressed); they may also turn to stimulants or illegal drugs such as cocaine and amphetamines to lose weight or overcome depression. Recently there has been an increase in the use of illicit drugs by women, as this pattern has become more ego-syntonic with being female. The National Client Data System, in a 1992 survey of female SAs who were admitted to treatment, demonstrated that alcohol was the most common primary drug abused by these women (alcohol only: 108,170; alcohol with a secondary drug: 80, 964). Following closely behind as primary drug of abuse was cocaine (103,631). Other common primary drugs were heroin (60,501), cannabis (19,315), amphetamines and other stimulants (9,732), and tranquilizers and sedatives/hypnotics (4,603). Thus, although tranquilizers and amphetamines are considered to be used more often by women, they account for only a minority of the primary drugs abused by women who enter treatment for substance abuse.

Female problem drinkers are more likely to use mental health services and other non-alcohol-specific programs than male problem drinkers are. In general, female SAs will often present for psychotherapy for issues not related to substance abuse.

GENDER-RELATED ISSUES

Female substance abuse is very much related to the general problems of women in our society. Issues such as age, social class, ethnicity, living environment, marital and relational issues, stage of substance abuse consumption, sexual and physical abuse, and the social changes brought about by feminism all have profound effects.

Low Self-Esteem and Sex-Role Conflicts

Lack of social power and external pressure to conform to sex-role stereotypes can create a level of stress that drives some women to substance abuse. These women are overwhelmed by the message many of them have been subjected to throughout their lives—that they are less worthy because they are women. Far from protecting them, the culturally defined behavior demanded of women actually contributes to much of the pain and conflict that leads them to substance abuse. Those who become addicts or alcoholics are further insulted because of the greater stigma of being female SAs, which only increases their difficulties (Sandmaier, 1980).

An essential feature of alcoholism in women is a preoccupation with what they perceive as their inadequacy, ineptness, and inability to establish themselves in their environment. Female alcoholics feel less socially competent and less effective in goal achievement than do women who are not alcoholics. They also experience more covert and overt anxiety, and often feel unworthy and dissatisfied with their purpose in life (Corrigan, 1980).

Women are more likely than men to begin problem drinking in response to a specific trauma, even with no prior history of alcohol abuse. These traumas most often involve losses that threaten their sense of self, such as divorce, desertion, infidelity, death of a family member, a child's leaving home, or health problems (especially gynecological or menopausal) (Beckman, 1975; Sandmaier, 1980). Many women begin abusing alcohol in middle age, when such traumas often occur, or when they conclude that they can never fulfill the dreams of their youth (Beckman, 1975).

Cocaine's capacity for increasing self-confidence and providing a sense of control would seem to earmark it for use by women who have low self-esteem and whose lives are controlled by outside forces. Cocaine gives an illusion of power in circumstances where a woman's experience of powerlessness is extreme (Walker et al., 1991). In addition, climbing the corporate ladder, with its attendant long hours and stress, puts women in positions of substantially increased risk for drug abuse and addiction. The additional bonus of weight loss for women obsessed with body image provides a frequent rationale for continued stimulant drug use.

Greater social stigma still attaches to drinking and drug abuse by women than to that by men. Women alcoholics often state that their husbands drink with them yet disapprove of their drinking (Corrigan, 1980). As a result, many women react with shame and attempt concealment. Even those who have lost control when drinking alone often manage to limit themselves to one or two drinks when dining with their husbands or women friends (Glatt, 1979). Women who stay home frequently drink and nap in the afternoon, hoping to look fresh and competent when their children and husbands come home. Their ability to conceal their drinking habits may account for much of the "telescoping" (shorter duration between onset of drinking and alcoholism) described in female alcoholics (Beckman, 1975). This denial of women's drinking continues because its feared consequences, such as overt sexuality and family neglect, violate traditional female taboos (Sandmaier, 1980).

A female alcoholic may abandon responsibility as a wife but cling desperately to her role as a mother. Her performance as a mother, even when it is somewhat impaired, minimizes the attention paid to her drinking (Corrigan, 1980). Fifty-seven percent of women alcoholics reported difficulties in their role as wives, whereas 42% reported such difficulties as mothers (Corrigan, 1980). Women who work sometimes hide substance abuse through non-challenging jobs and extensive absenteeism (Reichman, 1983), although younger women, especially those in challenging or part-time jobs, are drinking more openly (Reichman, 1983). Wilsnack et al. (1986) found slightly higher rates of heavier drinking among women in full-time employment than among full-time homemakers; however, again, women employed part-time had more drinking problems than women who were full-time homemakers or were employed full-time. These results varied according to the women's age: in the 45-to-54 age group, women in paid employment drank more than full-time homemakers, but in the 55-to-64 group, full-time homemakers drank more (Wilsnack et al., 1986).

Taking a job outside of the home does not decrease a woman's responsibilities in the home. A 1993 study performed by the Families and Work Institute (*New York Times,* 1993) reported that when both parents work, the wife still does 80% of the cooking and 70% of the child care. This helps us to understand why working mothers are so stressed and so highly vulnerable as a group to alcoholism. Their drinking may be related to the increased accessibility of alcohol, as well as to increasing responsibility and role realignments (Shore, 1992).

Women who are especially vulnerable to substance abuse can be divided into two groups: those who were functionally and emotionally overresponsible in their families of origin, and those who were underresponsible (Bepko & Krestan, 1985). Alcohol and drugs help overcome taboos against self-expression and self-gratification in overresponsible women, who were raised to take care of everyone but themselves. Substances of abuse let them be underresponsible, express anger and defiance, and have sex without intimacy. In treatment, these women strive to be perfect patients just as they have tried to be perfect wives and mothers. But they are willing to work on this overresponsibility, and respond well to reality-based interventions that help reverse their low self-esteem.

Underresponsible women have not developed sufficient knowledge of their own emotions or appropriate coping techniques. They deal with life incompetently, view themselves as special, and expect to be cared for as adults. In treatment they are defiant, look to others to meet their needs, and feel angry and vindictive when these others do not respond. They try hard to prove that no one can really help them; this sets them up to be rejected. They often respond best to paradoxical interpretations that predict and prescribe their resistances (Bepko & Krestan, 1985).

Middle-class women may drink as a result of two types of conflict over sex roles (Wilsnack, 1982): A woman's sex-role behavior may conflict with her own values; or the woman may not be conflicted herself, but her values and activities may clash with an environment that demands sex-stereotyped behavior. These conflicts (combined with other stresses) may explain the high rate of problem drinking among married working women, compared with unmarried working women or married women who do not work outside the home. Women from the poorer levels of society, in particular, often use alcohol to escape from conflict over sex roles; the more they drink, the more confident they feel (Sandmaier, 1980).

Some women develop substance abuse out of overaggressiveness, arising in part from rejection of stereotyped female behavior. Some women alcoholics—a minority in studies to date—reject all social pressures to be "ladylike" and are generally rebellious. Their defiance covers a broad range of activities, from problems at school to illegal activities, serious parental conflict, promiscuity, and early abuse of drugs and alcohol (Sandmaier, 1980). This contrast between "caretakers" and "wayward women" is evident in the results of research about both alcoholic and heroin-addicted women (Colten, 1980; Wilsnack, 1973). In their struggle to behave within rigidly proscribed roles, women who could not fit into the stereotyped "feminine ideal" seem to have chosen another rigid role ("bad, chemically dependent woman") as an alternative to the first.

Beckman et al. (1980) noted the following area of conflict in alcoholic women: They were rated higher on conscious femininity and somewhat lower on unconscious femininity than were nonalcoholic women. This finding supports other writings on addiction (e.g., Baldinger et al., 1972; Marsh, 1979; Miller et al., 1973; Wilsnack, 1973), which suggest that addicted women who tend to be "caretakers" have more traditional concepts of appropriate feminine behavior. As a result, assertiveness, independence, competition, and taking active control of their lives would tend to create conflict for these women. Their attempts to conform to traditional expectations would most likely be approved by their families and physicians, and drugs that would support these attempts would be encouraged until the drugs themselves become problems (Wolper & Scheiner, 1981).

In apparent contrast, Colten (1980) found that heroin-addicted women scored lower on both masculinity *and* femininity (i.e, showed lower androgyny) than nonaddicted women. Beckman (1975) noted that alcoholic women and women in psychiatric treatment scored lower on both masculinity and femininity than did women in a control group. Colten's (1980) study revealed that women addicts who endorsed traits traditionally considered masculine, such as competence, independence, and activity, had higher self-esteem. Although passivity and depression are more common in female than male SAs, a growing number of these women, particularly those who are younger, are very assertive (the "rebellious" or "wayward" subgroup).

Marital and Relational Issues

Substance use by male spouses or partners is an important factor in female substance use patterns. If both partners in a couple drink heavily, for example, they tend to support each other in continued alcoholism. Women are frequently introduced to alcohol and drugs by men (Reed, 1985), and alcoholic women are more likely to be married to alcoholic men (Beckman, 1975). Female cocaine use is also very much tied to the use of cocaine by spouses or significant others: Recent surveys indicate that 87% of women addicted to cocaine were introduced to it by men (Walker et al., 1991).

Estep (1987) discusses the influence of the family on both alcohol use and prescription drug use by women. From interview and questionnaire findings, she concludes that those women who seek treatment for their use of both alcohol and depressant drugs, when compared with controls, have companions who drink and take prescription sedatives more heavily and more frequently than the companions of non-SA women. Female SAs in treatment generally have also been through more marriages and have had more abortions, miscarriages, and childbirths. In addition, women who are in treatment have a higher incidence of arrests than do controls, which may create problematic separations from their families while they are incarcerated.

Alcoholic women frequently state that marital problems are the reasons they drink (Liepman et al., 1989). Alcoholic women have a high divorce rate and are left by their spouses more frequently than are alcoholic men (Corrigan, 1980). Sexual dysfunction in alcoholic women was found by Forrest (1982) to be quite common, but whether these problems are more causes or effects of alcohol use was not determined by this study.

In a national study conducted in the early 1980s, Wilsnack et al. (1986) found that only 8% of adult women reported being less particular in choosing a sexual partner while intoxicated, whereas 60% reported that another person who was also drinking had been sexually aggressive toward them. Thus the societal expectation that women are more promiscuous when drinking was not confirmed, but this expectation had sinister consequences in terms of behavior *toward* drinking women. Victimization through rape and domestic violence is also far more common among chemically dependent women than among other women in the same community.

Women entering drug treatment have been noted to be socially isolated—more isolated than male addicts, who are in turn more isolated than female nonaddicts (Tucker, 1980; Wallace, 1976). These women report having fewer friends, fewer romantic relationships, and greater feelings of loneliness than either of the two other groups. The relationships they do have seem to be more stressful and troublesome. When these women have partners, the partners are more likely to be involved in drugs also (Ryan & Moise, 1979; Tucker, 1980). In addition to feeling isolated, addicted women are more likely than nonaddicted women from similar backgrounds to have children and to have them at an earlier age, and they are less likely to be living with the fathers of their children or with any other sexual partners (Tucker, 1980).

The support female SAs receive in caring for children seems to come more from family members and from female friends than from spouses (Schwingel et al., 1977). About 30% of addicted women live with their families of origin or other relatives, and many others live close to relatives (Moise, 1979; Tucker, 1980; Wallace, 1976; Wolper & Scheiner, 1981). Binion (1980) found that women who were involved with drugs often ran away from home many times during adolescence, and that many quit school before graduation; adolescence has traditionally been considered a time when young people begin to separate from their families and develop identities of their own (e.g., Erikson, 1950). However, younger addicts are also often heavily involved (or overinvolved) with their parents, and either reside with them or see them frequently (Ellinwood et al., 1966; Moise, 1979; Stanton, 1979a; Tucker, 1980; Wallace, 1976; Wolper & Scheiner, 1981).

Women addicted to heroin can be divided into two very different groups, which correspond to age (Rosenbaum, 1981). Those over 25 appear passive, and have usually been introduced to and maintained on heroin by their mates. Younger women addicts tend to be more liberated and assertive; in addition, younger lower-class addicts may use drugs as part of a culture that is powerful, respected, and prestigious. My own studies of women heroin addicts, most of whom were over 25, revealed the majority to be quite passive, with their addiction fused to that of their mates (Kaufman, 1985). However, an impressive minority remained remarkably assertive. Most of the latter group maintained their own heroin supplies separately from their mates', and after completing treatment achieved a good deal of traditional success.

Women who are still under the "spell" and control of dominant male addicts/pushers are very difficult to treat, because these men often not only will not participate in treatment, but will undermine their mates' treatment and sobriety. These addicted males require individual treatment of their own, which they will sometimes accept if they are reached by family therapy.

Sexual and Other Abuse

Over the past decade, there has been growing awareness of the important contribution of sexual abuse, especially incest, to female substance abuse. It is these abused women who are often harder to treat than other female SAs, because their trauma has left them more likely to have suicidal ideation, self mutilation, borderline personality disorder, greater substance abuse, post-traumatic stress disorder, sexual problems, hospitalizations, and antisocial personality disorder than female SAs without sexual abuse (Barnett & Trepper, 1991; Weatherford & Kaufman, 1991; Bollerud, 1990). It has been estimated that 75% of women in drug treatment have been sexually victimized (Bollerud, 1990). Extreme and brutal physical and emotional abuse also may create severe psychological dysfunction.

Many sexually abused girls deal with their overwhelming anxiety, guilt, fear, and anger by suppressing their feelings rather than stirring up problems (Barnett & Trepper, 1991). When they try to talk about their having been abused, they are most often disbelieved, blamed, or punished. These abused girls develop several personality patterns that leave them vulnerable to becoming SAs, including low self-esteem, self-derogation, self-destructiveness, dissociation from their feelings, and distance from those closest to them (Barnett & Trepper, 1991). Sexually molested adolescent girls also generally lack factors that might protect them against substance abuse, such as loving, firm parenting, clear intergenerational boundaries, and open lines of communication. These girls are then often attracted to drug-using peer groups, and find that drugs and alcohol help suppress painful memories and affects. Substances also help continue the disassociation that began during the sexual abuse. Continued substance abuse perpetuates all these maladaptive defenses and behaviors, so that the solution causes as many problems as the initial trauma, if not more (Barnett & Trepper, 1991). Abuse of substances also leaves these young women vulnerable to date rape, gang rape, and illegitimate pregnancies, all of which perpetuate their traumas and difficulties with self-esteem and survival.

PERSONALITY TRAITS AND PSYCHOPATHOLOGY

A wide variety of psychopathology, personality styles, and personality disorders are seen among women who abuse drugs and alcohol. These disorders are probably of greater frequency and intensity than in similar men. However, it is difficult to separate pre-existing pathology from the social consequences of substance abuse, which are more severe for women. When women deviate from socially accepted "feminine" behavior, the consequences are far more serious than they are for men. Not only do these women face society's condemnation, but they frequently condemn themselves. This cycle lowers their self-esteem, which drives them further into substance abuse.

The high incidence of depression in female alcoholics has been well documented. Winokur and Pitts (1965) were among the first authors to link alcoholism in women to affective illness. Schuckit et al. (1969) found that 27% of 70 female alcoholics had suffered severe depression prior to their alcoholism (such individuals are called "secondary alcoholics"). More recently, data from the Epidemiologic Catchment Area Study, focusing on alcoholism and major depression, showed that alcoholism was primary and depression secondary in 78% of the male subjects with both disorders. An analysis of women subjects revealed a striking reversal of this relation: In 66% of the female subjects, depression was primary and alcoholism secondary (Helzer & Pryzbeck, 1988).

Winokur et al. (1970) described a "depressive spectrum disease," in which women with severe depression were found to have a high incidence of first-degree male relatives with sociopathy or alcoholism and female relatives with a high incidence of depression. Based on their genetic studies of depression and alcoholism, Winokur and Clayton (1968) speculated that alcoholism may have a different pattern of inheritance in women than in men, although this may only be true for the minority of alcoholic women with a strong affective component to their illness. Women alcoholics also show an overall higher incidence of suicide attempts than males; however, this may relate to the generally higher occurrence of these attempts in females (Winokur & Clayton, 1968). Recent findings (Merikangas et al., 1985) challenge the concept that depression in parents is genetically linked to alcoholism in progeny. Merikangas et al. emphasized a tendency of the conjoined factors of alcoholism and depression in parents to cause alcoholism and depression in children. However, even more recent studies show a direct relationship between parental major depression and female alcoholism (Kendler, Heath, Neale, Kessler, & Eaves, 1993).

Studies utilizing the Brief Psychiatric Rating Scale reveal high scores among chronic female alcoholics on Anxiety, Guilt, Tension, Depressed Mood, Hostility, and Neuroticism (Hoffman & Welfring, 1972). Bromet and Moos (1976) felt that these findings may relate in part to the higher proportion of married male to married female alcoholics, as married alcoholics of both sexes tend to be healthier than single alcoholics.

Studies of heroin addicts, however, only partially support the hypothesis that females demonstrate greater psychopathology. In a review of 15 studies of psychopathology in female drug abusers, 5 (33%) found that females functioned more poorly than males; no studies supported the opposite conclusion; and 4 studies made no comparison. Six studies (40%) did not report broad male–female differences, instead noting psychological difficulties in both sexes (Burt et al., 1979).

DeLeon (1974) found greater evidence of anxiety and depression, and DeLeon and Jainchill (1980) found more emotional disturbance and psychosomatic symptoms, in women addicts. Ellinwood et al. (1966) found that female addicts were more often diagnosed as neurotic (10%, vs. 1% for males) and psychotic (7%, vs. 0% for males), and that males were more often diagnosed as personality-disordered (77%, vs. 66% for females) and specifically antisocial (17%, vs. 3% for females). According to these studies, female SAs show a greater degree of Axis I and Axis II psychopathology than do male SAs. However, a recent tendency in U.S. society to condone certain substance use and abuse patterns among women has begun to normalize this behavior, as well as to equalize psychopathology between male and female SAs. This is based on the principle that the more out of keeping any behavior (including substance abuse) is from normal cultural practices, the more likely psychopathology is to be present. Thus we would expect female users of hard drugs (i.e., heroin, PCP, intravenous cocaine) to be sicker than male abusers of "peer-compatible" substances (Kaufman, 1976a) or female abusers of prescription drugs. Similarly, we would expect male SAs who use a drug out of keeping with their social background to be sicker than those whose substance use is compatible with their origins (e.g., upper- and middle-class male heroin addicts would be expected to have more psychopathology than addicts raised in ghettos, where heroin use is more normative).

Brook et al. (1992) review what they refer to as the "generalized female vulnerability hypothesis," which claims that drugs and alcohol will have a greater intrapsychic effect on females than on males because of physical vulnerability, social control and labeling, and internalized sex-role norms. Surprisingly, their research did not find a differential gender effect in the developmental path to delinquency. However, their studies did demonstrate *earlier* delinquency and drug use in males.

MMPI profiles of female addicts parallel the findings reported above. According to Hill et al. (1962), the typical female addict in the study had a "neurotic psychopath" profile, with high elevations on the Depression and Paranoia scales. Women alcoholics also scored higher than men alcoholics on the MMPI "neurotic triad"—the Neurasthenia, Hysteria, and Depression scales (Zelen et al., 1966). However, overall profiles of personality characteristics of male and female alcoholics resemble each other more than they do those of nonalcoholics (Beckman, 1975). Both men and women alcoholics scored high on Depression, Psychasthenia, and Psychopathy in Zelen et al.'s (1966) study. Rosen (1960) found that women's overall profiles were different from men's, but that women alcoholics and matched women outpatients showed marked similarities in MMPI profiles.

The personalities of female SAs have been separated into various subtypes. Mogar et al. (1970) described five personality subtypes in these women: normal–manic, normal–depressive, hysterical, psychopathic, and passive aggressive. Hart and Stueland (1980) classified six personality types of female alcoholics: (1) passive impulsive neurotic, (2) introverted obsessive compulsive, (3) paranoid, (4) schizoid, (5) trait disorder with psychopathology, and (6) extraverted obsessive compulsive. The two most common were normal–manic and normal–depressive, which are marked by hyperfemininity, strong masculine strivings, masochistic tendencies, and confusion over sex roles (Beckman, 1975).

These citations on differing forms and prevalence of psychopathology in female SAs are in no way meant to revive the myth that female SAs are sicker and/or more difficult to treat than males. Few experts would say that the antisocial personality disorder so prevalent in male SAs is a healthier psychological state than the depression prevalent in females. Not only is depression a healthier developmental adjustment, but it renders SAs much more amenable to treatment. Another factor that accounts for much greater psychopathology in female than in male SAs is the very high occurrence of sexual abuse (particularly incest) among females, as described above.

FAMILIES OF ORIGIN

One remarkably consistent finding has been the high prevalence of parental substance abuse in the families of female SAs. Winokur and Clayton's (1968) study of families of male and female alcoholics revealed fathers of alcoholic women were often themselves alcoholic (28%), as were mothers (12%) and sisters (12%). The same study showed similar but lower percentages in the fathers, mothers, and sisters of alcoholic men (21%, 3%, and 2%, respectively). In 1975, Beckman noted that 28% was the low range for prevalence of alcoholism in the fathers of women alcoholics, and estimates as high as 50% were common.

Evidence indicates that in the future, progressively more female alcoholics will be born to alcoholic mothers, as the incidence of maternal alcoholism is increasing. In 1980, Corrigan found that only 3% of women alcoholics over age 50 had ever seen their mothers drunk, whereas 55% of those under 30 had. Bromet and Moos (1976) noted that more female than male alcoholics had mothers who drank heavily.

Binion (1980) found that "drinking a lot" was more common in families of heroin-addicted women (59.7%) than in families of matched controls (42.9%). Parental condoning of the use of alcohol and drugs appears to lead to abuse, even when the parents do not abuse substances themselves (Kandel, 1975).

Families of female SAs show a high incidence of disruption. Sandmaier (1980) and Wilsnack (1982) both found that women alcoholics are more likely than men to have lost one or both parents during childhood through divorce, desertion, or death; psychosis is also frequently seen in parents or close relatives. Although rates of disruption are high in both alcoholic men and women, Gomberg (1980) noted that they are higher in women. Those who have experienced broken homes before the age of 10 are significantly more likely than men with the same history to become heavy drinkers (Boothroyd, 1980). Many female narcotic addicts have experienced early separation from or death of a parent, usually the father (Stanton, 1979a). Johnson (1968) found that 65% of female narcotics users had parents who separated during their childhood.

Many of the women alcoholics described by Beckman (1975) described their mothers as cold, severe, and domineering and their fathers as warm, gentle, and alcoholic. These fathers only rebelled against their dominant wives when drunk. Daughters preferred their fathers and felt that if their mothers had been more loving, their fathers would not have needed to drink. They gravitated to their fathers for the affection and support they did not get from their mothers. Their identification with their alcoholic fathers and lack of positive female role models left them without a clear sense of female identity, which made them directly vulnerable to developing alcoholism as adults or to marrying alcoholics in order to rescue them. This pattern of a weak father overinvolved with his prealcoholic daughter is common. An alternative scenario—the totally absent father—is also prevalent, as is the pattern of parental mental illness, particularly unipolar depression. Fathers of female alcoholics are more likely to be depressed, mentally ill, or absent than mothers are (Winokur & Clayton, 1968). Daughters of alcoholics are heavier drinkers when there is maternal alcoholism than when there is paternal alcoholism (Beckman, 1975).

Alcoholic women are more likely than nonalcoholics to have had unhappy childhoods with little acceptance and approval (Corrigan, 1980). An early study by Wall (1937) found that hospitalized female alcoholics had no particularly strong ties to either of their parents or to their siblings, compared to 37% of male alcoholics who had a strong attachment to their mothers. Williams and Klerman (1984) summarize the families of origin of female alcoholics as demonstrating marked impairment of parent–child relationships, with family homeostatic balance significantly damaged by separations, neglect, erratic discipline, and poor parenting.

Stanton et al. (1982) have observed, as have I (Kaufman, 1976a), that female addicts are often in overt competition with their mothers, in part because they experience them as authoritarian, controlling, and overprotective. Fathers of female addicts are often overly indulgent or sexually aggressive, particularly when intoxicated on alcohol.

Although single-parent families have often been equated with the kind of dysfunction that leads to substance abuse as well as to personality and social difficulties, there is also evidence to the contrary. Cashion's (1982) review of the literature concluded that female-headed families, when not plagued by poverty, are as successful as two-parent families in regard to adjustment and lack of delinquent behavior. Lindblad-Goldberg (1989) concludes that even poverty-stricken single-parent families are not inevitably dysfunctional. Factors in single-parent families that can favorably affect developmental outcome include lack of conflict, financial stability, good supervision, and positive role modeling. Other important critical issues are absence of maternal depression and the mother's sense of control over her environment, which lead to a feeling of mastery and well-being (Lindblad-Goldberg, 1989). The mother needs to be in charge of the family, with the children doing what they are told and the mother providing balance and discipline. When the maternal grandmother is also in the house, it is essential that she not assume primary authority, but maintain a supportive alliance with her daughter (Lindblad-Goldberg, 1989).

GENDER-SPECIFIC CONSIDERATIONS FOR PSYCHOTHERAPY

The stress-, loss-, and identity-related issues reported in the studies of chemically dependent women described up to this point suggest that psychotherapy would be particularly useful. However, therapists working with these women and their families will need to be sensitive to several gender-specific considerations in implementing therapy (Wolper & Scheiner, 1981).

Since female substance abuse is often precipitated by loss, therapists should be sensitive to these issues, and empathic understanding of these losses should be a focus of treatment. Likewise, the commonality of sexual abuse in their histories mandates that this be worked through. Inpatient and residential settings are excellent for processing sexual abuse, as these provide structure and support during the difficult release of painful feelings, which could easily lead to relapse without such protection. Thus, I advocate processing these issues either during the early residential phase of treatment, or later when sobriety is solidified. Former perpetrators can be brought into treatment and confronted by their female victims in the presence of a therapist who has sensitivity for all parties.

The single mother is in a difficult bind if child care is necessary in order to enable her to attend hospital or residential treatment. If there are no family members capable of caring for the children, then they may have to be placed; most often with the siblings separated from one another as well as their mother. In many settings, even brief residential treatment may cost the mother the housing that would enable her to bring her family together again. Thus a woman who is motivated to enter treatment and can afford it, or is offered a funded slot, may be at war with her maternal instinct if she is to receive the treatment she so desperately needs (Walker et al., 1991).

Another serious threat to a female SA's choosing to enter residential treatment is the potential loss of a significant other, particularly one who has any use of illicit drugs or alcohol. If the primary emphasis of treatment is on minimizing the risk of relapse, then the female SA is often strongly encouraged, supported, or even commanded to relinquish this relationship. This loss will deprive her of economic and social support as well as of her primary adult love relationship. The choice thus presents another difficult decision if a woman is to enter into and/or remain in treatment until completion (Walker et al., 1991). Of course, the ideal treatment plan would involve an intensive program for the significant other as well.

Still another problem is the fact that a female SA often lacks parenting skills. This issue and the substance abuse can be worked on simultaneously if a facility can accommodate the woman and her children. If this is not possible, then guided therapeutic visits could be part of the program, as well as psychoeducation that focuses on such parenting issues as communication, limit setting, and bonding.

Female SAs have more problems with employment than do male SAs (Kail & Lukoff, 1984). Treatment for women who do not live with family members should focus on vocational training and socialization with family members and non-drug-using friends. Treatment for single women with children should emphasize child care and parenting skills, whereas women with spouses can learn ways to achieve a better balance between employment and child care (Kail & Lukoff, 1984).

FEMINIST THERAPY

Many female (and some male) therapists have recently espoused a focus on a number of important issues, which have been grouped under the rubric of "feminist family therapy." Even the most enlightened therapist can benefit from considering and implementing these aspects of treatment. A basic concept is that the therapy of female SAs must "empower the disempowered" (Walker et al., 1991). Thus "women's gifts for creating and recreating communities of their own" should be utilized, rather than subjecting them to male-dominated hierarchies (Walker et al., 1991). Thus women are helped to "find their authoritative and authentic voices" and to "reauthor their lives so they are supported by webs of meaningful, nonoppressive relationships" (Walker et al., 1991). Empowerment is taught by giving women choices, involving them actively in treatment planning, giving them successful role models and images to hold on to, and helping them define a self.

Feminist theory reminds us of the need to work on several key psychodynamic issues. These include a variety of sexual problems that are often not addressed in treatment, eating disorders, depression, shame, and guilt (Forth-Finegan, 1991). Women's shame is often a result of their having failed to achieve the "idealized gender image" that is so strongly emphasized and taught by the culture. Feminist psychoeducation helps change this image to one that is more achievable and obtainable for women, thus relieving shame. Guilt is more difficult an emotion to work with; it is more amenable to in-depth psychotherapy with an understanding, empathic therapist. Lowering perfectionistic self-demands helps to relieve both shame and guilt. Woodman (1982; cited in Forth-Finegan, 1991) proposes that healing addiction involves "giving permission to the self to express and to own the full range of feminine energy, the energy of the wet, moist, earthy, strong, expressive and intuitive; by taking one's power and developing the power from within."

Barnett and Trepper (1991) emphasize the importance of empowering women who have been sexually abused to stop blaming themselves for the abuse that took place in the past, to put an end to all present abuse, and never let abuse happen again. These authors have developed a three-stage therapeutic model for work in a family therapy context with the female SA who is an incest victim.

In working with the families and networks of chemically dependent women, therapists must remember that drug and alcohol treatment programs have, for the most part, been organized for chemically dependent men. We now know that men and women in the same facility do not necessarily receive the same services. Therapists should become aware of the possibility that they themselves may have limiting cultural views of women's (and men's) appropriate roles, as well as diminished sensitivity to alternatives that might be more fulfilling for some women (Hare-Mustin, 1978).

Individual psychotherapy, in and of itself, will not counteract a setting that has different standards for women or a therapist who lacks gender sensitivity. But psychotherapy can, if applied with sensitivity to the chemically dependent woman and her family, make a unique contribution. The woman who is chemically dependent is likely to be pivotal in the family situation, because one of a woman's roles is to be responsible for the welfare of her family. If things go wrong, she is likely to be blamed and may be burdened by guilt. Women who are chemically dependent are thought to be "worse" than men in the same situation (Colten, 1980), and are less likely to be supported by others as a result. Thus, when working a chemically dependent female, a therapist must pay special attention to the potential of misinterpreting the problems forced on her as originating "in her." For this, the therapist may need additional training in gender issues. A therapist should also be vigilant about the sensitivity of the entire treatment program to gender differences, the consequences of stereotyped roles, and the implications of status differences between men and women.

WOMEN AND TWELVE-STEP GROUPS

Although the percentage of my female patients who have utilized AA, Narcotics Anonymous (NA) and Cocaine Anonymous (CA) to facilitate solid sobriety and personality change is similar to that of my male patients, there are some valid reasons why women may resist the Twelve-Step concept. Bill Wilson, the founder of AA in 1935, "was influenced by white, male, middle-class, Christian values of the 1930's" (Kasl, 1992, p. 5). He "based the 12 steps and the Big Book on experiences of 100 men and one woman" and his definition of personality traits are those of "white, upper-middle-class men who have power in the system." Thus AA (and, by extension, other Twelve-Step groups) was created to deal with "egocentric, arrogant, controlling, resentful, violent" men and not women, whose substance abuse so often develops out of struggling with or against the victim role that society often mandates for them. Thus, when women are told that questioning AA or other Twelve-Step groups means they are "deluded" or "lack humility" (Kasl, 1992, p. 5), it reinforces their dependence on the program in ways which leave them feeling quite impotent.

Some feminist critiques of Twelve-Step groups have attacked the concept of "powerlessness" as reinforcing the weakness of women in our society. Berenson (1991) challenges this criticism on the grounds that it involves an inaccurate perception of what powerlessness is all about in the Twelve Steps. He states that the experience of powerlessness is in fact a major source of empowerment and effectiveness. Berenson (1991) feels that once men and women can recognize the primacy of their feminine, accepting side, then they are better able to express their masculine, assertive side. He states that the powerlessness of the Twelve Steps provides "a foundation for an empowering, non-dogmatic, spiritual practice that is supportive of feminine goals" (Berenson, 1991, p. 79). He quotes the phrase "courage to change the things I can" from the Serenity Prayer as addressing the assertiveness necessary to take definitive action to correct external problems. The Twelve Steps can be differentiated into "surrender" steps and "action" steps, with the former setting the stage for the latter to occur. Berenson sums up his argument by stating that "the experience of powerlessness can lead to a new sense of empowerment from which gender, social and political inequities can be more effectively addressed" (p. 79).

Nevertheless, some women will find the sexist barriers to Twelve-Step work insurmountable. For them, there are workable alternatives as long as there is a commitment to working within a comprehensive program to achieve personality change. One organization that is particularly sensitive to these issues is Women for Sobriety (WFS). Its motto is "We are capable and competent, caring and compassionate, always willing to help one another, bonded together in overcoming our addictions" (Kasl, 1992, p. 165). WFS is a more holistic approach than the Twelve Steps, and thus encourages women to meditate, eat healthy food, smoke less, and treat their bodies with love and care (Kasl, 1992) — all ingredients of many if not most present-day comprehensive treatment programs for men and women. The steps of WFS are directed "to build up women's fragile egos and battered self-esteem through self-discovery, and to release shame and guilt through the sharing of experiences, hope and mutual encouragement" (Kasl, 1992, p. 167).

I have no argument with any comprehensive system that reinforces sobriety, as long as this method is sufficiently available to provide the same level of support that AA and other Twelve-Step groups do. Unfortunately, WFS is not available in many areas of the United States. Thus women who have the sorts of objections voiced in this section can work primarily through small women-only Twelve-Step groups, together with other comprehensive self-help and psychotherapy groups. However, as with male patients, my most successful results are with women patients who use the Twelve Steps as a supplement to pragmatic psychodynamic psychotherapy. I also attribute a substantial part of this success to a sensitivity to female gender-related issues as described in this chapter.

CHAPTER 3

Defense Mechanisms
in Addicted Persons

A separate chapter is included on the defense mechanisms, in order to emphasize the importance of an understanding of these mental processes in the psychotherapy of SAs. For example, some defenses are supported in the early phases of therapy and confronted later; for others the opposite is true. Although the different defense mechanisms are presented separately here, defenses are often used simultaneously or sequentially. This is particularly true of paired denial and projection or denial and rationalization. Defenses also often occur in specific groupings, which help to define personality styles (Bond, 1986).

In traditional psychoanalytic theory, "defenses" are defined as operations of the ego that protect the ego against either internal dangers (sexuality, anger, passivity, the death drive) or the imagined, unconsciously exaggerated aspects of realistic dangers (death, castration, obliteration, fusion, catastrophic explosion) (Fenichel, 1945). In this view the defenses work within a topographical model, serving to keep painful affects out of the conscious mind, and pushing them down into and keeping them in the unconscious mind. Thus the defenses can be seen as functioning horizontally. However, Kernberg (1967) has described the vertical evolution and function of splitting types of defenses (devaluation, idealization), which are quite common in SAs.

Defenses maintain an individual's sense of integrity and homeostasis. Alcohol and drugs are frequently used as substitutes for defense mechanisms. Thus, these substances provide a substitutive homeostasis, or an anesthetized/obliterated state in which conflicts are removed from awareness. Drugs and alcohol also prevent more adaptive defenses from being developed and lead to the atrophy of healthier defenses previously utilized.

47

Shapiro (1989) refers to defenses as "self-awareness-distorting processes," which are articulated automatically and with dimly conscious awareness of the self that is utilizing them. These processes prevent ideas, feelings, motivations, impulses, and entire subjective experiences from being consciously articulated or from reaching self-awareness. I agree with Shapiro that this formulation is closer to resonating with therapeutic clinical experiences than is the traditional concept based on a mechanical drive-based structure.

Substance dependence and abuse lead to more primitive utilization of defenses. It is appropriate to say that substance abuse results in the use of more primitive defense mechanisms in a less adaptive way, rather than that it totally replaces the defensive system. The denial of SAs is paradoxically superficial as well as primitive; it entails a distortion of reality that is quite superficial and almost conscious. Yet the defenses are considered "primitive" because developmentally they are used in this manner by young children and by individuals with relatively unformed, underdeveloped egos. In addition, alcohol and depressant drugs dampen powerful, primitive emotions and instincts when they threaten to overwhelm defenses.

Fenichel (1945) defines defenses as either successful or unsuccessful. All successful defenses are considered types of sublimation, because they permit instant gratification without leading to symptoms (e.g., passivity into activity, hostility into altruism, anger into art). Unsuccessful defenses may develop into neuroses because they lead either to continued anxiety or to symptoms. The defenses of SAs are unsuccessful, in that anxiety and depression recur when the substance is removed. Rather than leading directly to symptoms (as in neurotics), primitive defenses in SAs lead to dysfunctional personality types, frequently termed "character disorders." In the *Diagnostic and Statistical Manual of Mental Disorders,* third edition, revised (DSM-III-R; American Psychiatric Association, 1987), they are referred to as "personality traits" or, when they are more severe, "personality disorders."

The defenses of SAs that are emphasized here are denial, projection, and rationalization, but all customary defenses are discussed. Perry and Cooper (1986) have found that denial, projection, and rationalization cluster together within individuals, in addition to sharing a basic similarity: They allow the individual to disavow some aspect of himself or herself. These defenses are far more easily observed by others by the individuals using them. They permit individuals to minimize their problems, but do not in any way prevent the consequences of their behaviors. They offer a "temporary holiday" from conflict and pain, but ultimately the consequences are worsened.

DENIAL

Denial is considered the most common defense mechanism used by SAs. The word "denial" has many more meanings in the field of substance abuse than was intended by its original psychoanalytic usage. Each meaning or definition of denial makes a valuable contribution to the understanding and psychotherapy of SAs. Generally in the field of chemical dependence, "denial" is applied to the denial of obvious reality, as well as to a whole range of behaviors and statements that have a denying quality. These denying behaviors are used to justify, hide, and protect substance abuse; to deny responsibility for the consequences of behavior; to avoid treatment; and to preserve self-esteem in the face of negative consequences (Whitfield, 1982).

Thus SAs do not merely lie about how much they drink and use drugs. They deny both emotionally and factually deny how much they have manipulated and hurt their families and friends. They deny how self-destructive their past behavior has been, as well as their future potential for serious illness and early death. When this denial is confronted early, they become furious. If they accept the confrontation as valid, they easily become emotionally devastated and depressed, or attack in retaliation (hence the fury).

In order to maintain denial, SAs must continue to deny any aspect of their environment that contradicts their original reality distortion. They accomplish this by selective perception, which registers only information that conforms to their narrowed self-definition (Brown, 1985). They may also distort environmental input so that it conforms to their perception of reality. This obviously narrows their ability to take in environmental stimuli, leading to a lack of growth. For example, an AA member with 10 years of sobriety described how great his denial was before he became sober. He had shot one of his fingers off when intoxicated. He stated that he had not been concerned about the loss, but had begun eating starfish to grow back his missing digit (because echinoderms can regenerate missing limbs)!

One of my major points in this book is that although general characteristics of chemically dependent persons are presented here, there are many individual variations. Individuality often gets lost in the field of substance abuse, particularly when it comes to the label of gross denial, which is often assumed to be at least very similar if not identical in most if not all SAs. Denial, like all defense mechanisms, is used differently by each individual; it may also be used differently over time by the same individual. A large portion of denial may disappear after only a week or two of abstinence. Still, some denial usually remains, and this may take years to resolve in a twelve-step group or even in psychotherapy. This remaining denial rarely if ever resolves without some intervention and is often referred to as "secondary denial."

In order to convey the severity of the basic denial in SAs, it is usually referred to as "primitive denial," as opposed to more adaptive forms of this defense. Denial is not automatically a primitive defense mechanism; it becomes primitive when it severely impairs reality testing. Often several defenses are used simultaneously in order to facilitate denial. Denial is frequently used together with rationalization and projection, as in this common example: A male alcoholic or drug addict denies his excessive consumption, yet rationalizes that he drinks or uses drugs as much as he does only because his wife nags him too much or does not understand him. In addition, he may rationalize by stating that all of his male friends also drink or use drugs and all of their wives nag them. Any SA with shame about his/her use of alcohol or drugs will readily deny the extent of his/her problem. However, a gentle confrontation will often rapidly bring a much greater estimate of use. For instance, many individuals who say at first that they only have three drinks a night will admit by the end of the interview that each drink contains 3 to 5 ounces of alcohol or that they consume a 1.5-liter bottle of hard alcohol every few days. Yet they seem genuinely surprised when they realize how much they use.

Classic Psychoanalytic Views

Fenichel's (1945) book *The Psychoanalytic Theory of Neurosis* continues to be a classic and is used here as a reference point for the psychoanalytic definition of denial. Denial may be merely the wish to deny unpleasant realities (Fenichel, 1945). The gradual development of ego strength and reality testing should theoretically make this type of wholesale falsification of reality impossible; however, the denial process continues to exist in even the healthiest of adults, in the form of fantasy. Denial also exists in neurotics, who split the ego into a superficial part that knows the truth and a deeper part that denies it, or vice versa. Fenichel did not deal directly with denial in SAs, but he described an "oral regression" in SAs, which would explain their ability to use this defense mechanism in such a "childish" manner.

Anna Freud's (1966) monograph *The Ego and the Mechanisms of Defense* is another classic work in this area, as its title implies. In it, she stated that denial may utilize fantasy, word, or act to deny the existence of anxiety and pain. Here the fantasies are actually used to control, compensate for, or substitute for painful situations. This use of denial is supported from one generation to the next by children's play, stories, myths, and fairy tales. Many of these deal with a child's allaying anxiety by gaining power over a giant (a male authority figure) or winning over a princess (mother/dependence gratification). A. Freud (1966) recognized that even in adulthood, fantasy can be used to reverse (or escape from) a dangerous situation; however, if the ego overuses this defense, its relation to reality can be profoundly shaken. Excessive use of fantasy inhibits syntheses, a key adaptational operational mechanism. The more the ego chooses fantasy gratification, the more damage is done to reality testing. States of drug and alcohol intoxication invariably provide fantasied solutions, which, with constant use, replace reality testing.

Denial in word and act is similar to denial in fantasy, except that the fantasy is acted out through either words or actions. One area where this kind of denial is common in adult SAs is sexuality. Cocaine abusers often find that the drug stimulates them to talk "dirty" and become more responsive to "dirty" talk, as well as to act out their most primitive and varied sexual fantasies. These sexual acts are used to deny sexual fears. Sedative and alcohol abusers find that substances relax their sexual fears, so that they can function well sexually while denying their sexual difficulties. With cocaine or depressant abusers who continue to use drugs regularly, the solution misfires, and they rapidly become incapable of sexual performance. However, at this stage they deny that they have any sexual needs, or even at times that they ever did have such needs. When they first enter treatment, they refuse to acknowledge their primitive sexual activities. This is in part conscious withholding and in part unconscious denial. As they come to trust their therapists, they reveal more; as they do so, their denial lifts, and sexual acts are recalled that were denied and repressed.

The Chemical Dependence View

In addition to the classic psychoanalytic view of denial, there are many other ways that the term is used in describing the defensive structure of SAs. Conscious lying, particularly about substance use and related behaviors, is considered part of denial in the field of substance abuse, although it is too conscious a process to be considered a true defense mechanism. However, SAs may truly deny that they have lied, so that they do not know when they have told the truth or not; thus lying and true denial become woven together.

A biologically based type of denial is the "blackout" or alcohol anamnestic response. Blackouts are one of the critical signs distinguishing alcoholics from problem drinkers; they occur more frequently as the disease progresses. (Blackouts are also seen in abusers of depressant drugs.) A blackout consists of amnesia for all or parts of behaviors performed during intoxication. One frightening (though fortunately rare) example of a blackout is provided by the occasional airline pilot who flies cross-country under the influence of alcohol and subsequently cannot remember doing this. More commonly, parts of a prior evening's conversation are totally forgotten, particularly provocative statements made by the SA (which he/she would like to forget). It would seem, then, that even forgetting during blackouts is at least partially psychodynamically determined by the defense mechanism of denial. Other toxic effects of alcohol and drugs on memory, information processing, and judgment may also facilitate or mimic denial (Whitfield, 1982).

Denial may also influence selective recall of events, so that the patient only remembers the pleasant aspects of an intoxicated episode. This recall may be emotional ("euphoric recall"). For example, an alcoholic may remember only the warm, friendly glow of drinking with the gang at the neighborhood tavern, but may forget almost being killed while driving home (Whitfield, 1982).

Denial of being an SA is often reinforced by an individual's definition of what or whom a drug addict or alcoholic is: "I can't be an alcoholic—I go to work every day," "I'm not on skid row," "I can run a marathon or ride a bicycle 100 miles in a day," "I can hold my liquor." Probably the most frequent denial mechanism is the claim that because the individual has control of alcohol or drug intake most of the time, or functions well most of the time, he/she therefore cannot be an addict or alcoholic. This claim is such an integral aspect of the disease of alcoholism or drug dependence that it is often pathognomonic of the early and middle phases of the disease (i.e., a diagnosis can be based on this one symptom alone). It is only in the very late phases that individuals totally lose control of intake or become consistently dysfunctional. Other aspects of an individual's own uninformed definition of substance dependence can also support denial: "My liver tests are normal," "I drink no more than my friends or my doctor," "Everyone smokes pot or uses a little cocaine now and then."

Denial may also represent a magical wish that things had happened the way the SA wanted them to happen rather than the way they actually did. Or denial may be driven by the fear of the powerful stigma associated with the label of "alcoholic" or "drug addict." Denial is also used to describe the general inability of many SAs to examine or recognize even the most obvious psychodynamic aspects of their behavior; Wurmser (1987) calls this avoidance of introspection "psychophobia." This phobia can gradually be resolved with sobriety and long-term psychotherapy. Finally, there may be a specific type of denial in which the numerous difficulties experienced by the SA are thought to be totally unrelated to the use of drugs or alcohol. Whitfield (1982) attributes this to a genuine confusion, which he terms a "complex thinking quandary."

Wurmser (1985) proposes that denial may become so severe that it leads to a split identity, in which two personalities engage in sharp conflict with each other and then use denial as the main weapon against each other. He describes a case in which the denial evolved from the patient's "vanishing emotionally" by teaching himself to shut out feelings from infancy, and then later reinforcing this through drugs. In this case, one identity was that of a "good boy who [was] bending over backwards, giving in, compliant, well adjusted versus that of the defiant, arrogant, angry, even murderously furious man and addict" (Wurmser, 1985). Wurmser (1985) states that the denial of one's identity leads to the assumption of a part-identity or false self. This denial of idealization may lead to depersonalization as a result of such a great loss of the sense of reality. Wurmser emphasizes that the denial of drinking is only the most superficial version of the many layers of denial.

Denial may be strongly reinforced by the environment. Some family members and close friends of SAs deny the substance abuse and related behaviors because of their own substance use or other individual pathology. Other friends and relatives give up pointing out the consequences of substance use and abuse because they grow tired of not being heard or listened to. Still other family members may support denial because substance abuse and denial of it play a basic integrating role in the family's homeostasis (Kaufman, 1985). Even physicians and therapists may deny patients' alcoholism and drug abuse as a result of various needs of their own, particularly their own substance use.

Denial, when utilized with distortion and delusional projection, is considered the most primitive use of defense mechanisms, according to Vaillant (1986). Wurmser (1987) is of the opinion that denial is not innately a rather primitive defense mechanism, but that primitiveness is best determined by the extent of conflict, associated anxiety, and diminished ego integration. I would add the degree of impairment of reality testing as an important sign of evaluating the primitiveness of denial or any other defense mechanism. Individuals who continue to use primitive defense mechanisms in a rigid manner experience troubled lives characterized by lack of growth.

There is a hierarchy in the use of denial, from normal to pathological. Denial is a universal mechanism for dealing with misfortune or for encouraging assertion in the face of danger. After the situation has passed, a healthy individual can be honest about the real feelings he/she experienced and the dangers he/she survived. Denial is primitive and pathological when it involves the maintenance of a belief that is out of keeping with the person's environment and background, and when it compromises the individual's ability to deal with reality. When denial reaches this point in most individuals, it is considered psychotic. When it reaches this level of intensity in alcoholics or drug-dependent persons it is not considered psychosis; rather, it is considered typical of the psychological aspects of the disease of chemical dependence.

Metzger (1988) reminds us of the universality of the denial of death and its relationship to fear of death. The latter fear is related to threats to existence, which unconsciously becomes equated with any experience that causes anxiety. Thus denial of threatening external events or of anxiety occurs in all individuals, according to existential theory, as a denial of fear of death. SAs repeatedly deny their risk of dying, either from a single overdose or hypersensitivity reaction, or from chronic effects such as AIDS or liver disease. Once they have faced this aspect of their denial of death, they can then be helped to appreciate their death anxiety. Alcoholics and drug addicts are particularly vulnerable to fears of death, perhaps because of early childhood losses or because in losing control over their substance use and related behaviors, they are more prone to loss of a sense of self. This is one of many reasons (which will be discussed in detail in Chapters 5–6) why denial should not be confronted early on. That is, chemically dependent persons need denial to maintain their sense of self-integrity and their feeling of bodily and emotional intactness (Metzger, 1988).

A Note of Caution

One note of caution needs to be sounded about the use of "denial" as a label. Denial has become so widely acknowledged as a hallmark of alcoholism or drug abuse that to deny substance abuse is frequently considered diagnostic of the disease. Obviously, however, some individuals who deny that they are alcoholics or drug addicts do so only because they have been wrongly accused, not because they are SAs. Caution should also be utilized in not overlabeling a multitude of substance abuse behaviors as "denial."

PROJECTION

"Projection" is another very common defense mechanism in SAs. It is defined as falsely attributing one's own unacknowledged feelings, impulses, or thoughts to others (Vaillant, 1986). In using this mechanism, SAs blame others for their problems, usually those who are closest to them. They may also project the blame for their problems onto seduction by alcohol or drugs—for instance, beer is the best thirst quench-er, a bottle of fine Chardonnay and a few fine brandies are the perfect complement to an excellent meal, sensamilla is the best strain of mariju-ana, and so on. They may also blame their friends, feeling that they would be excluded from their group if they did not use drugs or alco-hol at social gatherings. Projection is often the flip side of self-blame: In order to avoid the lowered self-esteem or depression that results from blaming himself/herself, the SA blames others.

Wallace (1985a) points out that SAs engage in a unique form of projection, which he terms "assimilative." In assimilative projection, an SA assumes that others are like himself/herself and perceives them that way. This is utilized more often in regard to positive qualities than to negative ones. It is a valuable defense early in therapy, when the newly sober SA identifies with the healthy qualities of sober persons in his/her environment.

RATIONALIZATION

The third mechanism in the triad of common defenses is "rationaliza-tion." Rationalization is a defense in which the individual deals with conflicts or stressors by utilizing incorrect but reassuring or self-serving explanations for his/her own behavior or that of others (Vaillant, 1986). In the classic psychoanalytic view, the ego is afraid of impulses such as those that are aggressive and/or sexual, and thus attempts to vindicate and justify them as good or to provide imagined secondary purposes for them (A. Freud, 1966).

Typical rationalizations of SAs include the following: "I drink be-cause I need my sleep, and without sleep I couldn't function," "I drink to tolerate an oppressive job/marriage/society/social engagement," "I function better on cocaine." "I need cocaine because I have atten-tion deficit disorder with hyperactivity" (a very small minority of adult cocaine addicts have adult attention deficit disorder). The denial and projective aspects of these rationalizing statements are quite obvious; again, the three main types of defenses are very frequently fused.

OTHER DEFENSE MECHANISMS

All other defense mechanisms are used by SAs as well. Each is described briefly here, and their relevance to SA is discussed. Here the defini-tions of Vaillant (1986) are utilized as a basis for discussion, except where noted.

• *Acting out.* This mechanism is as common in SAs as denial is, since the very use of drugs and alcohol to avoid, soothe, or replace feelings is by definition acting out. However, when drugs and alcohol are first relinquished, other forms of acting out continue or replace the use of substances. This acting out can range from lateness and missing sessions to impulsive sexualized relationships and other chaotic situations.

• *Altruism.* Although this is generally considered a healthy defense mechanism, masochistic altruism may lead to maintaining destructive relationships or damaging self-sacrifices. In later sobriety, helping others to get and stay sober is an altruistic act that strongly reinforces sobriety and facilitates personality growth.

• *Autistic fantasy.* Autistic fantasy is the use of drug-induced daydreams as a replacement for effective action or relationships (particularly symbiotic fusion under the influence of narcotics, or ecstatic visions on hallucinogens). Excessive reliance on such fantasies makes it all the more difficult to develop the coping skills necessary to obtain reality-based gratification when sober.

• *Devaluation, idealization, and splitting.* These three mechanisms are grouped together because they are often part of the same process. In splitting, all significant persons are either "all good" (through idealization) or "all bad" (through devaluation); splitting also refers to the SAs self-view as either "all good" or "all bad." It derives from a failure to integrate the positive and negative qualities of self and others into cohesive images. The same individual, particularly the therapist or significant other, may be alternately devalued or idealized. However, once an idealized individual is devalued there may not be another chance to restore the relationship, unless there is an unusual amount of prior basic trust. SAs often repeatedly split individuals in their environment into playing the roles of punitive aggressors or benevolent protectors. Numerous vigorous disputes occur between the parties cast in these roles as they are manipulated by the SAs to meet certain needs. Although this mechanism is the *sine qua non* of borderline personalities, it is frequently seen in SAs who are "pseudoborderlines" (see Chapter 4 on personality disorders).

• *Displacement.* In displacement, a feeling about a person or thing is transferred onto another, usually less threatening object. Most conflicts are displaced to alcohol and drugs in SAs, so that the critical underlying issues are not addressed. This is one more reason why underlying issues cannot be dealt with until the use of substances is replaced with solid abstinence.

• *Distortion.* Distortions are severe misrepresentations of external reality to suit inner needs, including megalomania and wish-fulfilling delusions. Drug-induced hallucinations and delusions are also used to justify superiority or entitlement in narcissistic personality disorder (see Chapter 4).

• *Dissociation.* This mechanism involves dealing with conflicts or stressors by temporarily altering consciousness or one's sense of personal identity. It is a variant of denial that is often facilitated by drugs and alcohol.

• *Externalization.* Externalization is a more general term than projection. It refers to perceiving in others aspects of oneself, including impulses, conflicts, moods, attitudes, and ways of thinking.

• *Humor.* As a defense mechanism, humor is a means of dealing with conflicts or stressors by emphasizing their amusing or ironic aspects. It is a useful defense in all phases of recovery when it does not utilize gross denial. Humor permits SAs necessary balance when they are dealing with the inevitable consequences of their past behaviors (e.g., losses, legal difficulties, and tax consequences). Humor also permits expression of feelings without personal discomfort or uncomfortable effects on others.

• *Hypochondriasis (somatization).* Either of these terms refers to transferring conflicts, stressors, or painful affects into physical symptoms and preoccupations with pain and/or somatic illness. Somatization is a very common mechanism in patients who become dependent on pain medications. Here, the use of opiates to dull the pain perpetuates the problem: There is a hypochrondrical preoccupation with withdrawal symptoms, which leads to further excessive use of opiates. Hypochondriasis can also lead to the abuse of hypnotics to provide overvalued sleep, or of sedatives to prevent the tachycardia of anxiety or tension headaches. Most SAs in withdrawal show hypochondrical preoccupation with their symptoms. Indeed, hypochrondriasis may present problems in early recovery when an SA is dealing with the physical aspects of the prolonged abstinence withdrawal syndrome, or even in later recovery when conflicts are somatized. The societally sanctioned adage "Have a pain, take a pill" is a seductive and dangerous message for the recovering somatizing SA.

• *Intellectualization.* The excessive use of abstract thinking to avoid experiencing or expressing disturbing feelings is a very common defense mechanism in SAs, particularly alcoholics. At times this defense is so extreme that an SA presents with alexithymia (the inability to recognize and express feelings).

• *Isolation.* This mechanism is the inability to experience content and affect simultaneously; as either ideas or emotions displaced or kept from consciousness. Isolation is often an integral part of denial of feelings.

• *Passive aggression.* Passive aggression refers to dealing with conflicts, such as anger or feeling powerless, by indirectly asserting oneself or by appearing to comply with directives in a manner that undermines them (see the discussion of passive aggressive personality disorder in Chapter 4).

• *Reaction formation.* Reaction formation is the replacement of behaviors, thoughts, or feelings with their diametric opposites. This is seen frequently in SAs: When they do not receive something they want very badly, it is then perceived as worthless.

• *Repression.* In drive theory, repression is the key defense mechanism, as other defenses are utilized only after memories and affects are repressed (Kaplan & Sadock, 1981). Affects and ideas may be repressed into the unconscious before they have reached consciousness (primary repression), or after they have been experienced and are again attempting to become consciously present (secondary repression). Consciously, the repressed material may be symbolically expressed in symptoms, dreams, or fantasies. A good deal of repression is misidentified as denial in the field of substance abuse. This distinction is important, because repression is a much more unconscious mechanism than denial, and therefore less subject to conscious control.

• *Sexualization.* This term refers to transferring enhanced sexual significance to a feeling, person, or aspect of a person in order not to experience anxiety or guilt related to prohibited impulses. This is a very common mechanism in SAs, who frequently sexualize relationships as a substitute for feared intimacy, as an expression of power, or as a means of gratifying needs for dependence. Drugs often serve as the "currency" for these transactions; that is, they facilitate sexuality or are traded for it.

• *Suppression and anticipation.* These two mature defense mechanisms are linked because they function jointly, are relatively conscious, and require a healthy ego that can focus on future rather than immediate gain. Suppression involves keeping all aspects of a conflict in mind and postponing action, emotion, or preoccupation. Anticipation is the ability to be aware in advance of negative emotional and behavioral consequences and to take appropriate emotional preparation. Here anticipatory guilt and anticipatory anxiety are used to modify behavior in an adaptational direction.

• *Sublimation.* Sublimation is the channeling of conflicts, painful affects, or stressors into socially desirable behavior. In drive theory, instincts are sublimated into significant goals or relationships rather than dammed or diverted (Kaplan & Sadock, 1981). Thus sublimation is one of the healthiest of defense mechanisms, and its utilization is a goal of long-term recovery, particularly in facilitating creativity.

• *Undoing.* Undoing is the alleviation of conflicts, stressors, and painful affects, particularly guilt, by behavior that symbolically makes amends for or negates prior thoughts, feelings, and actions. As seen in recovering SAs, it involves the actual making of amends (see discussion of the Eighth and Ninth Steps in Chapter 7) to those upon whom pain has been inflicted (Chappel, 1992).

A CASE EXAMPLE

The patient described below was an SA in recovery who utilized a variety of defense mechanisms, many of which could be subsumed under the rubric of denial and/or projection. A closer look reveals the use of numerous other defenses, which were helpful to understanding and treating this patient. This patient's history is also utilized to provide case material for Chapter 4 on personality disorders.

Background

David* was a 45-year-old, single, successful executive at the time he entered treatment as the result of an urgent request by his employer. He was referred because he had become chaotically embroiled in a highly charged sexual relationship with his secretary, Sara. She had filed a sexual harassment suit against him; nevertheless, he was continuing to pursue the sexual relationship, and was also writing a job description for her to be promoted to the level of his assistant (denial). He stated, "I never feel good unless I'm in an addictive relationship (rationalization, sexualization). When I lose it I'm devastated" (devaluation of self).

At the time of his first meeting with me, David had 84 days of sobriety, had a sponsor, and was attending two to four AA meetings weekly, depending on whether he was on the road (which he was for 180 days a year) or at home. He had used drugs heavily as a youth, and had been in and out of difficulty with alcoholism for over 20 years. He had a history of five convictions for driving while intoxicated (DWI). He had been incarcerated for 6 months as the final consequence of these offenses, but had not had a DWI for 18 months at the time of our first meeting. He had recently seen a psychiatrist, who had diagnosed him as having bipolar disorder; he had been on lithium and Prozac for 6 months, without benefit. He had also received extensive

---

*Recognizable aspects of this case history have been changed to preserve confidentiality, and the material is used with the patient's permission.

psychotherapy after a prior, even more turbulent 3-year relationship had ended. "She was in jail for committing assault and battery on me. She got out and found where I'd moved and blew up my car" (devaluation of other). He retaliated by throwing beer bottles at her (acting out), and was involuntarily hospitalized for 3 days.

When David returned for his second session with me, he reported that he had just taken his chip to commemorate 90 days of sobriety. Still, he had not slept in the past 5 days because of a mixture of missing Sara and the chaos at work as a result of their relationship. He was becoming unable to concentrate at work, because he was so preoccupied with alternating thoughts of taking revenge on her and getting her back. She was spreading terrible rumors about him, yet she had sent him a Valentine (splitting) during the week. Their relationship had polarized the president and vice-president of the company into persecuting and rescuing him while exonerating and indicting her, respectively (environmental splitting).

Family History

Both of David's parents were still alive. His mother was 80 years old and was described as quite "depriving and nongiving." Yet David recalled that his mother repeatedly protected him from his father, which enraged his "rage-aholic" father even more. His father was 90 years of age and was a talented photographer. He had been married five times before he met the patient's mother, and he had kept this a secret from her and David for many years. When his paternal grandmother told this secret to the patient's mother, his father went "crazy." The father had been a successful athlete until David was 5, but his athletic career was ended by cancer, which he survived as a result of surgery. David stated that his father rejected his mother because she preferred him, and that his father even once left home over this. The father physically and verbally abused David, particularly when David cried, was weak, or had physical problems (asthma). David described his parents' frequent arguments as verbally violent, though never physical. He heard his mother cry hysterically, but she did not lash out for fear his father would kill her. The father once refrained from talking to David for an entire summer because David had had his hair cut in a way similar to the Beatles'. Even now, his father still called him derogatory names like "asshole." David was cared for by his grandparents substantially from birth and described them as nurturing, although David's grandfather physically abused him when he was 19. David was quite distant from his brother, who was 5 years younger. He described the brother as a conservative school teacher.

As he worked on his identification with his family of origin in the later stages of therapy, he stated, "I rage like my father and grandfather, and fall apart and play victim like my mother and grandmother." However, he played the former role mainly when intoxicated or in the devalued phases of a relationship.

Personal History

David had been born in the Midwest with his "head bones out of shape." He spent the first month of his life in an incubator. His mother rejected him because of this, and his grandmother moved in to care for him. Although he had almost no recollection of his first 5 years, he did recall one very early memory: "I was in a bassinet, and a big bug was buzzing my face. I wanted someone to make it go away."

He moved to California at the age of 3, and was there with his mother and grandmother for about 6 months until his father rejoined the family. At 4, he was left with his grandparents; he recalled crying for his mother and father. When he was 5, the family system changed drastically: His father was diagnosed with cancer and told that it was fatal. David recalled that his father cried and vomited in response to his diagnosis, and that when he returned home with his colostomy, "our whole life was fucked." David's asthma began at this time, and Tedral was prescribed. "I got high and addicted to Tedral by age 5. My father hit me and said he hated me because I was sick." After these incidents, David felt he "closed up and lived my childhood in my head."

David had a sexual relationship with a female cousin at the age of 13. He recalled being "ripped over the coals" for this, and he was never permitted to see her again. He felt a great deal of shame over this experience.

He traveled 2,000 miles to attend college and felt quite frightened and lonely away from home. After leaving home, he had many sexual and romantic relationships, almost all of which ended in chaotic torment for both parties. Most of his early relationships were colored by his and his partners' heavy alcohol and drug use, though the chaos continued even when they were not drinking or drugging. David had two, 3-year relationships in the 1980s, in each of which there was escalating violence during the relationship and obsessive preoccupation afterward. Part of the reason for the repeating scenario was his choice of partners: He sought women who looked and acted like Madonna, Sharon Stone, or Tracey Lords. Even in the rare instances in which the women were not themselves highly sexualized and/or angry, enough projective identification occurred (see Chapter 8 on Countertransference) that these women alternated between the roles of victim and abuser.

David began his third session with me by reporting that Sara had copied his personal diary and was passing his most intimate and self-deprecating statements to the other executives' secretaries. He was preoccupied with his sexual jealousy of her (sexualization of loss), as well as with his anger and desire to have her back. He had multiple dreams and fantasies about her having sex with other men (paranoid projection). In one, she was fellating a man's large penis. It turned into a huge worm and bit at the filaments of an open heater. He said to her, "Just bite it," and she did. In his associations he stated, "She makes sure I know about all of the guys she's giving blow jobs."

This behavior continued to escalate, and, as could easily have been predicted, David drank again after 4 months of sobriety (acting out). His slip lasted only one night, and he was actively back into his AA program the next day. However, his compulsive sexual relationship continued to escalate. He stated publicly in a jealous yet smug rage that Sara had had sex with four to six other employees and the carpet cleaner. He talked to the wives of several of these employees about her alleged promiscuity and the possibility that their husbands might have AIDS (acting out).

David's employer insisted that he enter the hospital after he left a note on a picture of Sara that was in public view at work (devaluation of other). The note listed several of the men she had supposedly slept with, and was seen by several other employees. At the time he entered the hospital, he stated that he was "almost over her," although he still "thought about her 12 times a day." He was already in a new relationship, which he stated was not sexual, had no addictive characteristics, and was helping him heal his wounds from Sara (displacement).

A battery of psychological tests was performed in the hospital, including a Rorschach and an MMPI. The examiner noted David's statement that projecting blame is not reasonable defense of one's actions, yet recorded that he lacked insight into the great extent to which he used this defense (intellectualization, in part learned from the AA slogan—"Take your own inventory, not someone else's"). The patient's personal isolation was noted, yet he was seen to be superficially gregarious (reaction formation). Exaggerated needs for attention and affection were noted. His lack of self-control and anticipation were also observed. The psychometrist warned that David "could terminate [treatment] prematurely, due to his lack of owning his own pathology and his general tendency toward defensiveness."

David remained in the hospital for 2 weeks, although he was told that he should stay longer to solidify his sobriety. He left to pursue his new relationship (which quickly became sexualized), and to deal with his employer's threat to relocate him to the Midwest with the rest of their California operation. He bitterly fought against the relocation, because it meant leaving Pat, his new, "angelic" lover (idealization), as well as leaving his own lovely home, his sober support network, his sponsor, and lastly his new psychotherapist.

He made several trips to the Midwestern job site and deprecated every aspect of what life would be like there (splitting, devaluation). He saw his only alternative to the relocation as going on disability and working in a gas station "off of the books" (splitting).

He became increasingly close to Pat, particularly after they sexualized the relationship. He left her for a trip to his new job site, feeling a great deal of pain and loss. He began drinking a few miles from her home and continued to drink until just before the California state line, where he was arrested for driving under the influence. He shared this DWI and his alcoholic history with Pat, who immediately terminated the relationship (she had previously divorced an alcoholic). He complained of severe insomnia, pounding headaches (somatization), and repetitive negative thoughts of Sara, Pat, and his father rejecting him. He awakened from a nightmare about similar rejections and became preoccupied with the blinking "0" on his message machine denoting no calls. He was also preoccupied with going to jail and with the idea that the correction officers would beat him every time he cried (as his father had done). He felt trapped by having to choose between his dependence on his employer and his reliance on his sober network. When he finally arrived at his new job site, an intervention was performed, and he was hospitalized in a chemical dependence unit in the Midwest. He managed to be transferred back to my care for a mandated full course of treatment.

When he was admitted he informed me that he had not drunk for the month since his DWI and that he was back with Sara, but she was now a totally changed woman as a result of her fine work in an Al-Anon program. They had made love again. "It was different. It wasn't a physical performance contest. It was slow and with feeling. We were both there." (There is no better word than denial to describe this behavior, but it is also an excellent example of splitting with alternation between devaluation and idealization.) I responded to his shift to a former lover and his current idealization of her with a confrontation: "David, you need to focus on yourself this time and not a woman, even if she were Mother Teresa."

David remained in the inpatient chemical dependence program for 1 week, followed by 3 weeks of attendance in a partial hospital program (6 to 10 hours daily). David then saw me for a month after discharge, during which he decided to leave his company, for which he had worked for 7 years. He subsequently touched base with me a few times, informing me about his progress and sobriety. He had stopped seeing Sara and was working successfully at his own business.

Ten months later he returned to see me, having 1 year of sobriety under his belt. He had again gotten into a difficult relationship, which had just broken up. Although this one was far less stormy and mutually destructive, he was again depressed and preoccupied with the woman. She had 4 years of sobriety and attended many of the same AA meetings as he did. Thus, although he eliminated several meetings where he was most likely to see her, he still saw her repeatedly, which delayed his ability to let go of her. We contracted for weekly psychotherapy to work on the underlying issues that led to his relationship problems. The differences this time included his requesting and paying for the therapy entirely on his own, and his having a reasonable sober core as a result of a year of sobriety. An anticipated critical issue was his continued commitment to psychotherapy after he got over his grief and preoccupation with his latest loss.

This is a poem written by David during his first hospitalization. It describes his splitting defenses.

People Always Say

People always say,
"I got over him,"
"Oh, I quickly forgot her.
It was just a sexual thing."

But they're all fools and liars,
those people who say
they can forget their lovers.
They really never do.

They spend too much time staring out the window,
and making senseless trips to the store
to buy greeting cards
for nobody.

In their deepest selves
they remember the sweetest parts
of the most selfish sex,
the bittersweet echoes of hope and disappointment
behind the angriest words of rejection.

They lay awake at night and wonder,
"Should I have tried harder?"
"Was it right to walk away?"
"Why was it so intense and so shallow
both at the same time?"

They turn to the wall
sleeplessly asking
why sex felt so much like love,
why they feel separation anxiety
over a person who was no good for them
to begin with.

It's because there is a sweet river
forever in the heart
that flows from an impossibly high mountain top
and you climb it every night in your dreams
hoping to find someone there.

THE USE OF DEFENSE MECHANISMS IN RECOVERY

As therapy and sobriety progress, a recovering SA learns to substitute defenses. Early in the therapy, many aspects of denial are not confronted, and some denial is replaced with suppression or self-pity. Reaction formation is used to transform alcohol from the most precious love object into a dangerous enemy (Metzger, 1988). Undoing is utilized in recalling the pain inflicted on others and making amends. Altruism is used in providing service to others, such as in the Twelfth Step of AA and other groups. Humor returns with sobriety and is often supported by the Twelve-Step group. Sublimation is used through artistic and other creative productions. With ego maturity, there is much less acting out and more capacity for anticipation (Chappel, 1992). The use of defense mechanisms in recovery is discussed at greater length in later chapters.

Personality Disorders in Addicted Persons

I have included a chapter on personality disorders in this book because an understanding of these disorders is extremely important in assessing and treating drug- and alcohol-dependent patients. By most diagnostic criteria, the vast majority of SAs have at least one diagnosable personality disorder (Craig, 1988). A close clinical examination over time will reveal that some aspects of personality disorders have developed secondarily as a consequence of substance dependence, whereas others are primary and stem from the interaction of early developmental wounds and experiences with biological predisposition. In many cases, therefore, personality disorders may have a primary etiological role in substance abuse, rather than simply being secondary to it. Genetic precursors may even exert their influence through specific neurochemical pathways, as Cloninger (1988) has hypothesized. The origins and diagnosis of personality disorders are also very much related to social class and gender.

Some personality disorders become more severe with abstinence, as a result of the removal of affect- or behavior-dampening drugs and alcohol, or the unavailability of substance-related behavior patterns. More commonly, SAs shed many of their disordered personality traits after they detoxify and remain off drugs. Some achieve healthier personality adaptations after months of abstinence, and even more integrated personalities often appear to develop after a year or more of sobriety. However, personality disorders that appear to be resolved can re-emerge rapidly after relapse. Regardless of the stage of recovery of a particular patient, a knowledge of personality disorders is essential to understanding and treating SAs, as these disorders and traits are ubiquitous and shift with each stage.

At the same time as we therapists espouse the importance of understanding personality disorders, we must remain aware that we do so at the risk of dehumanizing our substance-abusing patients. Personality disorders do not capture the essence of the human condition; in effect, they may blind us to the humanity of our patients. Thus, at the same time as we diagnose, we should tune into aspects of personality that go beyond personality disorders (and defense mechanisms; see Chapter 3).

PREVALENCE

In a study of 121 opiate addicts in Chicago, Craig (1988), utilizing the very sensitive Millon Clinical Multiaxial Inventory, found that 100% had at least one personality disorder and 27% had more than one. The most common diagnoses were as follows: antisocial personality disorder (ASP), 22%; narcissistic personality disorder (NPD), 18%; borderline personality disorder (BPD), 16% and dependent personality, 16%. Other researchers have found much higher rates of ASP in opiate addicts; Rounsaville et al. (1982) found 68%, and Kosten et al. (1982) found 55% (14% in the latter study were diagnosed as having BPD). Khantzian and Treece (1985) found that 65% of narcotic addicts manifested DSM-III personality disorders with 8% in Cluster A (paranoid, schizoid, schizotypal), 45% in Cluster B (histrionic, NPD, ASP), 35% in BPD (also Cluster B) or mixed, and 9% in Cluster C (avoidant, dependent, obsessive compulsive).

In a study of 76 lower-social-class cocaine abusers, Kleinman et al. (1990) found that 71% had at least one personality disorder and 40% had two or more. The four most common diagnoses were as follows: ASP, 21%; passive aggressive personality disorder (PAPD), 21%; BPD, 18%; and self-defeating personality disorder, 18%. The authors contrasted their findings with those of Weiss and Mirin (1986) with upper-middle-class subjects, which showed BPD and NPD to be most common. In a comparative study of lower-class addicts, Rounsaville et al. (1982) found ASP rates of 32.9% in cocaine addicts and 54% in opiate addicts. Their study also demonstrates the importance of choice of criteria. When the Research Diagnostic Criteria were used instead of DSM-III criteria (the former exclude drug-related adult antisocial behavior), the rates of ASP dropped to 26.5% and 7.7%, respectively. Griffin et al. (1989) compared male and female cocaine abusers, and found that 22.1% of 95 males and none of 34 females could be diagnosed as having ASP.

ASP is generally thought to be the most common personality disorder in male alcoholics; Meyer's (1986) review found a range between 15% and 49%. In a comprehensive study by Helzer and Pryzbeck (1988), ASP was found in 15% of alcoholic men and 10% of alcoholic women, in contrast to 4% and 0.8%, respectively, among nonalcoholics. A substantially higher association has been found between personality disorders and alcoholism when clinical samples are studied (Nace, 1989). Koenigsberg et al. (1985) found personality disorders in 61% of drug abusers and 46% of alcoholics, with BPD (43%) the most frequent diagnosis; next came ASP (21%) and mixed (17%). Hesselbrock et al. (1985) found that 49% of male and 20% of female hospitalized alcoholics were diagnosed as having ASP.

Kosten et al. (1982) further suggested that the 32% of opiate addicts who did not meet diagnostic criteria for a personality disorder might in themselves represent a unique character disorder for which no diagnostic category as yet exists. These addicts tended to be better educated and employed, to have less Axis I psychopathology, and to demonstrate higher social functioning. Further research should be done on all SAs who do not meet criteria for Axis II disorders, in order to determine whether they represent a previously unnamed personality disorder. Perhaps they follow several clusters of personality traits, with none sufficiently differentiated to meet criteria for a personality disorder.

To summarize, the vast majority of SAs have at least one personality disorder diagnosis. Opiate addicts, males, and lower-social-class SAs tend to be diagnosed as having ASP; middle-class SAs, females, and prescription drug abusers are commonly diagnosed as having NPD, BPD, histrionic personality disorder, and self-defeating personality disorder. Personality disorder characteristics are essential factors to be considered in the development of individualized treatment plans for SAs. Another critical reason for their importance is their association with greatly increased comorbidity, including greater prevalence of Axis I disorders, polysubstance use, and other personality disorders (Kosten & Rounsaville, 1986; Nace, 1989; see below). Personality disorders generally tend to occur in clusters, with most Axis II comorbidity occurring within the cluster.

RELEVANT FINDINGS FROM RESEARCH ON NON-SUBSTANCE-ABUSING SUBJECTS

Comparisons of personality disorder prevalence in a variety of populations find BPD to be the most common diagnosis: community samples, 1% to 29%; outpatients 8%; inpatients 15%; outpatients with a personality disorder, 27%; and inpatients with a personality disorder, 51% (Widiger & Rogers, 1989). Oldham and Skodol (1991) found that only 11% of all patients in New York State mental health facilities in 1988 were given Axis II diagnoses. Many patients who meet the criteria for one personality disorder will also meet the criteria for at least one other (particularly in inpatient settings). The most common personality disorders among patients meeting the criteria for other such disorders are (of course) BPD and histrionic personality disorder, which also have the highest comorbidity with each other (Widiger & Rogers, 1989). Widiger and Rogers have also found high co-occurrence of BPD with ASP, schizotypal and dependent personality disorders, and PAPD.

Because of the substantial degree of co-occurrence of other personality disorders with BPD, we might consider that this diagnosis is more an indicator of severe dysfunction than a distinct personality disorder. High general comorbidity also calls into question the distinctiveness of separate personality disorders. Perhaps we should focus on clusters of behaviors that have common developmental origins and common defense mechanisms. Several authors have suggested that personality disorders be divided into broad categories, such as active versus passive (Stone, 1980), or reward dependence versus harm avoidance versus fearfulness (DSM-III-R; American Psychiatric Association, 1987). Kernberg (1975) suggests that individuals with personality disorders be classified according to their usual level of functioning. Higher-level diagnoses would include all cases of hysterical, obsessive compulsive, and depressive masochistic personality. Intermediary diagnoses would include a few cases of NPD, some cases of infantile personality and all PAPD cases. Lower-level or borderline diagnoses would include most cases of NPD and infantile personality; all cases of schizoid, paranoid, hypomanic, and "as-if" (persons who behave "as if" they have feeling relations with others that are really only pseudo contacts); and all ASP cases (Kernberg, 1975).

Stone (1980) observes that even the most astute divisions into major clusters lose sight of the essence of the qualities they are attempting to describe. He proposes rating individual aspects of all personality disorders on a scale of 1 to 10 so that patterns of personality traits evolve, rather than limiting individuals to one or a few personality diagnoses. Stone warns, however, that even this more comprehensive schema will not depict such important personality attributes as courage, humor, or trustworthiness, or the importance of sociodemographic influences.

COMORBIDITY OF SUBSTANCE ABUSE, PERSONALITY DISORDERS, AND OTHER DISORDERS

Alcoholics with a personality disorder are more likely to have anxiety, depression, mania, schizophrenia, and chronic depression, according to Cadoret et al. (1984). They are also more likely to have suicidality, non-compliance, loss to follow-up, and a poor prognosis (Nace, 1989; Gold-smith et al., 1989). Hesselbrock et al. (1985) also confirm that alcoholics with ASP consume more alcohol and abuse other drugs than those without ASP; moreover, they begin to abuse alcohol at an earlier age.

As might be expected, opiate addicts with personality disorders have been found to have higher rates of alcoholism (two to three times higher, in fact) than addicts without personality disorders (Kosten & Rounsaville, 1986). These authors grouped personality disorders among their sample of 533 opiate addicts into four groupings: BPD, NPD, ASP, and "other." The BPD group (14.5% of total n) included subjects with schizotypal, schizoid, and paranoid personality disorders. This group had the most unemployment, least education, and highest rate of major affective disorder. (The common occurrence of depression in BPD patients has been attributed by Millon, 1981, to an extension of their personality style. Thus low self-esteem, overidealization, and rejection sensitivity inevitably lead to frequent depressive episodes.) When affective symptoms remitted in Kosten and Rounsaville's BPD patients, they often manifested impulsive violence and antisocial behavior; 66% of the BPD subjects also met ASP criteria.

Kosten and Rounsaville's (1986) NPD grouping (9.6%) included subjects with dependent and histrionic personality disorders. The NPD subjects were easily provoked by minor insults, which were experienced as grave assaults on their grandiosity. This group had four times as much hypomania as the rest of the sample and made very shallow relationships with their counselors. Moreover, 50% of the NPD group were alcoholics, apparently using alcohol in part to self-medicate painful aspects of manic or narcissistic disillusionments. Kosten and Rounsaville's (1986) "other" group (7.6%) included subjects with PAPD and with avoidant and mixed personality disorders. The ASP group was most prevalent (54.7%).

Khantzian and Treece (1985) noted that 49% of narcotic addicts had diagnoses in both Axis I and Axis II, with affective disorders being the most common Axis I diagnoses when there was also personality disorder. They also noted that subjects with any personality disorder had higher polydrug use, particularly those with ASP. In addition, the ASP group had a higher "heaviest narcotic episode index" and used more non-narcotic drugs.

Obviously, the high incidence of comorbidity of other personality disorders, Axis I pathology, and polysubstance abuse in SAs with personality disorders calls for various shifts in treatment approach.

GENERAL TREATMENT PRINCIPLES

The major reason why those who treat SAs need to achieve an understanding of personality disorders (or perhaps they should be termed "personality clusters") is to develop relevant modifications of therapeutic techniques. For the purposes of therapy, perhaps personalities may be better classified as to severity of impairment rather than specific disorders. There are three basic principles in the treatment of any severe personality disorder, all of which are relevant to most SAs (Freeman & Gunderson, 1989):

1. Intervene directly and actively to correct and interpret transference distortions.
2. Maintain a stable, consistent framework in regard to fees, schedule, interruptions (minimal or none), roles, limits and other boundary issues. These should be spelled out in a mutually agreed-on contract with clear expectations and consequences.
3. Connect actions with their underlying feelings so as to shift therapy away from action and towards more direct communication. However, borderline personalities will require the therapist to exert the greatest *limits* on self-destructive or therapy-threatening behaviors.

According to Freeman and Gunderson (1989), if deeper psychotherapy is to be done with any personality-disordered patient, he/she must have a fairly high-functioning superego, so that there is a minimum of conscious distortion and lying. In personality-disordered patients who are SAs, a stable core of sobriety will help strengthen superego functions, so that deeper therapy can take place. AA and other Twelve-Step groups are extremely helpful in providing powerful support for telling the truth, as an "honest program" is one of the cornerstones for sobriety. A daily taking of one's "own inventory" is one of the bases of the Twelve Steps.

A second critical criterion for in-depth psychotherapy is the patient's capability, based on prior object relations, for a neurotic transference as opposed to a primitive and/or annihilative transference. An annihilative transference can be resolved only if there is a basic capacity for trust or latent capacity for neurotic, higher-level transference. Many SAs can relate at this higher neurotic level effectively after long-term sobriety (2 or more years) is stabilized.

Though the reader should keep in mind the reservations I have stated earlier about overgeneralization of techniques based on specific personality diagnosis, I now discuss the three most common personality disorders seen in SAs—ASP, NPD, and BPD—in the context of diagnosis and relevance to psychotherapy. It is of interest that all three of these common disorders in SAs are in Cluster B; thus many SAs will have characteristics of all three disorders. Teasing out these interwoven characteristics and determining the predominant pattern constitute a difficult task. PAPD is also discussed briefly, although it may be more a frequent pattern of behavior in SAs than a true personality disorder.

ANTISOCIAL PERSONALITY DISORDER

ASP is the most common personality disorder seen in SAs. This is a lifetime diagnosis and, as defined by DSM-III-R, cannot be made unless an individual has demonstrated substantial antisocial behaviors before the age of 15. Yet even this diagnosis can change over time (Kosten & Rounsaville, 1986). Gerstley et al. (1989) have emphasized the importance of dividing antisocial individuals into a primary and a secondary group. The primary group has ASP (the *disorder*) as a result of genetic and early childhood experiences. The secondary group manifests antisocial *behavior* as a result of substance abuse or fears of loss or narcissistic injury, but does not have the underlying personality disorder. The primary group has three major underlying personality defects: the inability to (1) empathize, (2) experience guilt, and (3) develop meaningful relationships. Obviously, this group has a poorer prognosis in therapy than the secondary group. In addition, among opiate abusers diagnosed as having ASP, Woody et al. (1984) found that a codiagnosis of lifetime depression enhanced the ability to benefit from psychotherapy.

Behavioral Characteristics

The behavioral characteristics of individuals with ASP are well described in DSM-III-R (American Psychiatric Association, 1987) and should also be maintained in DSM-IV, as suggested by the *DSM-IV Options Book* (American Psychiatric Association, 1991). Before the age of 15, future ASP patients meet three or more of the DSM criteria for conduct disorder. That is, they are often truants, runaways, and fighters (who may use weapons); are physically cruel to people and animals; destroy property (by various means, which may include arson); have early sexual experiences involving use of force; lie often; and/or steal (with or without physical confrontation) (American Psychiatric Association, 1987). Some of these behaviors are highly rewarded by peers, so that these pre-ASP youths may receive a great deal of early acclaim. Some behaviors—such as substance abuse, charming ingratiation, ability as a fighter, early sexual prowess, getting away with forbidden pleasures, and defiance of authority—can bring great popularity to youths in most cultures, so that their potentially self-destructive behaviors are minimized or overlooked (MacKinnon & Michels, 1971).

As an adult, a person with ASP may be sufficiently cunning that even the most experienced therapist can be fooled initially, particularly without information from relatives, friends, or authorities. The opposite-sex therapist may be conned and enthralled on the one hand, or disgusted on the other. Competitiveness and anger, or fear and distancing, are more likely to be seen in the same-sex clinician. Individuals with ASP may have distinguished themselves either through a military act requiring emotional self-control and/or bravery, or the ability to perform a single or brief series of acts of brilliance not requiring follow-through (MacKinnon & Michels, 1971). ASP patients readily rationalize their behavior on the basis of past injustices done to them or the idea that everyone else gets away with worse travesties on society (e.g., under the guise of big business or government intervention). At times the projective focus can seem quite paranoid and immutable to psychotherapy.

The motivation of individuals with ASP may range from straight financial gain to the bizarre (before intercourse, one severely disturbed ASP patient of mine would fondle the money wrappers of cash he stole from banks, in order to enhance his sexual potency). Because of their inability to incorporate the existence of future consequences (lack of the defense mechanism of anticipation), they have difficulty postponing gratification, and thus punishment is often not an effective deterrent. ASP patients who are also SAs generally avoid violent crimes to get their drugs, unless they do not have successful con games or are neurophysiologically overactivated by stimulants (cocaine, particularly smokable "crack," or amphetamines, particularly smokable "ice"*) or withdrawal from sedatives. Vaillant (1975) emphasizes that the commonly described ASP characteristics of lack of anxiety, depression, and absence of motivation occur in outpatient settings. When appropriate

---

*Although smokable amphetamines or speed were called "ice" when first introduced in this country, the term has not quite caught on in general usage. However, the smoking of speed has become a common aspect of use among many southern California amphetamine abusers.

limits are set in residential environments, depression and anxiety become more available, and the ASP patient becomes more motivated for change.

Psychodynamics

Several aspects of the family histories of ASP patients are consistently reported. There is frequently a history of a father who himself would have warranted an ASP diagnosis or was an alcoholic (McGuffin & Thapar, 1993). Maternal deprivation in the first 5 years of life is commonly seen (Bowlby, 1963). Maternal inconsistency is described in the areas of care, discipline, and affection. Loss of a parent or a general lack of family cohesiveness, leading to a bereaved or neglected child, is also reported. In addition, there is a lack of any significant person who could compensate for the lack of nurturing and direct parenting. Often there have been frequent moves from one foster home or juvenile institution to another. Thus it is felt that the presence or intermittent manifestation of inconsistent, impulsive parents is more likely to produce an individual with ASP than is the loss of a consistent parent (Glueck & Glueck, 1970). When these individuals are offered even the best of mothering in later years, they are incapable of responding with the positive feedback necessary to maintain nurturing behavior. As a result of their lack of a consistent parenting figure, they learn that security must be derived from other than close human relationships. Their multiple early losses have taught them to extract love quickly and then leave relationships before they are left. Thus when they have the opportunity to relate to someone who is capable of loving, they "hit and run."

Their lack of consistent parenting also leaves ASP individuals without healthy figures for ego identification or for incorporation into a superego. Thus their consciences are generally described as resembling Swiss cheese; more technically, they have "superego lacunae" (Johnson & Szurek, 1952) with many weaknesses, yet some areas that are normal or overdeveloped. Wurmser (1974) has speculated that their consciences are overly punitive and harsh, and that although they frequently attempt to overcome them, they are too frightened of retribution to be able to do so. Superego lacunae develop when a message is communicated to a child to act out a parent's forbidden desires — for instance, when a parent slaps a daughter for suspected acting out while calling her a "slut" in a manner that is latently sexually exciting to parent and/or child, or when a son's acting out is condoned with a "boys will be boys" message.

Persons with ASP become frightened of the tension associated with awaiting the meeting of their needs, since early gratification occurred irregularly if at all. They grow to believe that others cannot tolerate their anxiety, so they learn to hide it. At times they project their anxiety onto significant others or therapists by projective identification. Since they feel deprived of love and security, they feel entitled to take whatever they can get from others (MacKinnon & Michaels, 1971).

Defensive Operations

The primary goals of individuals with ASP are to avoid tension, anxiety, depression, or feelings in themselves or others that are out of control. They do not have adequate defenses against their own anxiety, so they escape from it through acting out or through primitive use of defense mechanisms (MacKinnon & Michels, 1971). Their inner drives feel urgent and overwhelming, and delay or substitution seems impossible or intolerable. When needs are met, these individuals feel tension relief or satiation, rather than happiness or enhanced self-esteem. Thus drugs or alcohol are sought after, since they provide an instant relief ("oral orgasm").

Persons with ASP often primitively use denial, projection, and hypochondriasis (MacKinnon & Michels, 1971). They transfer their anxiety to others, particularly the "codependent" persons in their lives, and potentially to their therapists. They elaborately defend against guilt through denial of substance abuse and its consequences or social significance. They also often utilize reaction formation, rationalization ("Everyone else does it"), and entitlement (they are "professional orphans").

The case of David, described in the Chapter 3, would certainly fall into Cluster B. Although he demonstrated several characteristics of ASP (early sexual relationships, inability to maintain monogamy, criminal history, recklessness), this disorder would not have been the most valid personality diagnosis for him. David did experience considerable guilt and remorse; he maintained a job and a permanent residence; and he was capable of making a therapeutic relationship even when not coerced to do so by the law or employers.

Psychotherapy

The psychotherapy of ASP patients who are also SAs cannot begin until firm limits are set. Since they can transfer primary object attachments so readily, they can rapidly terminate a therapeutic relationship if it feels too intense or if a therapist demands the implementation of limits that they feel they cannot follow. Thus, the limits must often be reinforced by external controls or threats: loss of job, loss of income, conservatorship, loss of family members (this is not effective with more damaged ASP patients unless they are materially dependent), or incarceration. Often these controls are best implemented by persons other than a therapist, since when enforcing the controls is mainly the therapist's responsibility, they may be experienced as too punitive to be therapeutic.

ASP patients must be realistically but not punitively confronted with the consequences of their behavior. According to Vaillant (1975), once this is done, an individual with ASP then resembles an individual with BPD. In my own experience, this is not always true, as a number of other personality styles may also become evident or are already present but became more overt; these may include masochistic, obsessive compulsive, narcissistic, hypochondriacal, dependent, and passive aggressive styles. Some of these may have been already diagnosed as part of comorbidity patterns, but become more predominant when antisocial behavior is blocked.

The behavior of the ASP patient must also be controlled, in order to prevent self-destruction and to provide a contained environment that does not facilitate flight from therapeutic intimacy. A critical but difficult task for the therapist is to separate control from punishment. Most often the therapy of the ASP patient needs to begin in a totally controlled environment, such as a residential treatment community, a long-term hospital, or a flexible penal institution. This is because sufficient limits can only be implemented in these types of controlled settings. At times a less restrictive environment, such as a comprehensive outpatient program (20–40 hours a week), can provide sufficient control and stabilization. Other comprehensive long-term outpatient environments and/or intensive Twelve-Step programs can accomplish similar stabilization when participated in fully. Some individuals with ASP who successfully work a Twelve-Step program do so through the zeal of religious conversion. These approaches have the advantage of not limiting the psychotherapy to one helping person or one hour per day; they can provide structure, support, and/or psychotherapy for up to 24 hours daily. A therapist should bear a patient's anxiety and most often should not relieve it. The therapist may share his/her own anxiety, particularly as it relates to this patient or his/her projective identifications (Vaillant, 1975), but only after a therapeutic alliance has been established (see Chapter 8).

Once limits have been set and most manipulative defenses removed, the nurturing, reparenting part of the therapy can take hold. New, more adaptive defenses and coping mechanisms are gradually taught and practiced. Identification with healthy role models gradually takes place, and peer group support reinforces new skills and identifications. Practicing helping others (the Twelfth Step of AA and similar programs) and taking a daily moral inventory strengthen the superego. Jobs and therapeutic roles of long-term members of therapeutic communities are also critical to developing healthier egos and building self-esteem in persons with ASP.

Many of the above-described therapeutic techniques are also appropriate and indicated for patients with NPD and BPD who have severe personality pathology, particularly those who act out. Thus these points are not repeated, but differences are emphasized.

NARCISSISTIC PERSONALITY DISORDER

The therapist who works with severely damaged and primitive NPD patients may often lose sight of the healthy aspects of narcissism, which were first presented by Freud (1915/1957)—for example, self-esteem, self-assertion, and the pursuit of one's own interests, standards, ideals, and ambitions. Masterson (1981) views NPD as a result of narcissistic defenses against an underlying feeling state of emptiness, rage, and intense envy.

Behavioral Characteristics

NPD-patients present with grandiosity, extreme self-involvement, and a lack of interest in and empathy with others (Masterson, 1981). However, they pursue others for admiration and approval. They strive for perfection, wealth, glory, power, and beauty (often in return for the least effort possible), and seek others who will admire their grandiose achievements in a mirroring way. They may function at three different levels, ranging from (1) effective functioning, with neurotic problems (the "phallic narcissistic character") to (2) severe difficulties in object relations to (3) borderline functioning with weak ego strength (Masterson, 1981). Kernberg (1970) emphasizes more the excessive self-absorption, intense ambition, grandiosity, entitlement, and inordinate need for tribute from others. Underneath these compensations, Kernberg emphasizes emotional shallowness, defective empathy, and inability to tolerate mourning and sadness when faced with loss.

Kohut (1972) has contributed the important concept of "narcissistic rage" which is a severe angry response to anyone who injures an NPD individual's self-esteem. Components of this type of rage include a need for revenge, preoccupation with righting a wrong, and attempting to undo a hurt by whatever means.

Clinically, SAs with NPD may exhibit one of five patterns (Masterson, 1981). They may be (1) self-absorbed in the physical aspects of addiction, such as withdrawal symptoms, complications, and related somatic disorders (hypochrondriasis); (2) manipulative and antisocial, but in a grandiose way; or (3) needy, clinging, and demanding, with a strong feeling that everything is due to them (entitlement). Or they may be (4) "phallic narcissists." This pattern is particularly seen in flashy, wealthy cocaine addicts who may be extremely successful in cocaine sales or legitimate business pursuits, but who need to use cocaine to drive themselves even harder to achieve more and more. Finally, they may be (5) "closet narcissists," who present themselves as timid, shy, and ineffective, but who reveal themselves later in therapy as having a richly grandiose fantasy life. These fantasies may be acted out during intoxication, particularly on hallucinogens or stimulants. Closet narcissists may also project their own grandiosity into idealized love objects, so that they idealize others who unconsciously represent themselves; thus they often present with highly "codependent" relationships. This was quite true in the case of David, described in Chapter 3.

SAs with NPD expect to be noticed as special without warranting it. They feel that their problems are unique and will be appreciated if only they can find a special person who will understand and mirror them. They feel justified in exploiting others to meet their needs and alleviate their frustrations (American Psychiatric Association, 1987). Again, this behavioral cluster was clearly evident in David (Chapter 3). Since *every* SA in an intense state of craving or withdrawal will demonstrate many of the narcissistic behaviors described above, it is important to take a careful history from collateral sources of prior ability to receive and give empathy, and to observe the patient over time after withdrawal is complete. DSM-III-R (American Psychiatric Association, 1987) notes that many features of the other disorders in Cluster B (histrionic, BPD, and ASP) are often present, and multiple diagnoses may be warranted.

Individuals with NPD eventually drive everyone away who can provide gratification, or devalue those who remain. This real-life emptiness reinforces their empty internal world, which is devoid of positive object relations, and leads to their experiencing an internal void. They then desperately attempt to fill up the emptiness by gaining endless admiration from others and by controlling others to avoid feeling envy (Kernberg, 1989) for their successes. If they maintain conscious contact with their inner void, they will then have "bottomed out" sufficiently for psychotherapy to be effective (once again, see the case of David, Chapter 3).

Psychodynamics

According to Masterson (1981), the fixation of the individual with NPD comes before the stage of self-differentiation or rapprochement (15–22 months). The evidence for this is that these patients behave as if their primary objects were part of themselves, "an omnipotent dual entity" (Masterson, 1981, p. 13). Thus they feel they have not lost their blissful unity with their all-giving, mirroring, idealizing mothers. Then they must seal themselves off from the reality of the external world, which disputes this illusion; they do this by avoidance, denial, and devaluation of any reality input to the contrary (Masterson, 1981). David was only able to do this early in his relationships with lovers; but when his bliss dissipated, he medicated himself with alcohol. David would laugh longingly when he spoke of his fondness for Sutter Home wine. NPD patients can also induce this fused bliss artificially through drug experiences, such as opioid dreaminess, sedative oblivion, or stimulant euphoria (Masterson, 1981).

Some mothers of individuals with NPD are cold and exploitative; they ignore their children's need to individuate in order to gratify their own needs. David described his mother as quite cold, using him mainly to meet those needs that were not gratified by her husband and to express her hostility to her spouse. Other future NPD patients identify with their mothers' idealization, which manages to preserve their grandiose (but very hollow) sense of self (Masterson, 1981). Yet another possible dynamic is that a child experiences a depression as a result of feeling abandoned by the mother and shifts his/her symbiotic attachment to the father. If the father himself has NPD and the shift occurs before the child is fifteen months of age, then the child will have little choice but to develop NPD likewise (Masterson, 1981).

The false feeling of uniqueness in persons with NPD conceals the underlying pathological core, which is aggressive or empty and/or capable only of very fused object relations. Their internal fused object is harsh, punitive, and attacking, and their self-representation is consequently humiliated, attacked, and empty. They are vulnerable to experiencing depression as a result of feeling abandoned by the inner object whenever they attempt an individuated self-expression, or as a result of the external object's failure to provide perfect mirroring (Masterson, 1981). This depression is rapidly projected and denied, so that it appears that a person with NPD obtains ample supplies from within. The person's free access to aggression often enables him/her to coerce the environment into resonating with the narcissistic projection. When this fails, the person will attempt to deal with the lack of mirroring through avoidance, denial, and devaluation. The facade of in dependence and sadistic power is often quite attractive to dependent potential mates, who are "set-ups" for NPD individuals' hit-and-run relationships.

The extraordinary need for mirroring in NPD evolves from defective mirroring from the mother, which, according to Kohut (1977), evolves from the mother's own depression, narcissism, or psychosis. Defective mirroring also occurs in mothers who are frequently under the influence of drugs and/or alcohol. Masterson (1981), in contrast, emphasizes the mother's emotional withdrawal in reaction to the child's grandiose, exhibitionistic self. The mother withdraws because she is frustrated that the budding NPD patient's self-expressions do not resonate with the projections she has placed on him/her in order to shape him/her. Although this matches David's description of his mother, he may have been protected from even more severe narcissistic pathology by his grandmother, who was described as a relatively constant and loving presence.

Defense Mechanisms

The defense mechanisms seen in NPD individuals as described above include projection (particularly of depression and low self esteem), denial of their emptiness and wounds, and devaluation of those who hurt or abandon them. Since they may have great narcissistic investment in their bodies, persons with NPD are quite prone to somatization.

Psychotherapy

An essential aspect of the psychotherapy of SAs with NPD is the provision of a corrective emotional empathic experience, which helps to compensate for their early empathic failures. This empathic stance is a very difficult one to maintain, because of the many ways NPD patients distance themselves from others; however, it provides the patients with a healing internalization, which bolsters self-esteem. A patient also introjects other positive aspects of the relationship with the therapist. There is controversy as to the extent to which the idealized transference should be encouraged as opposed to confronted, particularly as a defense against rage and envy (Kernberg, 1975). The need for careful consideration of a delicate balance between interpretations that are experienced as providing nurturing growth and esteem, and ones that are felt as inflicting severe, life-shattering wounds, is most prominent in the psychotherapy of patients with NPD. In the early phases of psychotherapy with an NPD patient, I maintain a constant internal dialogue with myself, in which I make every effort to resonate empathically rather than confront the patient's demanding entitlement and provocative bravado.

These patients will often idealize or devalue their therapists, and test them to the limit to determine whether the therapists meet their grandiose expectations. It is important to resolve early devaluations, as they may lead to premature termination. Idealization should be interpreted over time, but rapidly enough to prevent the inevitable frustration of needs whenever a therapist is endowed with special powers. Eventually, according to Kernberg (1975), the idealization is interpreted as masking fantasies of rage and envy. Kohut (1971) prefers to permit these defenses to flourish, in order to avoid the empathic failure involved in confrontative interpretations.

As described in Chapter 3, David showed many more characteristics of NPD than of ASP. However, the constant failure of his grandiose narcissistic defenses led to borderline splitting, which led in turn to a low self-image most of the time. In the early phases of his love relations he presented in a manic narcissistic way, which rapidly deflated. This alternation between characterological manic narcissistic defenses and a depressive borderline presentation was undoubtedly the reason why he was placed on lithium by a prior treating psychiatrist.

BORDERLINE PERSONALITY DISORDER

BPD is often considered as a level of personality organization rather than as a distinct disorder. Thus borderline individuals may present a rather broad range of maladaptive behavior on "general dimensions of impulsivity, affect turbulence, and inconsistent self-representations" (Hurt & Clarkin, 1990). Kernberg (1975) refers to a "borderline personality organization," which includes most cases of NPD and infantile personality; all cases of schizoid, paranoid, "as ifs," and hypomanic personality; and cases of ASP. These patients share the primitive use of such defenses as splitting, denial, projective identification, and omnipotent idealization. They also manifest an unstable or diffuse self-identity and impaired reality testing, based to some extent on field dependence. Thus BPD is most often seen in association with other concurrent personality disorders. There is good evidence that many SAs who are diagnosed as having BPD are really "pseudoborderline" (Widiger et al., 1986). This occurs because characteristics inherent in SAs—such as (1) unstable and intense interpersonal relationships; (2) inappropriate, intense, out-of-control anger; (3) affective instability; and (4) physically self-damaging acts—will provide the five criteria necessary to diagnose BPD, when combined with substance abuse.

This will occur even in the absence of such basic BPD characteristics as identity disturbance, intolerance of being alone, and chronic feelings of emptiness or boredom. Thus we often see a "pseudoborderline syndrome" manifesting itself in SAs. We also see, however, that David met all criteria for true BPD.

The term "borderline" has a long history in psychiatry. Originally, it literally meant a disorder "on the borderline" between psychosis and neurosis. At present the variety of patients diagnosed as "borderline" is so great that, particularly at opposite ends of the spectrum, many patients with this same diagnosis appear to be extremely different. Stone (1990, p. 9) describes the typical or least confusing borderline patient as "stormy, unstable, overanxious, anger-prone, compulsive and destructive of self or others." Stone (1990, p. 9) lists additional typical personality traits as follows: moody, extremely emotional, alternating between adoration and contempt, irritable, manipulative, clingingly dependent, lacking depth, and vulnerable or fragile (again, David met all of these criteria). These symptoms should not be taken lightly, as the suicide rate in BPD is as high as that seen in the major psychoses (Stone, 1989).

Behavioral Characteristics

DSM-III-R emphasizes a "pervasive pattern of instability of self-image, interpersonal relationships and mood" in BPD (American Psychiatric Association, 1987, p. 346). The comorbidity of BPD with other personality disorders has been discussed previously. However, brief psychotic episodes and major depression are also both quite common, particularly in reaction to drugs of abuse. Often the individual with NPD is viewed as having a similarly, disturbed underlying core, but is able to present a cohesive, grandiose self that hides the inner identity diffusion (Kernberg, 1970); this was true of David only temporarily, in the early stages of a relationship. Stone (1980) notes the common occurrence of narcissistic traits in borderline patients (e.g., envy, attention seeking, exploitativeness, oversensitivity to criticism, and preoccupation with compensatory fantasies of power and success.) These are basically sufficient to permit most BPD patients to be diagnosed as having NPD as well, yet the two groups present quite differently. The fact that David had all of these traits helps us understand how he could be diagnosed as primarily a BPD patient, despite his narcissistic traits.

McGlashan and Heinssen (1989) constructed three subgroups of patients with BPD: those with narcissistic features, those with antisocial features, and those with neither comorbidity. They followed these patients over many years and found that BPD patients with antisocial traits were less likely to harm themselves and more likely to direct aggression outwardly. David would of course fit into a fourth very common group, which McGlashan and Heinssen did not define—those with both antisocial and narcissistic features.

Psychodynamics

Kernberg (1975) espouses what has been considered the classical view of the development of "borderline personality organization": namely, that it results from failures in development occurring during the phase of differentiation of self-representations from object representations (a phase that begins at about 8 months of age and is completed normally by the age of 18 to 36 months). Kernberg (1975) and others (Hedges, 1983) note that the future borderline's difficulties begin even earlier than 8 months of age, in that most of the first year of life is characterized by extreme feelings of frustration and aggression (as was David's first year).

This finding has recently been validated empirically by Perry et al. (1990), who, in blind ratings of patients with formal diagnoses of BPD, found 81% with histories of major child trauma, 71% with history of sexual abuse, and 62% who had witnessed serious domestic violence. They found that abuse histories were much less common in patients with borderline traits, and significantly more rare in nonborderline patients. Perry at al. also found that abuse began significantly earlier in those with BPD. Their findings support my own finding with Weatherford, in a study of adult children of alcoholics (Weatherford & Kaufman, 1991), that childhood abuse (particularly sexual abuse) was highly correlated with a diagnosis of BPD. In addition, the greater the extent of personality disorder pathology, the more the parents of alcoholics were perceived as drinking heavily and earlier in life. Thus we see the intergenerational heritability of borderline personality organization through parental substance abuse and more frequent and severe child abuse.

According to Kernberg (1975), the mother of the future BPD patient is seen as so dangerous that the dangerousness is projected onto both parents, and then later onto all sexual or significant relationships. Kernberg has hypothesized that the future BPD patient has an excessive amount of aggression, which may be attributable to constitutional intensity as well as to extreme frustration and abuse. As a result of excessive aggression and/or deprivation, the pre-BPD child experiences inadequate containment and incomplete absorption of troubling aspects of self by the mother. This leads to the infant's experiencing of the mother and other objects as frightening, dangerous or persecutory (Hedges, 1983). Because of the power of their own rage and the viciousness they experience in their external world, persons with BPD are unable to integrate the good and bad aspects of individuals in their environment into any coherent single identity. Thus all objects are ultimately seen as either "all bad" or "all good." They are unable to integrate ambivalence or contradictory mental states, so that all objects are "split" (Hedges, 1983). The lack of integration of good and bad ego states damages future development, as it prevents the differentiation of self from object and the integration of good and bad self- and object representations. Thus, in borderlines, ego states are composed of "contradictory, oscillatory internalizations," which are comprised of "good, bad, self and object experiences" (Hedges, 1983, p. 112). The inability to integrate good with bad prevents the expression of a spectrum of healthy affects and an experience of the self as differentiated from other constant objects. Thus individuals with BPD exhibit a protective shallowness in emotional relationships. David demonstrated these extremes and this "pseudodepth" in all of his close relationships, but in a most exaggerated way with his lovers. His projective identifications and/or object choices were enacted in relationships that went rapidly from highly sexual and adoring to vicious and sadistic. Feeling justified, David then retaliated in kind—providing distance from the closeness that was so overwhelming, but devastation at still another loss and failure.

The persistence of early internalized object relations in a toxic, "nonmetabolized" condition leads, according to Kernberg (1975), to pathological superego formation as well. Disturbed superego development arises from the presence of object images that are either "all good" or "all bad." Sadistic superego forerunners in turn distort parenting figures and prevent superego integration. The superego is personified, not abstracted and projected onto the external world, which is viewed as "all bad." When individuals with BPD are unable to achieve their aims aggressively, they attempt to control their environment by manipulation. When this fails, they regress to fantasied gratification. Thus they may cover up their inferiority with grandiose fantasies. Their many partial identifications lead to identity diffusion or "as-if" personalities, in which they pretend to be what other persons want.

Adler (1985) has described as an essential aspect of BPD a developmental failure in the formation of self-soothing capacities, as a result of the child's inability to recall comforting memories of significant caregivers even when they are not present. This and the need to self-soothe with drugs and alcohol has been noted in all SAs by Khantzian and Treece (1985).

Defense Mechanisms

The defense mechanisms of individuals with BPD are inextricably interwoven with their developmental psychodynamics; they include splitting, primitive idealization, extreme projection and projective identification, primitive denial, and devaluation (Kernberg et al., 1989). They have been discussed in Chapter 3, but are described again here in relation to BPD.

1. Splitting is the keeping apart of introjections and identifications of opposite quality, so that external objects are "all good" or "all bad." In BPD, when splitting is excessive, neutralization of aggression cannot occur; an energy source for ego growth fails, and a weakened ego falls back on splitting (this becomes a cycle). Another direct manifestation of splitting is selective lack of impulse control through splitting or ego control, which leads to impulsivity and addictions (Kernberg et al., 1988).

2. Primitive idealization refers to seeing some individuals as the "all goods" who will provide protection against the "all bads." BPD patients are unable to acknowledge any aggressive feelings toward the "all goods."

3. Projection and projective identification refer to the transfer of the "all bad" self-images onto external objects. Thus BPD patients see or project onto others the behaviors of dangerous retaliatory objects against which they must defend. At the same time, the patients empathize with the objects, which increases the fear of their own projected aggression. (See Chapter 8 for a detailed discussion of projective identification.)

4. Denial in BPD patients is of a very primitive type: There is mutual denial of two main areas of consciousness, which permits the same individual to be "all good" or "all bad." Thus the denial reinforces splitting.

5. Omnipotence and devaluation are linked to splitting and the use of introjection and identification. BPD patients shift between magical omnipotent introjection and magical objects; thus they feel the right to expect gratification and homage from others. When they fail to receive it, they feel devalued.

Psychotherapy

Kernberg et al.'s (1988) recent book on the psychotherapy of BPD patients is an excellent handbook for this difficult therapeutic challenge. All of the principles described in their book can be utilized, once the

SA with BPD has developed a method to facilitate abstinence. Kernberg et al. advocate developing a clear treatment contract, which, in the case of an SA, spells out how abstinence will be achieved and how slips will be dealt with. Kernberg et al. also advocate the use of the least restrictive measures possible, with full knowledge that when limits are set with BPD patients, they will be tested.

One specific aspect of psychotherapy with BPD patients is integrating the part-self and part-object representations. The underlying representations are identified by the therapist, labeled for the patient, and traced as they contribute to interpersonal relationships in the present. The internalized object representations of BPD patients are caricatures. They are fragmentary distortions that exaggerate certain traits and ignore others. The therapist identifies the predominant part-self–object dyads, to help the patient coalesce them into more realistic and balanced internal representations of self and object.

This is done in the transference. The therapist clarifies the patient's attitude toward and expectations of the therapist and himself/herself from moment to moment. Some representations of the self in others have been disowned. The patient learns to accept these through interpretations of the defenses described above. The maintenance of an idealized transference (which David held at his return to therapy after a year of sobriety) makes it difficult to interpret these defenses in the transference. Thus they are interpreted with significant others until sobriety is more stabilized and it is safer to work in the transference.

Steps for the therapist include the following:

1. Experiencing and tolerating the confusion.
2. Identifying the actors. Inferences are made about the representations of the patient's internal object world, based on recurring patterns with others (particularly the therapist).
3. Naming. Interpretations are best made while the patient is emotionally involved in the session but the intensity of affect is decreasing. The therapist may also need distance from the intensity to make a succinct, evocative comment.
4. Attending to the patient's reaction. The patient's associations and changes in interaction with the therapist are more important than his/her overt agreement or disagreement.
5. Interpreting primitive defenses. These defenses avoid intolerable conflict by creating sharp, unrealistic separation between loving and hateful aspects of the self and others. Even if they occur in consciousness, they are separated.

Regardless of the orientation and experience of the psychotherapist, BPD patients will switch therapists often. Perry et al. (1990) found that BPD patients who entered their study had a mean of 6.1 previous outpatient therapies. These authors noted the proclivity of these patients to re-enact traumatic patterns and regressions with therapists, which led to multiple premature interruptions. There is the possibility that current treatment techniques have not evolved or are not practiced so that BPD patients can be treated with fewer interruptions. Perry et al. (1990) feel that a key to successful therapy with BPD patients is to validate the reality and the impact of traumatic experiences, and to acknowledge the appropriateness of the patients' emotional reaction to the terrifying past experiences (Perry et al., 1990). Another key is a therapist's ability to withstand and contain projective identifications.

PASSIVE AGGRESSIVE PERSONALITY DISORDER*

One additional personality disorder, PAPD, is often diagnosed in SAs and is described briefly here. In my opinion, it is more a defensive style than a true personality disorder; moreover, its criteria (possibly even its name) are to be changed in DSM-IV. The key defense is the turning of outward anger against the self, but generally in ways that rather obviously demonstrate the individual's latent hostility. The behaviors are often passive, but nonetheless oppositional and obstructive, resistances to demands for performance, assertiveness, or intimacy. DSM-III-R (American Psychiatric Association, 1987) requires five of nine behaviors for a diagnosis, including: (1) procrastinates; (2) becomes sulky, irritable, or argumentative when asked to do something he/she does not want to do; (3) works deliberately slowly or poorly; (4) protests unjustly about demands made; (5) forgets obligations; (6) believes he/she is doing a much better job than others think; (7) resents useful suggestions about productivity; (8) obstructs efforts of others by failing to do his/her share; and (9) unreasonably criticizes or scorns those in positions of authority. In order for a diagnosis of PAPD to be made, these behaviors must be chronic and inflexible — not situational reactions to stress or a particular life situation in which there is perceived helplessness, such as military service or incarceration.

Individuals with PAPD find fault with the people they depend on, yet they are unable to remove themselves from these relationships. They are not assertive and express their needs and wishes indirectly. They do not ask questions about what is expected of them, so that they often feel overwhelmed. They become anxious when they are pushed to succeed or when their defensive pattern of retroflexed rage is removed.

---

*Note added in proof: Eliminated as a personality disorder in DSM-IV.

Because of frequent life failures, stormy relationships, and driving others away, they lack self-confidence, are pessimistic, and appear to hold on to their resentment rather than seek external satisfaction.

Many SAs use passive aggressive techniques with those they depend on, and if PAPD is truly a personality disorder, they often qualify for the diagnosis. Through their substance use and related behaviors, they exert powerful passive control over others in intimate relationships with them. Thus they provoke their loved ones to buy drugs and alcohol to prevent withdrawal; to pay for gas to get them to work; to provide money so that they will not be beaten by drug suppliers; to undress them and put them to bed; or to call employers and make excuses for their being late or unable to work. When sober, they continue to deal with situations that require assertion in a passive manner. This all seems familiar, as persons with PAPD often become involved with individuals with codependent behaviors. Yet the PAPD individuals themselves exhibit a codependent pattern, including constantly blaming others for their difficulties.

Passive aggressive behavior evolves in a family setting in which the child's parents are aggressive in their blocking or punishing the child's assertiveness. The child reacts to this by appearing obsequious, undemanding, and polite, but punishes his/her parents by subtly disobeying and undermining requests (e.g., doing almost everything but omitting one critical aspect, so that the project is undermined). Other explanations for the development of PAPD include a temperament disorder as described by Thomas and Chess (1977), in which the infant is born with such characteristics as frequent negative mood, negative responses to new stimuli, and slow adaptability to change.

Still another formulation is that PAPD emerges from parent–child interactions characterized by inconsistent demands that are poorly internalized and by inconsistency of gratification, which generate a lifetime of unresolved ambivalence (Esman, 1986). The child does not submit or defy; he/she maintains an ambivalent, inconsistent posture that generates hostility in others. This evoked hostility confirms the sense of injustice, which in turn justifies the feeling of injured innocence. The child thus develops the quality of an injustice collector (Esman, 1986). As the child enters adolescence, he/she learns that provocative, indirect behaviors may be the best way to obtain parental recognition, so that the behaviors become reinforced.

In psychotherapy, these patients often double-bind their therapists as to how to deal with their demands in much the same way that NPD patients do. To meet their needs is to support their pathology, but not to meet them leads them to feel quite rejected or to run from therapy. They will repeatedly frustrate their therapists by agreeing to utilize more adaptive behaviors, yet undermining the results so that the new behaviors also backfire. They will enter treatment during an acute decompensation, and attempt to leave as soon as they obtain minimal relief and before any work can be done on their defensive system. Vigorous confrontation will increase their resistance, yet giving in to their withdrawal or negative behaviors is seen as lack of concern. At times group confrontation by peers is more effective in shifting their responses than is individual therapy. As is true of most SAs, many of David's maladaptive ways of dealing with the world could be labeled as passive aggressive.

Beck et al. (1990) suggest that cognitive therapy is particularly helpful with PAPD patients. The first step they suggest is to engage such a patient actively in a collaborative therapeutic process. That is, the patient should feel that he/she is actively making choices, rather than being manipulated by the therapist. Thus the therapist can ask the patient to choose from several issues to work on, and several tasks for dealing with the problem when a problem is chosen. Another strategy is to teach the patient to recognize the feelings that precede automatic passive aggressive responses, so that he/she can alter these responses. In my experience, aggressive responses will always become manifest in the transference, often in regard to issues of time, money, or attendance at Twelve-Step meetings; they afford the therapist the opportunity to deal in the here and now with such responses.

The first requirement on the part of the therapist is consistency in his/her own policies and behaviors concerning time, money, interruptions, limits, and so forth. Once a trusting relationship is developed, a PAPD patient can be helped to see that passive aggressive ways of getting back at others are more destructive to himself/herself than to the others (Beck et al., 1990).

CONCLUDING COMMENT

This chapter does not deal in detail with personality disorders and traits other than the most common triad of ASP, NPD, and BPD. Dependent personality disorder is often seen in association with BPD, as is self-defeating personality disorder. Aggressive types of PAPD are often seen in ASP, as are some forms of paranoid personality disorder. Histrionic personality disorder may be little more than a higher-functioning form of BPD. As can be seen from the general comments on the psychotherapy of personality disorders, and the individualized sections on each of the three major personality disorders seen in SAs, modifications of psychotherapy based on the presence of personality disorders or traits constitute an extremely important aspect of treatment.

Phase 1 of Treatment: From Assessment to Achieving Abstinence

The method of psychotherapy described in this book can be divided into three relatively discrete phases (Kaufman & Reoux, 1988): (1) achieving abstinence, (2) early recovery (sobriety), and (3) advanced recovery. I am aware that several authors continue to espouse psychotherapy with alcoholics or addicts without requiring abstinence. At the same time, the vast majority of psychotherapists, particularly those whose practice includes many SAs, advocate the establishment and continuation of abstinence as a prerequisite for ongoing psychotherapy (Brown, 1985a; Chappel, 1992; Wallace, 1985; Washton, 1989; Zimberg, 1985). Those rare SAs who are "cured" while they continue to drink or use drugs are often individuals whose use of abusable substances is secondary to underlying psychopathology and/or who were not truly addicted over substantial periods of time. I do not doubt that in the hands of some therapists (though never myself), a few "genuine" addicts or alcoholics have been helped to achieve substantially happy, healthy lives while they have continued to drink or use drugs moderately, and have been able to use substances in a controlled manner for long periods of time after the termination of psychotherapy. In my opinion, the major problem with a controlled-use approach for SAs is that it will be wrong 99 times out of 100. Thus, in helping that one SA to drink or use drugs moderately, the therapist may be tempted to utilize moderate use as a goal for the 99 patients for whom it is totally inappropriate and in fact quite dangerous. Addicts and alcoholics who continue to use drugs and drink have a substantially higher death rate than the moderate-drinking segment of the general population.

After the treatment that demarcates the end of Phase 1, I advocate two discrete, separate phases of psychotherapy. Although these phases are stepwise and sequential, the first four chapters of this book have repeatedly emphasized the importance of an individualized assessment of each SA. Obviously, then, each individual will progress through these phases differently. In addition, the therapist guides the patient through each phase flexibly and according to the patient's needs and ego strength. The patient's acquisition of self-knowledge (including an understanding of feelings and related underlying issues), even early in the therapy, is one important way in which the patient can take control over his/her addiction (Dodes & Khantzian, 1991).

ASSESSMENT

Assessment with SAs must of necessity be more thorough and detailed than with other types of patients, because substances of abuse have such pervasive effects on both psyche and soma. Substance abuse and addiction can be dangerous even in their early phases. In addition, they substantially shorten an individual's life span over time.

Assessment is only one of several key aspects of the initial interview. The major goal of the initial evaluation is for the patient to end up committed to appropriate, workable treatment. Thus other functions of evaluation include initiating a working therapeutic alliance and orienting the patient to the components of his/her individualized program (Washton, 1989). Assessment is the beginning of treatment, and most patients will bond strongly to the first therapeutic person they meet, including their evaluator.

Assessment is always a process that continues throughout treatment, but this is particularly true of SAs; as their commitment to abstinence as well as their psychological state must be constantly re-evaluated. In the early phases of treatment, other critical information is often revealed that appreciably alters the assessment of the patient, as the therapist learns of previously withheld facts (e.g., loss of job or spouse, legal or financial crises). During this process it is essential that the therapist be exploratory without being judgmental (Dodes & Khantzian, 1991). The patient may project a harsh authoritarian image onto the therapist, and gentle confrontation of the projection will permit the evaluation to continue.

The first step in assessment is to determine the nature and extent of the substance abuse. Finally, a medical examination that delineates the specific physical effects of the substance(s) involved is important (Pattison, 1986) and is discussed below in more detail. The pattern of use of every type of abusable substance is determined. Many individuals will minimize the importance of their abuse of a secondary drug that is not their substance of choice (e.g., alcohol or marijuana use by cocaine addicts, or occasional cocaine or alcohol use by heroin addicts). Documentation of use of these secondary substances is quite important, as their continued use predisposes an SA to return to his/her substance of choice. Some important specifics are quantity, quality, duration, expense, ways in which intake was supported and prevented, physical effects, tolerance, withdrawal, and any drug-related complications. The circumstances under which the patient began to use and abuse drugs or alcohol and the current substance of choice are reviewed for their psychosocial and psychodynamic significance. Direct and indirect psychological sequelae—particularly psychotic disruptions, paranoid or suicidal ideation, and violence—are assessed.

Early effort is also devoted to why the patient is entering treatment at this specific time. Is a spouse finally so fed up and/or empowered that he/she is clearly communicating readiness to leave? Is the individual seeking treatment because an employer is mandating it as a condition of continued employment? Or is he/she attempting to obtain leniency in a pending court case? The understanding of immediate motivation tells us a great deal about true treatment needs as well as sincerity of commitment. Working with the judicial system can provide necessary leverage to motivate a difficult patient to enter and stay in appropriate treatment.

The past history of treatment is reviewed during the initial interview. What was helpful and what was not? How long did the patient stay sober? Did he/she work a Twelve-Step program, and, if so, with what level of commitment? Was the individual in ongoing psychotherapy, and, if so, what orientation did the therapist have? Did the patient lie to or con the therapist? What precipitated relapse? Is the patient willing to sign a consent form so that the present clinician can communicate with the prior treatment team, hospital, or therapist? How aware was the patient of earlier signs of relapse that preceded the major precipitant? Other important indicators of potential relapse include continuing related but nonchemical compulsive behaviors, such as gambling, promiscuous sexuality (including perversions and high-risk behaviors), binge eating, extreme exercising, food restriction, frequent rages, violence, loss of temper, and self-mutilation.

Exploration of how the patient obtained the money for drugs and alcohol is often quite revealing. To what extent are these activities indicative of underlying antisocial personality? How self-destructive, risky, or sensation-seeking were these activities? The family history of substance dependence is also gathered early, because such a history conveys a powerful risk for substance dependence as well as greater severity of illness (Kaufman & Reoux, 1988). The family and other collateral sources are interviewed in family sessions to provide their view of substance abuse and related behaviors. Many SAs will minimize the extent of their abuse of drugs and alcohol until confronted by their families. Others will be more honest in individual sessions, and later will use family visits to share their substance abuse history with their families in an open way, which opens up communication about other issues.

Peer relationships are also explored. Do most or all of the patient's friends, relatives, fellow employees, or supervisors use or abuse drugs and alcohol? To what extent does a supportive network of nonabusing or sober associates exist?

The psychological aspects of substance use are explored by asking what the patient is like on drugs or alcohol, what happens under the influence, and what effects are sought (Dodes & Khantzian, 1991). In addition, what fantasies are experienced before, during, and after drug use? What are its effects on family, friendship, work, and recreational performance? What feelings are stimulated by drugs and alcohol? What feelings are relieved or soothed by these substances? The patient's psychopathology is also evaluated, and a preliminary assessment of defense mechanisms and personality disorders is made (see Chapters 3 and 4).

The consequences of substance abuse pervade all biopsychosocial spheres and include unemployment, violence, divorce, financial and tax problems, family disruption, and legal difficulties. Assessment should include the specific events and situations that are the consequences of the problem; these, when and if the SA recognizes and accepts that he/she has a disease, are identified and labeled as part of the disease. However, for many if not most individuals, the disease is named or confronted only gradually at first — particularly if they are in massive denial of their substance dependence. Thus the clinician begins with questions such as "How do you use alcohol?" or "How does your use of drugs affect you and those who are close to you?" As assessment progresses and it becomes apparent that the patient is resistant to workable treatment, the therapist may need to become quite confrontative, to utilize a formal intervention (see "Motivation for Abstinence and Treatment," below), or to employ other similar techniques. However, some patients may need to demonstrate their ability to abstain from alcohol and drugs their way, "just one time," before they are motivated to accept a comprehensive and workable program. Therapists should be flexible but should not become enablers as they decide how many "one more times" to permit.

For many clinicians, patients in whom substance abuse initially goes unrecognized present particular difficulties. Such patients may include ones who present with a problem apparently unrelated to substance abuse, who minimize or deny abuse, or who escalate from controlled use to abuse, or dependence during the process of treatment. As time goes by while the therapist continues to treat this type of patient, and the problem is denied or ignored, it becomes progressively more difficult to confront the substance abuse—and even more problematic to require abstinence. It then requires considerable therapeutic objectivity or outside consultation to step back from the ongoing process of treatment and require the patient to deal with substance abuse before psychotherapy can continue. If this confrontation is done with empathic concern, the patient can actively participate in the shift of emphasis. Thus the therapist may say something like this: "It seems that our recent inability to make progress, particularly in regard to intimate relationships, is related to your drinking and how it affects those who are close to you. Let's talk about how you can stop drinking, so that we can again focus meaningfully on your relationships." With patients in ongoing treatment, therapists should first be willing to let them stop "their way" before requiring a detailed method for abstinence.

Another important aspect of assessment is laboratory testing. Tests of liver enzymes and a complete blood count are very helpful in confirming the diagnosis of alcoholism and the extent of liver and hematopoietic (blood-forming) damage. Many alcoholic patients who are strongly questioning their diagnosis or need for intensive treatment may be persuaded to accept diagnosis and treatment when they are confronted with definitive laboratory confirmation of their disease. However, therapists should not rely solely on these tests, as many alcohol-dependent persons may have normal or near-normal values. Urine screens for drugs of abuse may also be helpful in diagnosing substance abuse in resistant patients, particularly adolescents. These must be obtained under monitored conditions and carefully assessed for contaminants that can interfere with testing.

The medical sequelae and related complications are evaluated, and these are also used to confront resistant patients with their need for treatment. A patient is asked to accept appropriate medical treatment for any complications (e.g., hypertension, anemia, syphilis, hepatitis, AIDS, etc.), and the circumstances of this treatment are made a part of the contract.

Many chronic pain patients seek psychotherapy to deal with associated depression and/or drug and alcohol dependence. Those who have prior histories of substance abuse, or who currently abuse their pain medications and/or alcohol, need to be dealt with initially in the same way as any other addicted patient is treated. That is, they need to be given a thorough medical evaluation and detoxified. When a drug-abusing chronic pain patient is detoxified, he/she generally finds that the pain is much less than when he/she were using narcotics. With the drug-free state as a baseline, the patient's pain can be relieved with safer modalities, such as nonsteroidal anti-inflammatory drugs, transcutaneous electrical nerve stimulation, physical therapy and massage, acupuncture, relaxation, and imaging techniques.

MOTIVATION FOR ABSTINENCE AND TREATMENT

It is of interest that over the past 10 years, psychotherapists working with substance-dependent patients have become more and more insistent on maintenance of abstinence as a prerequisite for psychotherapy. Although they cite different reasons for their insistence, Bean-Bayog (1986), Brown (1985), Khantzian and Schneider (1986), Vaillant (1978), Wallace (1985a), and Zimberg (1985) all agree on requiring abstinence at the onset of treatment. Thus, during an evaluation, I will convey to the patient that I feel that in order for treatment to be successful, he/she must choose a method to reinforce abstinence. I inform the patient that although medications like Antabuse or methadone maintenance may provide that method, the best method in my experience is a Twelve-Step program. I also emphasize that since addiction has destroyed so many aspects of the patient's life, a holistic approach that develops the whole person is most helpful.

As the therapist points out the dangerousness to the patient of his/her potential self-damage, and facilitates abstinence with its protective qualities, "the therapist's caring concern may be internalized by the patient, providing a nucleus for the introjection of a healthy self-care function" (Dodes & Khantzian, 1991, p. 397). At times the therapist's confrontation may lead to abstinence, which then is perceived as the much-longed-for message of caring that had been so absent in the patient's childhood. At other times, the patient may see the therapist's requirement for abstinence as punitive, threatening, or unempathetic.

Some patients will refuse to enter treatment, particularly if abstinence is required. Several techniques that the therapist can use to motivate such patients have been described above (gradual persuasion, confrontation, laboratory tests). The patient's network provides many important sources of motivation for treatment. Spouses, parents, children, and work-related individuals (such as employers, supervisors, peers, and employee assistance personnel) may, individually or in concert, motivate an unwilling patient for treatment. Attorneys, judges, and probation officers also carry considerable weight in motivating patients if they are involved. One difficulty here is balancing the need for treatment with laws about confidentiality. If the family or significant other is seen in the initial interview, then a clear, mutually agreed-upon contract about what will be shared can be clarified. At that time, the family can be worked with to support or demand necessary treatment, as appropriate. Many employee assistance personnel and supervisors are presently quite well educated about substance abuse and can be strong motivators for treatment without any urging from the therapist. Experience has shown that SAs who are externally motivated do as well as or better than those who profess only internal motivation (Liepman et al., 1989). This is an important contradiction to those therapists who tell SAs and their families that they are unable to treat SAs who are not personally motivated.

Resistant patients in whom the methods noted above have failed, particularly if they are involved with their families and employed, may be good candidates for a formal intervention. This technique, developed for the treatment of alcoholism at the Johnson Institute in Minneapolis, Minnesota, is readily adapted for use with all addictions. (V. E. Johnson, 1980). In this technique, all available family members and the most meaningful support network members (e.g., employer, neighbors, friends, and clergy) are coached to confront the addicted person with the facts of his/her substance use and related behaviors. This is done with deep concern and without hostility. The participants list specific incidents and behaviors consequential to substance use and present them in a nonjudgmental fashion at the intervention meeting.

Family members can be immobilized by their fear and their love, and may find the idea of an intervention intimidating. They need to be educated about the deadly consequences of their inaction, and they need instruction on how to say, "We love you and because we love you, we will not continue to live with you while you abuse alcohol or drugs. If you accept the treatment being offered and continue to work at recovery, we will renew our lifetime commitment to you." The family needs to agree in advance about what treatment is necessary; insist on it in a firm, consistent manner; and follow through with the limits set, including the consequences of return to substance use and/or refusal to enter treatment.

As many family members as possible should be included. In addition, involvement of the employer is crucial, and in some cases may be sufficient of itself to motivate the addicted individual to seek treatment. The employer who clearly makes treatment a precondition for employment, who supports time off for treatment, and who agrees to continue support for the patient in aftercare offers a helpful model for the family and is a valuable ally.

In a nonrandomized study to evaluate the impact of family intervention, Liepman et al. (1989) examined the impact an alcoholic's social network could have on treatment. The two groups were differentiated by whether or not a formal intervention by the family occurred. In the cases in which intervention did occur, 86% entered treatment, and a higher rate of continued abstinence was seen in comparison to cases in which the alcoholics' social network received counseling but no formal intervention occurred. This study also counters the myth that an alcoholic cannot be "forced" into treatment.

DETOXIFICATION

Outpatient versus Inpatient Detoxification

Detoxification is not described in detail here; the reader is referred to several excellent sources (Gessner, 1979; Greenblatt & Shader, 1975; Liskow & Goodwin, 1987; O'Connor et al., 1992; Rosenbloom, 1988) for descriptions of this process.

Previously, I have written about the difficulties of outpatient detoxification and the need to utilize a comprehensive program (which reaches into the patient's home, network, physicians, and pharmacies) when attempting this (Kaufman & Reoux, 1988). Recently, I have encountered several case managers who have only been willing to approve outpatient detoxification in certain patients. If a patient is addicted to sedative drugs and/or alcohol, and inpatient detoxification is not available, I only perform the detoxification in a highly structured intensive outpatient setting (partial hospital program) in which the patient's vital signs and activities can be monitored for up to 14 hours daily if necessary. Urine drug screens and blood alcohol levels can also be monitored daily and provide immediate feedback about nonprescribed substance use.

Although cocaine addicts require little medical detoxification, and Washton (1989) has described excellent intensive outpatient programs, I prefer initial inpatient detoxification and stabilization for at least several days. This is particularly true with heavy cocaine users (i.e., those using over 5 grams weekly), and even more so in those who primarily smoke it. In these patients, there is often a prolonged sleep of up to 3 or 4 days, which is interrupted by bizarre, paranoid, impulsive behavior and followed by powerful cravings. Hospitalization accomplishes containment from drug use and other destructive behaviors, as well as nurturing motivation during periods of wakefulness.

Pharmacological Adjuncts to Detoxification

Again, the use of pharmacological adjuncts is not described here in detail, but the reader is referred to several excellent texts and articles in this area (Kosten, 1989; Banys, 1988; Jaffee & Ciraulo, 1985).

Many pharmacological adjuncts have been recommended for cocaine addicts. In the first few days after drug cessation, they may require neuroleptics for extreme paranoia and/or destructive behaviors (Kosten, 1989). Note that neuroleptics are contraindicated in acute cocaine overdoses in which there is agitation and hyperthermia, as they may worsen the latter symptom. Oxazepam or other benzodiazepines may provide active relief of agitation, irritability, and anxiety, which will help motivate the cocaine addict to become engaged in treatment. Several dopaminergic agents have been suggested to alleviate early cravings and withdrawal; these include amantadine, bromocriptine, L-dopa, and methylphenidate (Kosten, 1989), as well as carbamazepine (Halikas et al., 1991). L-Tyrosine and other amino acids have been used to enhance new dopamine production. Buprenorphine has been found to diminish cravings for cocaine and opiates (Kosten et al., 1989). Desipramine has been advocated as reducing longer-term craving by reducing dopaminergic receptor sensitivity (Kosten, 1989). Despite studies showing little if any benefit from Antabuse in large treatment groups of alcoholics (Fuller & Roth, 1979), I have found it very helpful in individuals who must leave hospital treatment early or who have otherwise tenuous sobriety (Banys, 1988).

DEVELOPMENT OF A PLAN
FOR ACHIEVING ABSTINENCE

After detoxification, it is necessary to develop a plan that enables the SA to stay off drugs and alcohol. The specific methods employed may vary according to the extent of use, abuse, and dependence. Effective, clear parental expectations and limit setting may occasionally be sufficient to stop adolescent drug abuse. Awareness through education about the physical and psychosocial consequences of substance abuse may motivate some SAs to stop. In general, however, greater efforts will be required.

Outpatient versus Inpatient Treatment

Individuals with moderately severe or intermittent substance abuse may need brief hospitalization to initiate a drug-free state. This may be followed by a variety of individualized approaches, including traditional 28-day inpatient stay; evening treatment 5 to 7 days per week; partial day hospital; intensive 20-hour weekly outpatient settings; and/or recovery homes. If the abuse pattern is severe—that is, if intake is excessive, social or vocational functioning is grossly impaired, or physical dependence is present—hospitalization may be set as a requirement early in therapy. Other criteria for initiation of inpatient treatment include low internal or external motivation; inability to abstain, particularly during therapy or other outpatient treatment; heavy peer and family substance abuse; potential for serious withdrawal; severe toxic overdose; severe comorbid medical or psychiatric condition; and presence of severe violence, suicidality, or other self-destructiveness. Relative conditions for outpatient treatment include (in addition to the absence of the preceding factors) lack of child care; potential devastating loss of employment as a result of absence from work; and other financial factors.

Well-motivated patients who require inpatient treatment and cannot afford it should receive this treatment from the onset and be permitted to pay for care through a payment plan. Comorbid disorders that require hospital initiation of treatment may include Axis II disorders such as ASP and BPD when necessary, as well as major psychoses, severe anxiety disorders, and severe depression with suicidality. Inpatient treatment provides an intensive orientation and stabilization that may provide the impetus for abstinence, particularly if effective, comprehensive aftercare programs are initiated. Most patients who are seriously addicted to drugs or alcohol will require intensive, high-impact programs at the beginning of therapy, whether these are inpatient or daily outpatient programs. A therapeutic milieu that is supportive of recovery can motivate very resistant SAs.

Methods of Reinforcing Abstinence:
Twelve-Step Groups, Pharmacotherapy, and Others

The patient is asked to choose a method to reinforce staying off all substances of abuse. The establishment of a method for maintaining abstinence is made a condition of the psychotherapeutic contract; the therapist engages in psychotherapy only if the patient has such a system for staying substance-free. Patients can choose one or more of the following: a Twelve-Step group (e.g., AA, NA, CA), pharmacotherapy (e.g., Antabuse, methadone maintenance, naltrexone), or other methods (e.g., acupuncture has been used for detoxification as well as abstinence; Whitehead, 1978). A lifetime commitment to abstinence is not required. Rather, the one-day-at-a-time approach is recommended: The patient commits to a method of maintaining abstinence for only one day at a time, but renews this commitment daily using the basic principles of Twelve-Step programs.

In a study of four different AA groups from the same Southwestern U.S. city, Emrick et al. (1993) concluded that there was homogeneity on some issues and diversity on other subjects. The commonality across groups was found in the areas of (1) encouraging spirituality and (2) discouraging innovation while a person was unsure about individual expression, independence, and self-discovery. However, two of the groups differed from the other two in that they had lower cohesion and higher aggression. This study of a few AA groups is just a beginning in quantifying the vast differences among the many different Twelve-Step groups available in any large community. Many patients who are uncomfortable in the first few meetings they attend will eventually find meetings where they feel quite supported. Thus I encourage them to try several different locations and types of meetings. Many recovering SAs will find a "home base," where there are several meetings daily from which to choose and where they attend all or most of their meetings.

Patients attending Twelve-Step meetings may have to try different groups and shop around for the most appropriate types of meetings for them. Initially, patients may find large meetings with speakers more comfortable; such meetings also provide successful role models for identification. Once SAs are engaged with a program, smaller groups, men's and women's stag, and/or "Big Book" study groups requiring a more active role by participants are more beneficial to personality change. Patients are also encouraged to obtain a sponsor. If a recovering person begins participating as a speaker, larger groups may again become desirable, with an active leadership role substituted for the earlier passive participation. It is often very helpful for a therapist to meet with a patient's sponsor at an early point in the patient's treatment, to facilitate their working together as a treatment team rather than being split into "good object" and "bad object" by the SA.

The particular aspects of AA that have been shown to be related to positive outcome as documented by quantitative research include having a sponsor, engaging in Twelfth-Step work (see Chapter 7), increasing participation as time goes by, and leading a meeting. Other determinants that are significant but less profound statistically include sponsoring others and working the Sixth through Twelfth Steps (Emrick et al., 1993). Emrick et al.'s review of the research literature also shows that AA involvement during and after professional treatment enhances improvement over treatment without AA involvement.

Many patients will elect not to work with a Twelve-Step program, particularly during their early attempts at sobriety. Some will drop out of treatment because of this inability and/or as a result of difficulty in maintaining abstinence, but will return later, more willing to adopt the principles of the Twelve-Step movement. Some patients never work the Twelve Steps. Thus it is often helpful to provide a wide variety of methods to maintain abstinence. For the Twelve-Step-resistant patients other groups with a more secular orientation (e.g., Recovery, Inc., or Secular Organization for Sobriety) can be helpful, but they are much less widely available than AA, NA, or CA. My preference with these resistant patients is to refer them to a colleague for group psychotherapy, one to three times weekly (see Chapter 9). Preferably, this colleague is one who has solid recovery from substance abuse himself/herself, as well as extensive training as a mental health professional. Ongoing, random urine screens for drugs of abuse may also help some individuals stay off drugs. Some patients who agree to none of these ancillary measures may be worked with if they agree to reenter hospital or residential treatment whenever they "slip" into substance abuse or dependence.

Drug treatments such as Antabuse, methadone maintenance, and naltrexone may also be helpful, either alone or in combination with other measures. Many alcoholic patients who are newly sober may be offered Antabuse for additional support, particularly if their situations are in any way shaky. Such situations would include (1) early discharge from inpatient treatment; (2) highly stressful work or family environment; (3) early travel to distant places; or (4) unavoidable contact with substance abuse in the social, familial, or work setting.

Treatment of Psychiatric Disorders and Cognitive Deficits

The next step is to obtain the patient's cooperation in treating any underlying primary psychiatric disorder(s), as well as acute and chronic cognitive deficits. Evaluation of such disorders or deficits will of course have begun during the initial assessment, but final assessment and definitive treatment should await the completion of detoxification. As reviewed by Grant and Reed (1985), long-term cognitive consequences may or may not resolve totally; moreover, resolution typically takes weeks to months, depending on the particular substances involved. The most rapid improvement usually occurs during the first 3–4 weeks, but, maximum return of function may not return for several years. Acute problems such as suicidality and hallucinations may require immediate evaluation and intervention. In all cases needing pharmacological treatment, agents with little or no abuse potential (e.g., BuSpar, Benadryl, Vistaril, neuroleptics, or lithium) are preferred. Sedative/hypnotic drugs and benzodiazepines should be avoided because of the danger of dual abuse and dependence. A new hypnotic, Ambien, is alleged to have less addictive and abusive potential than the benzodiazepines. Artane, Cogentin, and even sedating antidepressants and clonidine can be abused by these patients. Recently, a few of my patients have reported abuse of selective serotonergic reuptake inhibitors. Pharmacological treatment of clearly primary psychiatric illness (e.g., bipolar disorder) is often as essential as abstinence from drugs and alcohol.

Development of a Contract

Although it is not my own style to utilize a written contract with adults, an oral contract is developed at the end of the evaluation and/or detoxification period. Every attempt should be made to obtain the patient's and family's active participation in creating and agreeing to the elements of the contract. These elements include the following:

1. Agreement as to where, when, and how detoxification will take place (if it has not already done so).
2. Agreement as to what method of maintaining abstinence the patient will choose and related specifics (e.g., number and type of Twelve-Step meetings, monitoring of Antabuse or naltrexone, etc.). This component is generally postponed until after detoxification. Agreement to monitoring of substance abuse with random urine drug screens is obtained.
3. Agreement as to therapy for Axis I psychiatric or Axis III medical conditions (e.g., taking of lithium for bipolar disorder; plan for treatment of epilepsy or diabetes; appropriate treatment with non-narcotic drugs and drug-free modalities for chronic pain).
4. Agreement as to the family's participation in the patient's treatment, as well as to the family's participation in its own therapy. The latter may include treatment for substance abuse or a certain number of Al-Anon or Co-Anon meetings weekly for each family member.
5. Agreement as to the patient's and family's participation in a comprehensive program of education about the psychological, familial, and physical effects of alcohol and other drugs. This should include education about such key issues as the disease concept, cross-

addiction, the prolonged abstinence withdrawal syndrome, relapse prevention, and so forth.

6. Agreement as to beginning a commitment to a drug- and alcohol-free environment. The family agrees to eliminate all abusable drugs and alcohol from the house. The patient agrees not to associate with known SAs and "pushers," and to build a sober network of associates. The patient further agrees not to return to a work setting that is heavily laden with SAs (or the employer begins to "clean house"). Finally, the patient agrees to avoid geographical locations (general areas where he/she frequently bought or used drugs), as well as specific places such as bars or "crack houses" where he/she drank and/or used drugs. It must be emphasized that this is an initial commitment at this phase; enduring commitment will take considerable time and effort to achieve. Failure to develop this aspect of the contract will make outpatient induction of treatment impossible and will require the substitution of hospitalization or residential treatment. This commitment needs to be re-established after the patient leaves the hospital and/or returns home.

CASE VIGNETTE: DEVELOPING A TREATMENT PLAN WITH A DRY ALCOHOLIC

At the time Bob* entered treatment with me, he was 32 years old and was employed as a midlevel executive. He presented with the following history.

Bob, a fraternal twin, was born and raised in Ireland. His father and grandfather were alcoholics, and his mother was probably one as well. He initially stated that he had never seen his mother intoxicated. He was presently married to a woman named Carla, and they had a four-year-old son together. Carla also had two children, ages 9 and 11, from a prior marriage, who lived in the home. Bob had two other children, ages 5 and 8, living in Ireland with his first wife.

Bob had entered an outpatient program 6 weeks prior to seeing me, because his drinking had been out of control for about a year. He stated that he had left that program before treatment completion because he felt the therapist was patronizing. He admitted that the therapist had helped him get in touch with his feelings, but so fast that he felt overwhelmed by them. He stated that he was entering treatment now mainly because Carla had lost trust in him and had demanded that he do so.

---

*Recognizable aspects of this case have been changed to preserve confidentiality, and the material is used with the patient's permission.

Initially, Bob stated that he had three issues he wanted help with: (1) how to cope with his alcoholism and live life without alcoholism; (2) how to understand and learn to manage the parts of him he could not face; and (3) how to rebuild his own life, his wife's trust, and his confidence in himself as a total person.

Bob had already begun to attend a few AA meetings, even though he initially felt quite resistant to attending them. He was, however, "amazed and astounded" by how much he related to the people in AA and how encouraged he felt by not being alone with the problem. He was surprised to find "that they were not a bunch of degenerates," but people like him who were trying to figure out how to live life without alcohol or any other substance. As yet, he had no real concept of the Twelve Steps or of the role played by an AA sponsor.

At the end of our first session, Bob and I developed a contract specifying that he would continue to attend at least three AA meetings weekly and that I would meet with him once weekly. I suggested that he also regularly attend a specific type of meeting that focused primarily on the Twelve Steps of AA (referred to as a "step study meeting"). I also requested that his wife join him for our next session. Because Carla had provided the initial impetus for Bob to seek treatment, I felt it was important that she be involved in our sessions.

I liked Bob because he was quite intelligent, displayed an Irish wit, and had a rather poetic grasp of his struggle. However, since he did not start with a 30-day inpatient program, I realized that the psychotherapy itself would have to provide a lot of education about alcoholism and AA. His commitment to AA would probably be more gradual and tenuous than if he had begun his treatment in a 30-day, 24-hour-a-day immersion in a residential or hospital setting. These facts were reflected in his goals. Hence he would have to learn to live his life with alcoholism, not without it. I also realized that he would have to deal with emotional issues very slowly, because they were so frightening to him and his sobriety would have to be quite stable to permit much uncovering. On the basis of the information gathered thus far, it seemed that Bob was duplicating dynamics with his wife that were very much like his mother's nagging relationship with his father. But there were also crucial differences, as his own wife was not alcoholic and openly demanded that Bob enter treatment. In contrast, Bob's mother had generally nagged and provoked his father about most things, but denied any need for him (or herself) to receive treatment.

The negotiation of a workable treatment contract with Bob was relatively easy. This was so because both he and his spouse were high-functioning in many areas and adequately motivated. In addition, Bob's ego functioning was relatively well integrated, and he was psychologically minded. He also had prior initiation into treatment, which helped him articulate his needs in this therapy. The course of Bob's treatment is described in Chapters 6 and 7.

Developing a treatment contract is often much more difficult than it was with Bob. Problem patients will have many relapses in the first phase of treatment, even though they have overtly agreed to attend Twelve-Step meetings and present themselves physically at the meetings. Patients who choose methadone maintenance, naltrexone, or Antabuse as their method of reinforcing abstinence may continue to drink or use drugs problematically. These patients may need a more restrictive method of maintaining abstinence, such as hospitalization or residential treatment. Relapses are an integral part of the addictive process, yet permitting treatment to continue during too many or too frequent relapses puts the therapist in the position of being an enabler who condones substance misuse, which could be dangerous if not lethal. If family members or employers have fiscal or emotional controls over the patient, and they are a part of the treatment process, they can be asked to tighten constraints on the patient. This pressure is utilized to facilitate a return to meaningful therapeutic involvement. At times, the most therapeutic intervention is to ask the patient to leave treatment and return when he/she is more motivated. The therapist may continue to work with sober members of the family after the identified patient has left, as described in the final chapter of this book.

EARLY PSYCHODYNAMIC ISSUES IN TREATMENT

Following the confrontative phase of motivating the patient for treatment, and the negotiations (with help and support as necessary) involved in developing a treatment plan, the therapist shifts to providing support, direct assistance, and information. When the patient is involved with a therapeutic team, manipulative and splitting activity must be kept to a minimum, so that the patient will learn newer and more adaptive ways to get needs met. A split treatment team undoubtedly replicates the patient's divided or disorganized parents. This should not be interpreted at this point; rather, the team should understand the patient's projective identifications and/or splitting, and work together to present a unified approach. The treatment team must be consistent and cohesive, while providing a safe environment that is neither too giving nor too withholding (Khantzian & Schneider, 1986). A psychodynamic understanding of splitting and of how the patient uses this mechanism is very helpful to the team in working together and providing adequate treatment.

If the patient has completed detoxification and is feeling nurtured by the protection of a hospital setting, he/she may be able to make substantial progress toward catharsis of grief from early losses or expression of rage at early sexual, physical, or emotional abuse. These feelings may be facilitated by techniques such as family sculpture, psychodrama, or guided physical expression in the safety of residential settings.

Patients will often report unusual dreams during this phase, in part as a result of the rebound of dreaming sleep, which was suppressed by drugs or alcohol. They often dream of their substance use and related activities. Although the therapist empathizes with the cravings expressed by these dreams, they are often interpreted as part of the mourning process, which is necessary as SAs grieve for drugs, alcohol, substance-abusing peers, and associated behaviors.

A 34-year-old male patient who had been off cocaine for 3 weeks reported the following dream, complicated by hypnapompic and hypnagogic phenomena: "I saw a brownish-colored bird on the ground which looked wilted. Later I saw the same bird elevated in the sky. It was pure white. I felt a pulling sensation which took my breath away. I saw my roommate move and tried to call for help but I couldn't. I stopped breathing and then I felt my heart stop beating. My whole life passed before me." He was able to understand that the bird represented two sides of himself, his "dirty," addict side, and his now "clean," purified, sober aspect. He felt that his near-death experience in the dream was a warning of the consequences of his addiction, as well as a representation of the "spiritual awakening" that often occurs in newly dry addicts who commit to Twelve-Step work. Working with a dream at this level and in a manner that reinforces the commitment to sobriety is an example of appropriate utilization of psychodynamic principles in early treatment.

The early availability of this type of material presents a paradoxical problem, however. Psychodynamic constructs such as dreams, fantasies (particularly during intoxication), primitive transference, and regressive behavior are often readily apparent in newly withdrawing substance-dependent persons; however, their diminished cognition and/or psychosocial immaturity does not permit them to utilize this type of material appropriately. They form intense transferences, with rapid swings from clinging attachment to hostile rejection. These transferences must be interpreted at this phase in such a manner that helps to dissipate rather than to foster them; either the intense dependence or the hostility can drive the patient out of treatment if needs are not met. In general, an evaluation of the psychodynamics of drug use, intoxication, and dependence is helpful at this stage, although the content of the psychodynamic formulation will still be used minimally (Kaufman & Reoux, 1988).

The concept of drugs and alcohol as objects that provide self-soothing in the relative absence of other forms of nurturance in the present or great deprivations in the past can be demarcated in this phase, and is dealt with superficially but empathically here (Dodes & Khantzian, 1991). This concept is worked with more intensively over time, as feelings and fantasies are explored in more depth in later phases of treatment.

Many addicts and alcoholics have a "receptive stimulus barrier" (Krystal & Rankin, 1970), which leads to their being flooded by painful affects when they first become abstinent. This is pointed out in a cognitive-behavioral, educational fashion; the patient is encouraged to recognize each feeling and its antecedents, and to develop behavioral alternatives. The patient may also be flooded by excessively powerful affects, which he/she is helped to identify, differentiate, and verbalize (Dodes & Khantzian, 1991).

The narcissistic vulnerability to helplessness and powerlessness, which has been defended against by activating and/or dampening drugs, can be recognized just after detoxification and pointed out in order to avoid the patient's being overwhelmed by helplessness without having the anodyne of chemicals. When narcissistic SAs feel out of control of their inner (emotional) experience or feel criticized or confronted, they experience narcissistic rage. This rage is defined by an "insistent, compulsive, unrelenting quality" (Dodes & Khantzian, 1991, p. 395), which is unresponsive to reality and which corresponds to and may fuel many aspects of the addictive personality style. This rage needs to be soothed or ameliorated in the early aspects of this phase, or it will drive the newly abstinent addict out of treatment, self-justified that he/she has been wronged again.

ASPECTS AND FUNCTIONS
OF TWELVE-STEP WORK IN PHASE 1

In each of the three phases of psychotherapy with an SA, certain aspects of the Twelve Steps of AA and similar groups are emphasized by the patient and his/her sponsor. If the patient is sober but is not in a Twelve-Step program, then the therapist's work is more difficult, as much of the work that is so well done in such programs will have to be done in the therapy. It is helpful to the psychotherapist to understand which areas his/her patient will be working on in a Twelve-Step group during each phase of psychotherapy.

The key to the initiation of this proposed model of psychotherapy is a successful initial working of the First Step. In AA, this step is as follows: "We admitted we were powerless over alcohol—that our lives had become unmanageable." (The wording is changed as appropriate for other Twelve-Step groups.) This step requires a reduction in denial to the point that the patient is willing to admit that his/her life has become unmanageable as a result of substance use and that he/she cannot control this substance use. Patients may be helped in working this step by making lists of the times they were unable to control their substance use and the consequences of doing so. They may list all relevant drug-and alcohol-related problems (friends, family, job, health, legal consequences) in a way that helps them to be faced with all of the many difficulties their substance use has created. This helps the patient to assume the identity of an SA and to introduce himself/herself at meetings as an alcoholic or addict (Chappel, 1992). Presenting the First Step in detail to a group of peers, as is often done in inpatient settings, greatly facilitates getting beyond the primary denial of being an alcoholic or addict.

Chappel (1992) cites a very relevant AA saying in this context: "For many years I was not an alcoholic, but I was drunk all the time. When I became an alcoholic, I stopped drinking and I haven't had a drink since" (p. 413). Many individuals will seek psychotherapy in order to avoid accepting their powerlessness over drugs and alcohol, even though they are close to their "bottom."* These patients enter therapy in the hope of raising their self-esteem, in order to prevent it from becoming sufficiently low that they would have to face the primary nature of their addiction (Brown, 1985).

At this phase, patients often change meetings or sponsors quite readily, but these contacts often become more important than those with their therapists. This should not be used as a failure to establish an appropriate dependent transference, as these patients require multiple dependences. Twelve-Step meetings, sober peers, and sponsors are much safer, more supportive, and more readily available than dependence on a single therapist can possibly be (Brown, 1985).

The Second Step is also begun in this phase, but is generally not fully worked until years of participation in a Twelve-Step group. This is as follows: "[We] came to believe that a Power greater than ourselves could restore us to sanity." Many patients, particularly atheists

---

*The "bottom" is the level of failure, loss, shame, and humiliation an individual must reach before he/she can accept his/her powerlessness over alcohol or drugs. Some individuals have "high bottoms"; that is, they can be motivated by threat of loss of job or income. Others have "low bottoms"; that is, they must hit skid row before they are motivated.

and agnostics, have difficulty with this step because they have come to believe that the Higher Power can only be experienced as God or a god. It is most unfortunate when patients are so rigid about this idea that they cannot utilize the great potential helpfulness of AA and similar groups. Patients can be helped to see that a belief in God is not necessary, but only "a belief that something greater than and different from self can be of help" (Chappel, 1992, p. 413). The patient is encouraged to choose their own formulation of the shape of this belief. I encourage my patients who resist this concept to choose the power of the Twelve-Step program itself, which has helped more individuals stop using drugs and alcohol than any other program in history, as their Higher Power. The Second Step simply requires that the recovering individual acknowledge, "I cannot deal with this problem myself and need help from whatever it is that keeps me alive."

At times, a patient may have to work on psychodynamic issues of narcissism and entitlement before he/she can accept the common human experience that there is in the world a force greater than ourselves. Following this, the patient may begin to give up the unrealistic self-image that requires him/her to solve every problem alone (Chappel, 1992). The patient is helped to see that even though the Twelve-Step program is a spiritual program, it is not a religion. It is helpful that the patient accept and acknowledge that "something unaccessible to our five senses and different from the person" (Chappel, 1992, p. 415) may help the healing process. Spirituality is also helpful in moving the recovering person from self-centeredness toward a capacity for humility and self-love.

Nevertheless, many therapists and patients will feel that Twelve-Step spirituality has a powerful religious base, and therefore will resist involvement. There are many similarities between Twelve-Step groups and organized religion. These include "a moral and transcendent perspective, an emphasis on repentance, ultimate dependence and a conversion experience (termed a 'spiritual awakening' in AA), scriptures and a creed (The Big Book and the 12 Steps and 12 Traditions), rituals and a communal life" (Peteet, 1993). Other commonalities with religion include charismatic speakers, altruistic doing for others, and limiting close associates to those in the same group. Thus many individuals will rebel against Twelve-Step groups as their view of such groups in a religious context reinforces their resistance based on their atheistic or agnostic beliefs. Others may resist because of uncomfortable childhood experiences with being forced to participate in organized religion or being subjected to rigid, authoritarian religious dogma. The latter reasons, which can be quite heavily laden emotionally, may be more amenable to modification through abreaction of childhood memories than the former, which are fixed, basic ideological/intellectual constructs.

Before abstinence, alcoholics and addicts invest their belief in other dependence objects, such as alcohol, drugs, or their spouses. Yet they deny the powerful unconscious aspects of their psychological dependence, believing that they are self-sufficient and needful of no one. Underlying this denial is an inner introject or selfobject of a very punitive parent who sadistically abused a patient whenever he/she expressed dependent needs. Thus such patients fear dependence on a Higher Power. As this fear gradually resolves, the patients may accept the notion of a Higher Power as they see it (Brown, 1985).

Many patients may also reject the use of the word "sanity" in the Second Step, because "insanity" feels too out of control or involves more acceptance of the unmanageability in their lives than they are willing to admit (Brown, 1985).

Working the Second Step permits the members of a Twelve-Step group to move beyond an ego-centered position in the world. Individuals became more independent through accepting their dependence. They gradually learn (in contrast to many nonalcoholics and nonaddicts) that dependence is not a bad thing.

Twelve-Step work is extremely valuable to the newly sober individual, in that it relieves the painful alienation of the solitary aspects of substance abuse and recovery. It instills hope, provides mutual concern, and furnishes a basis to regain control of one's life. Here, according to the self-psychological view of Khantzian and Mack (1983), self-regulation and self-care become a multiperson phenomenon. Listening to the terrible damage that other SAs have done to their lives will often put patients in touch with the potential serious damage to their own lives. Others, of course, will use these stories as part of their denial: "I'm not that bad, I can't be one of them."

Galanter (1993) emphasizes the emotional well-being experienced by new members as they become involved in Twelve-Step groups. This well-being encourages continued involvement with the program as compliance with operant reinforcement. This positive reinforcement is then given for further participation: Members are given warm and enthusiastic approval when they share, when they receive anniversary chips and birthday cakes to commemorate days and years of sobriety, and when they speak more formally about their histories of addiction and recovery. They are also reinforced when they discuss their avoidance of cues that could lead to slips or relapses. Galanter (1993) attributes the function of Twelve-Step mottos and phrases to their serving as cognitive labels for avoidance of problem behavior, affects, attitudes and situations.

In Phase 1, a Twelve-Step group may function as a valuing, idealizing selfobject that provides almost perfect narcissistic mirroring. On the other hand, this explains, for instance, why newly dry individuals at an AA meeting are devastated when they are told by rigid old-timers they do not belong there because they are primarily drug addicts or because they are taking prescribed drugs (even nonabusable ones). The attachment to a Twelve-Step group provides needed internalization of self-care and self-valuing. Thus aspects of the narcissistic transference are assigned quite naturally to the group. Here again, the therapist should be comfortable with this form of healthy splitting. At this phase of therapy, the patient's sobriety often depends on his/her idealization of the group. Challenging this defense may lead to the loss of sobriety (Dodes & Khantzian, 1991). The fear of losing this idealizing transference to the Twelve-Step group, and consequently sobriety, is one reason why many members of such groups fear psychotherapy. A patient will begin to work more freely in psychotherapy when he/she is reassured by the therapist's knowledge of the Twelve-Step program and respect for all aspects of the program, including the idealized transference.

In the self-psychological view, the individual is helped to recognize and accept his/her powerlessness over alcohol and/or drugs as an impairment in self-governance. In most segments of our society, this admission is an inacceptable defeat; it can only occur with the aid of the moral principles of a closely knit group that unconditionally accepts anyone who admits that he/she only has the desire to stop drinking and using (Khantzian & Mack, 1989). One Twelve-Step saying used to counter resistance in this phase is "Bring the body and the mind/spirit will follow."

When individuals give up the idea that they can drink or use drugs, they suffer a narcissistic injury. As they incorporate this belief over time, they give up their pathological narcissism and replace it with the healthier self-knowledge that they are in charge of themselves. The latter represents a healthy form of narcissism. Some Twelve-Step sayings as reported by Khantzian and Mack (1989, p. 74) help to "puncture" this narcissism: "He suffers from terminal uniqueness," "Leave your ego at the door," and "No one is too dumb to get into the program but there are a lot of people too smart."

Khantzian and Mack (1989) emphasize that accepting a Higher Power helps the recovering individual shift from self-love to object love as the Higher Power becomes a selfobject. As this selfobject is internalized, more authority and structure within the self are provided.

END OF PHASE 1

Phase 1 ends for outpatients after they have been off drugs and alcohol for a week or two, have had the opportunity to put the treatment contract into effect, and have reached agreement with their therapists as to how the contract will be workable at that point in the therapy. Patients who have been in hospital, residential, partial hospital, or intensive outpatient programs (20 hours weekly) generally end Phase 1 when they graduate from these structured programs. This usually involves about 1 month of abstinence from drugs and alcohol.

Phase 2 of Treatment: Early Recovery (Sobriety)

Phase 2 begins after the patient has been detoxified and the treatment contract established. The major initial focus is on methods for maintaining a drug- and alcohol-free state. In the first 6 months to 2 years of psychotherapy, the emphasis is on directive, supportive, and cognitive-behavioral techniques, with more of a focus on safety and control than on uncovering therapies. At this stage, patients require direction and support because they have not yet developed adequate self-care and self-protection to avoid engaging in self-destructive behaviors and/or returning to substance abuse. However, psychodynamic techniques should always be kept in mind and should be further developed as a patient demonstrates unconsciously motivated behavior in transference, acting out, dreams, fantasies, and daily maladaptive activities. Powerful countertransferences continue to be evoked during this phase and require a high level of therapist awareness (see Chapter 8). Knowledge of these unconscious forces is used to help the patients understand self-destructive behavior and the underlying determinants of stressors that render recovering SAs vulnerable, so that the patient can learn to avoid these stressors or deal with them without regression. Successfully enacting these behaviors requires a great deal of practice by the patient and support from the therapist. Some individuals will need to come terms with painful experiences from the past and to achieve catharsis before they can establish secure sobriety. This can be done more safely in residential or hospital settings in the early stages of therapy, or later when a sober core is solidified.

McDuff and Solounias (1992) suggest that early in the patient's hospital stay, the therapist and patient choose a central psychodynamic issue that is integrally related to the loss of control over drugs and alcohol. In working together on this issue, the therapist and patient begin to develop a meaningful therapeutic alliance, which is sustaining in this early phase of treatment. This focus not only helps to keep the patient involved in therapy, but also provides valuable understanding that facilitates sobriety. McDuff and Solounias focus on one of six central issues that they find surfacing repeatedly (although any of the key points described in Chapters 1 and 2 could be similarly developed): negative affective states, traumatic events, character pathology, unresolved grief, developmental arrest, and persistent denial. They have found that a focus on any of these issues enriches the addiction treatment without detracting from sobriety. I would also suggest sexual issues, codependence problems, and psychodynamic aspects of relapse. When a focus on one issue is maintained, substantial resolution can be achieved through the techniques of short-term psychodynamic psychotherapy.

COGNITIVE-BEHAVIORAL STRATEGIES
FOR MAINTAINING SOBRIETY

Maintaining sobriety is still the goal of therapy in early recovery. Interventions to achieve this goal include cognitive and behavioral measures to prevent return to substance abuse. Encouraging drug-free behaviors and presenting opportunities to practice such behaviors help the sober patient to build up a repertoire of coping strategies.

Brownell et al. (1986) describe their relapse prevention approach in phases that bear some resemblance to the ones described in this book. In their stage 1, which they entitle "initial behavior change," they emphasize four areas: (1) decision making, (2) cognitive restructuring, (3) training in coping skills, and (4) cue elimination. These are compatible with the behaviorally based aspects of Phase 2 as I conceive of it. Decision making prepares the individual for analyzing the determinants of relapse. Cognitive restructuring teaches patients to interpret events, attitudes, and feelings in a rational way, and to practice adaptive responses in crisis. Training in coping skills provides the patient with specific strategies to utilize for each stressful situation. I do not personally use cue extinction, but it has much promise in the hands of therapists experienced in these techniques.

Washton (1989) identifies five "essential steps" to abstinence with cocaine abusers, which are helpful with all SAs. These can be paraphrased as follows:

1. Educate about the role of conditioning factors in producing relapse.
2. Identify external cues and internal feelings that trigger drug and/or alcohol cravings. Develop an action plan to avoid them.
3. Establish a support system, daily structure, and alternative rituals as substitutes for substance use and related activities.
4. Develop an action plan for handling urges and cravings.
5. Formulate strategies to prevent early dropout from treatment.

I tell patients a simple story about a former cocaine-addicted patient that illustrates the strong effects of conditioning factors in relapse. He said to me one day, "I understand now. I can't eat pizza pie because it makes me want to drink beer. If I drink beer, I'll use coke."

To apply this relapse theory to a specific case, we can examine the elaboration of a slip* by Jim,† who had a past history of many treatment failures and relapses. His psychotherapy included considerable relapse prevention training so that he was able to understand his cocaine lapse quite well, 48 hours later. He stated with minimal guidance:

1. "I spent three full days painting my old condo, in which I had repeatedly used cocaine."
2. "I had several extended conversations with a recently multiple-relapsing female addict."
3. "I rescued a very disturbed woman I had met at the hospital who was threatening suicide."
4. "One of the men at my recovery home is using crack, and another has asked me to get it for him."
5. "I went to a bar where I had previously bought crack, although with five sober CA members, so I thought it was safe."
6. "When I saw a former dealer there, my mind went on autopilot."
7. "I shut off all my relapse prevention techniques and bought crack."
8. "I then called the woman I mentioned [in 2 above] to help me not use it."

---

*A "slip" refers to a brief use of drugs or alcohol, generally no longer than 24 hours, which is rapidly followed by a return to sobriety and compliance with the treatment contract and/or a comprehensive program. A "relapse" refers to a longer and more destructive episode and includes a return of denial about powerlessness over drugs or alcohol.

†Recognizable aspects of this case history have been changed to preserve confidentiality, and the material is used with the patient's permission.

9. "She came over and we used together. She was the worst choice I could have possibly made."

10. "With the first hit I cried; I became depressed; I knew I couldn't use—yet I continued to use."

Unlike Jim's previous relapses, this slip was followed by sobriety, which has lasted for almost a year at this writing.

The relapse chain is often much more complicated than the simple "pizza leads to beer, which leads to cocaine," or even the more detailed sequence involved in the case of Jim. As described by Washton (1989), the relapse chain (which, although most readily applicable to cocaine, can occur with any abusable drug or alcohol) follows a scenario such as this:

1. There is a buildup of stress caused by positive or negative changes and life events (e.g., promotion, childbirth, IRS audit, threat of probation violation, alimony payments from prior marriages, divorce, spouse away for a weekend, therapist on vacation).

2. The stress activates excessively negative or positive thoughts, moods, and feelings.

3. Inability to tolerate these thoughts, moods, and feelings leads to confusion, bewilderment, irritability, depression, dissociation, or hypomanic elation (this affect intolerance has been well described by many of the psychodynamic theorists cited in Chapter 1).

4. Failure to act, or impulsive and excessive reaction, leads to a paralysis of withdrawal response and to perpetuation and escalation of the problem.

5. The individual denies the seriousness of the problem, and fails to utilize tools of recovery or using them inappropriately or in a "sham" way.

6. The person withdraws partially or totally from attendance at or active participation in meetings and therapy.

7. The problem escalates further, with maladaptive solutions worsening the problem (e.g., substituting alcohol or amphetamines for cocaine, compulsive sexuality, borrowing money).

8. The person experiences helplessness and inability to cope.

9. Drug preoccupations and cravings increase, as drugs appear to be the only solution that at this point will provide relief.

10. The person experiences increased isolation and alienation from support systems, as well as frustration, despair, hopelessness, and obsessive preoccupation with substance abuse.

11. Cravings become irresistible, and one or more substances are used. The relapse chain is completed.

This chain can be reversed by a sober peer group and/or a therapist with whom there is an excellent therapeutic alliance—quite readily at points 1–6, and with difficulty at 7–9. By point 10, hospitalization or another type of residential treatment setting may be necessary to avoid a relapse. The psychological craving for cocaine in particular is so powerful and so easily triggered by minimal stimuli that at times the craving alone appears to trigger a relapse. Generally, a careful look will reveal other factors.

AA and similar groups teach that people, places, and things associated with substance use can trigger relapse. Group members are taught to tune into and recognize those painful feelings that lead to cravings, and how these feelings develop (generally from exposure to people, places, and things). One of the strongest cues is an exposure to the actual preferred substance of abuse. Patients are encouraged to go on a "search and destroy" mission with a sponsor, trusted friend, or relative for that last bit of alcohol or drug in their car, clothing, home, or other favorite spot. A burning or flushing ritual helps to consolidate the giving-up process.

As mentioned briefly in connection with the development of a therapeutic contract (see Chapter 5), the most difficult cues to give up involve the network of drug- and alcohol-using friends and relatives. Most individuals who are successfully sober have given up all of their former drug- and alcohol-using friends, unless these friends too have become sober. The best way to do this is to develop an entire new network of relationships with sober associates. On the other hand, some recovering individuals are better able to balance recovering and nonrecovering friendships. Parents and spouses are often the most painful cues to substance abuse, and many patients require a great deal of individual and/or family psychotherapy in order to visit or live with family members. Family members who are active SAs themselves are highly problematic, and every effort should be made to have them develop a workable treatment contract involving their own abstinence (or, at the very least, their not drinking or using in the presence of the identified patient).

Places and settings (e.g., bars, restaurants, discos, parties, spectator sports, and fishing and hunting trips) that were previously an integral part of substance abuse are powerful triggers to be avoided. AA and other Twelve-Step groups tell the newly sober members to stay away from "slippery places" in order to avoid "slipping," or "falling." A new environment that does not contain all the old cues to substance use can provide a sense of safety, particularly if the anxiety about the newness of it can be overcome (Brown, 1985).

Many patients will be vulnerable to using drugs if they come near certain geographical areas where they purchased drugs. In big cities these may be certain street corners; in southern California, such an area may be an entire small city like Downey or Santa Ana. Some work settings are very strong relapse triggers. One patient of mine who was a car sales supervisor smoked marijuana at work, as did all of his employees. Another car salesman sold most of his cars to cocaine dealers, who often negotiated coke as part of the payment. Relapse prevention in individuals such as these should include a job change or substantial reconstitution of the work environment.

As noted above, feelings that are triggers for drug and alcohol use are generally produced by associated people, places, or things. Boredom, a common emotional trigger, is overtly more related to the absence of these three. But often individuals experience boredom when they feel helpless in coping with people, places, or things. Drugs and alcohol are tempting because they rapidly replace the painful void of boredom with euphoria or relieve the underlying anxiety and helplessness.

Cocaine is often used to treat depression or obliterate anxiety. It rapidly turns passivity into activity, impotence into polymorphous perversity, or mania into ecstasy. As Washton (1989) reminds us, "the desire for cocaine can be triggered just as easily (if not more so) by positive as well as negative moods" (p. 100). Cocaine is often so closely associated with sexual excitement that any sexual arousal may lead to the desire to use cocaine, particularly if the sex is at all out of the ordinary or perverse. Cravings for other drugs are also linked to sexual performance and excitement but not as powerfully as is cocaine. Desires for cocaine may be provoked by the positive emotions of others such as love (which may evoke underlying fear of intimacy), tenderness (which may bring out fears of vulnerability), or closeness (which may evoke fears of being engulfed or swallowed up). Cocaine does not just work by causing euphoria; it may cause a mental numbing that leads to an obliteration of concern with difficulties.

Patients can be asked to share lists of potential triggers in individual therapy, group therapy, or relapse prevention training. Peer contributions can be quite useful in helping each group member determine sensitive areas that he/she should avoid. Patients can be coached about effective ways to say "no" to triggers or to substances themselves in group or individual therapy, and these can be rehearsed and supported.

McAuliffe and Albert (1992) have divided triggers into three types: (1) those that should be avoided permanently from the beginning, (2) those that cannot be avoided, and (3) those that should be avoided early but must be dealt with eventually if an SA is to achieve full recovery. Type 1 triggers include active users, drug dealers, bars, and "shooting galleries." Type 2 triggers include losses, deaths, need for pain medication for surgery, as well as feelings such as stress, depression, and anger. Type 3 triggers include sex, intimate relationships, life cycle changes (e.g., childbirth), and major decisions (e.g., changing to a more demanding job—many SAs will require *less* stressful jobs, but employment is an important aspect of recovery). Each of these types of triggers is dealt with in the appropriate phase of therapy as described in this book. Thus, therapy in Phase 2 focuses on understanding and expressing feelings while continuing an emphasis on staying away from Type 1 triggers. Patients are advised to avoid Type 3 triggers until they have developed adequate coping skills in Phase 3. Thus in Phase 2 they are asked to postpone sexual relationships, intimacy, marriage, geographical moves, or major job changes until they have at least a year of sobriety and/or therapy. This resembles Freud's (1920) admonition against major life changes during the psychoanalytic process, but it may be even more necessary here.

Washton (1989) suggests several factors that are helpful in establishing a basic non-substance-abusing routine to replace daily preoccupation with cocaine or other drugs. He emphasizes, as have a colleague and I (Kaufman & Reoux, 1988), the importance of a comprehensive program, since substance dependence affects the lives of our patients so pervasively.

Washton (1989) sets a week of abstinence from cocaine as an obtainable goal. He emphasizes the importance during this week of frequent individual counseling sessions, which stress how to get safely through the 24 hours until the next day's therapy sessions. A fully planned and structured schedule is developed for each day of the week, including (and particularly) the weekend. Other external controls include having frequent urine tests, placing income and other financial assets under the control of a neutral third party, and obtaining a commitment to be hospitalized should a relapse occur.

Patients are encouraged to begin to weave their new network of support with their peers in group therapy and Twelve-Step meetings. In both situations, patients are free to contact one another and are encouraged to provide lists of names and phone numbers of sober peers who are readily available. Premature dropout is avoided by presenting realistic expectations about the pain of early sobriety. Patients are warned about "honeymoon" feelings of cure during early abstinence; these may occur as a result of positive physiological rebound or of a spiritual awakening related to acceptance of a Higher Power or other aspects of spirituality.

Washton (1989) also emphasizes teaching patients behavioral alternatives to deal with cravings. These include leaving the situation, getting involved in diverting activities, talking to one's sponsor or a fellow group member, increasing attendance at Twelve-Step meetings, focusing on the negative effects of alcohol or drugs, and detaching from the urge as if one were an outside observer.

Slips are often features of early abstinence. The therapist should accept slips as part of the disease of substance abuse, although without becoming an enabler who encourages patients while they slide into progressive deterioration as a result of their substance abuse. Each therapist should decide on how many and how severe slips he/she can tolerate before termination is necessary. Within these personal limits, slips should be viewed nonpunitively; they can be used as opportunities to help patients understand psychosocial stressors and the ways in which these may lead to substance abuse.

THE ROLE OF THE THERAPIST IN PHASE 2

Krystal (1978) has proposed a preparatory stage of psychotherapy much like the early recovery phase described here, in which the patient's affects are labeled and explained with the goal of increasing ego function. The use of affects as signals and the ability to tolerate painful affects is also taught. McDougal (cited in Dodes & Khantzian, 1991) has described the importance of a consistent holding environment that may last for years before patients can understand and appropriately express emotion. Even the most psychoanalytic therapist is called upon in this phase to work more directively in order to teach affect recognition and tolerance.

As Phase 2 progresses, a patient begins to shift from externalized behavioral controls to internalization. The patient learns to recognize anxiety or other internal discomfort; then, rather than acting out these feelings, he/she learns to reflect on them. At first patients may automatically utilize AA or other Twelve-Step cognitive slogans ("Put a plug in the jug," "Avoid being hungry, angry, lonely, or tired [HALT]," "You're only two dimes away from help," etc.). Later they use more critical self-examination, individualized insights, and more sophisticated coping devices to achieve behavioral control (Brown, 1985).

The therapist first supports the patient's reaching out to multiple objects of dependence and this dependence is not analyzed until sobriety is secure. The therapist initially often works through the patient's transferences to others rather than through those to the therapist. Very often, the transferences employed are those to the patient's sponsor, who is often viewed as either a godly savior or a terrible tyrant.

Brown (1985) emphasizes the importance of an individual's attaining a sober core identity as an alcoholic/addict if any uncovering therapy is to occur. Her concept is that the stronger the core, the further the individual can cycle beyond it; yet he/she may have to return to it again and again. Brown describes the functions of this core of sobriety as providing relief, a sense of control, a period of consolidation, and a strengthening of identity.

Replacing maladaptive and dysfunctional activities with behavior that maintains sobriety is a treatment goal of early recovery. Less destructive substitute objects and behaviors of all kinds are helpful and should not be confronted. Cigarette smoking was addressed much later in sobriety until the late 1980s, when there was a movement in the field toward encouraging or requiring early cessation, because smoking is a strong paired stimulus for the use of alcohol and other drugs. The use of medications such as Nicoderm, Nicorette, or clonidine can facilitate nicotine abstinence. Presently, I suggest that patients consider a program to stop smoking as part of their abstinence. I do not require it, however, because as I am sensitive to the need for some patients to maintain their nicotine dependence, lest their cravings and irritability lead them back to drugs or alcohol. The therapist may encourage active alternatives, such as regular exercise, recreation, or education; these not only minimize loss, but support the concept of a healthier total life adaptation. Object substitution may also prevent, or at least lessen, the grieving that SAs sometimes experience while mourning the loss of the substance of abuse itself, as well as associated activities and relationships.

In the concept of treatment I propose, psychotherapy during early recovery should not confront defenses too rapidly and should not prematurely remove them. These defenses are instead redirected and supported to help maintain abstinence and continued treatment. If long-term sobriety is to be maintained, defenses must ultimately be removed, but only gradually—over periods of time often ranging from 2 to 5 years of abstinence (Wallace, 1985b). Prematurely reducing or removing preferred and effective means of coping with anxiety can result in relapse of substance abuse or in patients' terminating therapy. Confronting and interpreting defenses, as well as having the patients own more responsibility, come later in successful psychotherapy of SAs (Kaufman & Reoux, 1988). In other words, therapeutic interventions that are appropriate later may be inappropriate during early sobriety.

Phase 2 also requires a dual shift for the average therapist—namely, from confronter of denial to motivator and supporter, and from nondirective listener to active teacher of new strategies and coping behaviors (Brown, 1985). The ability to adapt to an active, directive stance is necessary for the psychodynamic therapist who wishes to include SAs in his/her practice, particularly SAs who do not already have a sober core.

Treatment of intrapsychic conflicts and forces with dynamic approaches can be used to reinforce the principles of AA or other Twelve-Step groups. For example, unresolved conflicts over issues such as omnipotence, narcissistic entitlement, power, control, or dependence conflicts may prevent a patient from obtaining a sponsor and/or using a Twelve-Step group fully. Psychodynamic therapy of such conflicts may help the patient to accept the principles and practices of a Twelve-Step program more readily.

Paradoxically, the need for grandiosity can be met by "surrendering" to a group such as AA. This need is sublimated through the helping of other SAs. The group or fellowship itself can become the Higher Power, and the patient shares in this power. A Twelve-Step group provides a forum for demonstrating verbally and behaviorally the personal power and control that can be achieved through its principles. Unresolved dependence needs can also be met through meetings and sponsors, as well as the program's 24-hour-a-day availability. By becoming a sponsor oneself, the advanced member of a Twelve-Step group enhances self-esteem and reduces anxiety through helping others, using the more mature defense of altruism (Kaufman & Reoux, 1988). A Twelve-Step saying that illustrates this is "You can't keep it if you don't give it away."

Although a powerful therapeutic alliance may begin in Phase 1 of the treatment as the patient begins to trust the therapist who has helped him/her get sober, the concept of the alliance has more validity here in Phase 2. Many of the therapist's feelings and attitudes that are conducive to a workable therapeutic alliance are described in the discussion of countertransference in Chapter 8. However, the therapeutic alliance is a separate entity. As I utilize it, it consists of the patient's underlying trust of the therapist's humanity and concern. This trust overrides the patient's powerful transferences and permits them to be analyzed and understood. Thus, no matter how angry, hurt, or wounded he/she feels, the therapeutic alliance permits the patient to maintain the underlying basic belief that the therapist is working in his/her best interest. Thus the patient is willing to work toward self-understanding rather than blaming the therapist or abandoning therapy.

It is critical that the therapist have a basic belief that drug- and alcohol-dependent patients can benefit from psychotherapy. The therapist must also feel comfortable with addicts and alcoholics if a therapeutic alliance is to occur (Forrest, 1982). The therapeutic alliance will be aided still further if the therapist has a liking for addicted and alcoholic patients. Often the therapist's comfort with a personal, workable, integrated method of therapy is necessary before he/she can develop a belief, in the likability of these patients and comfort with them. On the other hand, the therapist who likes these patients innately (and many do not) will be more likely to seek out methods of psychotherapy that work well with addicted/alcoholic patients.

The therapeutic alliance develops and deepens as a result of mutual trust, respect, and concern. The therapist must understand the SA's deep, powerful anxiety about annihilation in close relationships, and then, particularly through nonverbal responses, must gradually reassure the patient that this will not happen in the therapy. The exploration and interpretation of this anxiety are begun here, but it will not be resolved with the therapist and significant others until Phase 3. Yet the anxiety should be alleviated through support, interpretation, and modified therapist distance, so that the patient feels some comfort with his/her interpersonal anxiety with the therapist.

Forrest (1982) emphasizes the importance of the therapist's genuine warmth, and empathy in developing a therapeutic alliance. Forrest states that these qualities are developed by the therapist's ability to (1) offer unconditional acceptance, (2) be affectively and cognitively attuned to the patient's feelings, (3) communicate this attunement to the patient, and (4) be a real person who is present and able to express his/her own feelings about what is going on. The therapist communicates a sense of dignity, respect, and worth to the patient, which helps rebuild the patient's self-esteem as well as develop the therapeutic alliance. At the same time, the therapist should care enough to confront the patient consistently and rationally about whatever self-damaging and therapy-destructive behaviors he/she continues to exhibit.

Brown (1985) presents an approach to the treatment of alcoholics that integrates psychotherapy with AA. Using a developmental perspective, she likens the period of early sobriety to infancy and states that it is characterized by extreme dependence and a corresponding need and reliance on external structure and support. Transference manifestations of intolerable anxiety about feelings of dependence are easily misinterpreted as resistance. Defenses against this anxiety should not be confronted as resistance, but supported as allowing the patient to continue in treatment. The conflicts about dependence that threaten to end treatment prematurely should be addressed directly.

Khantzian and Mack (1983) emphasize early developmental impairments in the ego structure of SAs. Substances are used to mute or contain threatening and potentially overwhelming effects. Thus in early recovery the therapist should provide a secure environment—one that places a premium on safety and adequate control of such affects as depression, rage, anger, and anxiety. Proper, enforceable limits are necessary; without them, the violent tendencies of antisocial patients or the manipulations of all addicts/alcoholics can make treatment impossible. It is only in a cohesive, unified treatment program that these patients can feel safe in dealing with their anger and adequately nurtured, so that they can experience and "verbalize painful affects such as depression, shame, loneliness, hurt and fear" (Khantzian & Schneider, 1986, p. 329).

Khantzian and Mack (1989) state that external sources of narcissistic sustenance are gradually transferred into intrapsychic resources. The therapist can initially meet some of this need while taking care to avoid indiscriminate overgratification. Extremes of being too withholding or too giving are avoided. Narcissistic needs are met to help improve the patient's sense of self-esteem and self-stability. The therapist provides care and security until patients can obtain these on their own — at first through identification with the therapist, as well as with their sponsors and other members of Twelve-Step groups.

Patients' self-preservative skills result from internalization of program rules and development of an "observing ego." As patients internalize these rules, they begin by thinking about them before, during, and after their destructive behaviors. As each behavior is met with caring imposition of limits and consequences for transgressions, new, more adaptive skills develop (Khantzian & Schneider, 1986).

CASE VIGNETTE: BOB'S EARLY RECOVERY

For a time, Bob (the patient described in Chapter 5) continued to attend three AA meetings weekly, according to the terms of our initial contract. Carla, his wife, came to his third session because she had reportedly been too angry at him to come the week before. She still did not trust him and felt that he was emotionally withdrawn. She demonstrated little overt anger in our meeting and was supportive of his AA program. She stated that since Bob started AA, he was more flexible and tolerant. But she continued to have trouble trusting him and was still checking up on him to see whether he was drinking.

Carla was angry at Bob for not taking more of a role with the children (their 4-year-old son and her two children by a previous marriage), yet she tended to exclude him from parenting. I suggested that she attend Al-Anon, but she was quite resistant, although she did not share this in the joint session. According to an earlier report by Bob, she felt that the problem was entirely his and that he was the one to be "fixed."

In the following individual sessions, Bob began to deal with several themes. One was his feeling of guilt, its basis in his religious and familial roots, and his need to be punished for his transgressions (particularly those relating to alcohol). Another theme was his resistance to choosing and working with an AA sponsor. This was explored from several bases, including his relationship with his father and his own projected perfectionism. Bob felt that his sponsor, when he selected one, should be his father's age. He stated, "My father put everything in one basket, so the basket always broke. He disappointed me so much, yet I wanted to be like him." Thus his ambivalence about his father presented another difficulty in his obtaining a sponsor.

One of Bob's major fears was that a sponsor would be so demanding that he would lose his job because of the time spent with the sponsor as well as in other AA activities. Bob related this fear to his need to be perfectionistic with himself and his expectation that others would be as hard on him as he was on himself: "A sponsor might require me to do so much it would stop me from the perfection I need in every other aspect of my life."

He also saw how his fears of a sponsor applied to his difficulties in achieving close relationships with men in general: "To have close friends feels intimidating. I would have to open up. They wouldn't like me if I bared my soul. Yet I feel more comfortable now in thinking about making friends in the future."

Bob could see that the moral inventory of AA's Fourth and Tenth steps would be helpful to him in taking stock of who he was, and would help alleviate the guilty feelings about himself that made him push everyone away before they could reject him for his perceived immorality. However, he saw dealing with these feelings as yet another source of his fear of a relationship with a sponsor.

Here we see how Bob's inability to obtain a sponsor was related to psychodynamic themes of control, obsessional perfectionism, projection, ambivalence, fear of father and authorities, and fear of fusion with a father/twin.

Ten weeks into his psychotherapy, Bob began to recall that while growing up he had indeed seen his mother intoxicated several times. He was becoming more "comfortable and tolerant of the concept of someone being an alcoholic and realizing that a lot of good people are alcoholics." His layers of denial about his own and his family's alcoholism and their related behaviors began to peel away.

As he began to look at the members of his family more clearly, he became more in touch with the distance between them all, and even with his sadness about this: "I'm comfortable being 6,000 miles away from my parents. I'm not comfortable with my parents."

He and his twin were overtly separated. "We're like chalk and cheese. We look the same but we're fundamentally different. We had totally separate friends. I'm 2 minutes younger, but I had all of the responsibilities of being the oldest. I was a year ahead of him in school. I went to the university and he became a plumber." (Yet they had announced their weddings on the same weekend.) The distance Bob felt both from his family of origin and from the children of his first marriage, and his guilt about his absence in each case, were apparent.

He began to look at his sadness about all of his losses, as well as his own role in his difficulties. For the first time, he was experiencing his grief and his own responsibility for these losses without drinking his feelings away. He began to achieve a new kind of closeness with his present wife and family. His stepdaughter asked to be allowed to use his last name, which "had a powerful effect on me. It gave me a warm feeling. Yet it bothers me that this family is the only one I ever miss."

I supported Bob in experiencing these warm feelings. However, I felt that he was not yet ready to deal with the grief over the loss of his family of origin and first nuclear family. His underlying and deep ambivalence toward his mother, father, sisters, twin brother, first wife, and first two children was not tapped at this time. My plan at that time was that these feelings might be better resolved in the transference later, or perhaps that Bob would come to terms with them through the steps of AA, particularly through taking his personal inventory and making amends.

After the session that focused on dealing with Bob's feelings for his family, he returned to Europe on business and visited his family of origin in Ireland. While there, he participated in his family's conspiracy of silence. Upon his return from his trip, Bob lost some of his commitment to AA. He was experiencing more guilt and was losing ground in his struggle to project his difficulties onto the disease of alcoholism and accept the disease concept. He was denying his progress toward taking an honest moral inventory, and felt that he was "sugar-coating" his problems with the rest of the world just as he had done with his family.

I told Bob that his denial of his alcoholism was attributed to his emotional isolation rekindled by his contact with his family, where all feelings were powerfully denied (or dissolved in alcohol). He felt supported by this comment and replied, "I've been looking away from the absolute that I'm an alcoholic and I need help. I've been trying to take six of the Twelve-Steps all at once. You've refocused me. It's not my job to take on more and more. It is my job to work the steps so I can be in a position to make more of my life." I ended the session by pointing out that it was becoming easier for him to understand how and why he resisted AA.

Bob then eliminated some of his business pressures, sought reassurance in his list of phone numbers of AA members, and felt his "sanity" return. He realized that he was not feeling part of his family out of his own choice. He also became aware that his tensions on the job were related to his need to control people and events, which led to his inability to delegate tasks and responsibilities.

I positively reframed the experience by saying that he had done great relapse prevention for himself and that these were tactics he could use again and again. I outlined for him what he had accomplished:

1. He recognized the problem and its underlying themes.
2. He was aware of his desire to drink as a way of coping.
3. He used a symbolic extension of AA as a talisman to ward off anxiety.
4. As the anxiety began to diminish, he then resolved or lessened the impact of the stressors.
5. Lastly, he used the experience in order to learn about living life more deeply and working AA more fully.

We developed these issues in depth throughout the session, and he ended with a great deal of relief: "I feel better about the last few weeks now. I see it more positively."

This session is a good example of the educational, cognitive-behavioral approach at this level of therapy. Still, the psychodynamic issue of giving up control continued to be explored.

In subsequent sessions in what was now the fourth month of therapy, we continued to work on his need to be in control and how it led to his resistance to AA and psychotherapy. Bob spoke of the anxiety he experienced when he had no preplanned topic for a session, because this left him feeling out of control and afraid of spontaneity. "I'm trying to control the whole process. I'm not willing to say who I am; then even I will reject me. To go all the way to self-understanding is very frightening."

Shortly after this session, Bob's parents traveled from Ireland to visit him. His first response to their visit was guilt about his taking his problems out on them for their role in his past. I supported him about learning to understand his past without laying blame and dwelling on it, yet expressing the painful feelings arising from childhood. When we were thus able to sidestep his guilt, he began to speak of his issues with his parents.

He spoke of his desire to talk with his father but avoid his mother.

"She'd be so accusatory. Her 'How could you's' about my becoming an alcoholic." I asked whether he felt that his mother would prevent him from speaking with his father. He replied, "No. I despised him for his drinking. If I say we're both alcoholics it generates a lot of emotions. Then I'll despise myself and feel guilty for having despised him. I'd be confronting that and him. I blame him for his drinking. He was so weak. Yet I feel ashamed of how I treated him through my judging. Now that I've had the same personal experience, I can empathize with my father. I know what a blow it would be for him for me to be critical since he's had enough suffering already."

I suggested that he bring his parents to a session while they were here in order to deal with these difficult issues in a neutral environment. His immediate response was "No." Then, "I don't want to violate the general conspiracy of silence. I'm their son. I want to seem successful." I encouraged him further by replying, "The time is right to talk to your father." He responded, "If only I could lose my sense of wanting to control everything. If I opened up he'd be hard on me."

He ended the session by saying, "I feel good about talking about my guilt—more at peace. Yet my inner voice tells me to protect myself, even from you." He continued to be quite ambivalent about becoming dependent on me, and to back away from the dependence and distance himself from me when he felt it.

In the following session, Bob reported that Carla was getting quite angry with his father and mother because of their selfishness and denial. After this session, Bob was able to tell his parents about his recovery and psychotherapy. His mother asked to meet me, but Bob refused at first. His mother repeated to him that she was not herself an alcoholic. He feared that if he brought his parents to a session he would have to be brutally honest in confronting them, as he felt Carla was urging him to do. He was dealing with his parents by shutting down and isolating himself from Carla, and the children, and felt confronted by her about this. Yet he expected praise from Carla because he had finally told his parents about his alcoholism. He felt relieved when I identified this sequence, and further relief when I supported his level of honesty and openness as appropriate for his present level of sobriety and psychotherapy. I also supportively said, "You're becoming progressively more honest, but you can't expect that your parents will too." Patients like Bob require a great deal of support and encouragement as they gradually give up their defense of intellectualization and begin to recognize and express feelings. Since initial efforts to let out feelings may be condemned by significant others who are surprised and reactive to these expressions, it is particularly important that the therapist be supportive.

Both of Bob's parents attended the next session. His father began by saying, "I am an alcoholic. I'm some way to blame." I explained about genetics and the uselessness of blaming self or others. Bob's mother responded with a predictably powerful statement: "I thought Bob would never drink because he saw his father drink. He drinks because he's unhappy—because he's stressed out from his materialism." Bob ignored his mother's anger and spoke to his parents about what he was obtaining from AA. He stated that he was learning about new perspectives and coping strategies, and experiencing the safety of being with other alcoholics. He explained that he was also learning to give up his need to be in control and beginning to face his emotions. His mother responded by saying that Bob had better control of his anger now, and that if AA and psychotherapy were helping, she was all for them. In the session, the family shared a myth: that Bob looked like his father and acted like his mother, while his twin was the opposite and very laid back. I was struck by how much Bob did look and speak like his father, and how torn he was between the two identifications.

He cut down on AA meetings after his parents' visit. He was confronted with his resisting positive, necessary involvement in AA; he replied, "I don't want a sponsor. I don't want to have a friend." I interjected, "You say that because you desperately want one and are afraid to have one." He responded to this by talking about his fears of opening up and being rejected for it. "If they knew me, they wouldn't like me. I don't want to be tied into the lives of others. I recently changed AA meetings. As long as I don't have a sponsor, I can stand at the door of AA and not come into the room."

When Bob returned, he stated that our last session had removed his blocks about AA and he was again feeling rejuvenated by AA; yet he was still hesitant to being open and honest in any aspect of his life. I responded by saying that it would take more effort and practice to do this, as well as further exploration of his fears.

Bob reported that things had settled down at home, as he was letting Carla know about his likes and needs and getting positive feedback for it. He had also shared at an AA meeting and gotten supportive feedback, which he felt, however, was too patronizing. At the same time, he was becoming willing to reveal his lack of perfection to his boss. As he was becoming more open about his needs with Carla, he was still finding it difficult to express his anger with her. I interpreted that anger was particularly difficult for him to express, because he felt that all anger was like that of his "barking, harsh, critical" mother; hesitating to express anger as she did, he held back all anger. I stated that he was also intimidated by Carla in the same way he was by his mother. I supported Bob for taking these steps toward getting in touch with and expressing his feelings directly to his wife, boss, and AA peers, particularly since this was never done in his family of origin.

ASPECTS AND FUNCTIONS OF TWELVE-STEP WORK IN PHASE 2

During the second phase of therapy, patients who participate in AA or similar groups will work all of the Twelve Steps, but with an emphasis on the Third and Ninth Steps. The First and Second Steps are still continued on a daily basis, because of the need for continued acceptance of powerlessness over alcohol or drugs and the concept of a Higher Power. The Third Step is the most difficult and anxiety-provoking for most new group members, but much more so for those who have resisted a spiritual/religious aspect in their lives: "[We] made a decision to turn our will and our lives over to the care of God as we understood Him." This step requires a conscious surrender of one's will and life to the Higher Power. Even though the phrase is "God as we understood Him," most newly abstinent individuals who are atheists or agnostics powerfully resist this step. Even those who believe in God fight the idea that they do not have control over their own lives. The Twelve Steps help them to realize that even when they desire to let go, they cannot will it. Letting go can result from surrender of the "primitive fantasy that God is humanly parental and primitive" (Chappel, 1992, p. 413). This loss of control is similar to that experienced in meditation, in which the mind is open and cleared until inner control is ultimately achieved. Patients who have difficulty with this process are advised to trust their close colleagues and their sponsors for guidance until they begin to experience this healthy inner control (Chappel, 1992).

The Fourth and Fifth Steps are the cornerstones of Phase 2 of recovery and are most helpful to psychotherapy. The Fourth Step is as follows: "[We] made a searching and fearless moral inventory of ourselves." Chappel (1992) agrees that recovering SAs who have worked the Fourth Step are more comfortable with and responsive to psychotherapy than are those who have not. He also feels that this step enhances the development of an observing ego. Brown (1985) suggests that individuals should list their assets as well as their liabilities, so that they are not overly focused on the negative. The Fourth Step begins the ongoing process of psychotherapy of oneself, which is an important aspect of Twelve-Step work. This step teaches our patients about how to look at themselves honestly, and encourages recognition of strengths and character depth (Brown, 1985). In performing the Fourth Step, SAs come to recognize the degree of their denial and the types of defenses they use to maintain self-deception. Many individuals will experience hope and release after doing this step (Brown, 1985). Many describe a tremendous cathartic relief. Few are discouraged; many feel a mixture of good and bad feelings, as well as surprise that it was not as bad as they had suspected it would be.

The Fifth Step is this: "[We] admitted to God, to ourselves and to another human being the exact nature of our wrongs." The human being to whom the wrongs determined in the Fourth Step are presented is usually the patient's sponsor. However, some individuals will choose to work the Fifth Step with their therapists and this is certainly an appropriate utilization of psychotherapy. It is essential and most reassuring that whoever hears the moral inventory respond in a manner that is accepting and noncritical. Often, the person presenting the inventory feels a great deal of fear that he/she will be responded to in a punitive manner. This is based on a lifetime of projectioning of punitive selfobjects and/or living under the control of a harsh superego. When the SA's worst behaviors are shared with another human being who is accepting, the SA generally experiences tremendous relief. Performing this step helps the patient find great support in his/her former social network, so that he/she can return to it as it becomes safer to do so. I have not found that patients use the Fifth Step for catharsis of material that they then keep away from their therapy. If anything, it helps them recall and shape material that they have denied, withheld, or repressed and have not shared previously.

The Sixth Step—"[We] were entirely ready to have God remove all these defects of character"—omits (as does the Fifth Step) the "as we understood Him" qualifier after "God," but this is still implied. The purpose of this step is a readiness for further change. However, here the problems to be changed are characterological; as all therapists know, these types of problems shift only very gradually. This readiness to change carries over from the Twelve-Step work to the psychotherapy, particularly when both therapist and patient have characterological change as a major goal (Chappel, 1992). The major attitude achieved in working the Sixth Step is a readiness for the development of openness and willingness (Brown, 1985). Yet the Sixth Step emphasizes the partnership among the group member, his/her Higher Power, and the therapist. The patient is aware that he/she must be ready if change is to occur. An appropriate Twelve-Step saying here is "Do the groundwork and turn the results over to God."

The Seventh Step, "[We] humbly asked Him to remove our shortcomings," directly follows the Sixth Step and continues to develop the concept of surrender. The humility in this step is applied to acknowledging the difficulty in change, yet wishing for change in regard to relinquishing adverse characterological traits. As this step is worked successfully, behaviors such as selfishness, blaming, and narcissistic indifference may change.

The Eighth and Ninth Steps also form a natural pairing. The Eighth is "[We] made a list of all persons we had harmed and became willing to make amends to them all," and the Ninth is "[We] made direct amends to such people wherever possible except when to do so would injure them or others." Becoming willing to make amends moves a person past resentment and blaming to a point of being mentally prepared to act. As part of the Eighth Step, the individual develops a capacity for empathy, which is used to reduce the likelihood that his/her behavior will hurt others (Chappel, 1992). This step develops relational skills that help the patient participate more fully in psychotherapy. As with the earlier steps, there is a progression from acknowledgment of wrongs and a change in attitude to action. In working the Eighth Step, the individual lowers denial, recognizes the harm done in the past, and assumes responsibility for the damage done to others. As this list evolves, there is a great release from guilt. The acknowledgment of these truths helps the individual to move forward in his/her psychotherapy and life program (Brown, 1985).

In the Ninth Step, the person moves from admitting and accepting responsibility for past wrongs to performing restitution where possible and in ways that do no harm. It is the doing, the action that is critical; it demonstrates that the individual is "walking the walk and not just talking the talk" (Twelve-Step saying). Not just acknowledgment and apology, but also correction and undoing, are involved (Brown, 1985). The individual assesses when an open acknowledgment would or would not be harmful and acts accordingly. Often in working this step, Twelve-Step group members will repay old financial debts (including those to therapists). This is of course appropriate, but it may be too easy. Thus individuals are encouraged to work at paying off emotional debts as well as monetary ones.

An example of harming another person through making amends is a former spouse's revealing a multitude of affairs. An example of making powerful emotional amends is making whatever reparations are possible to a child whom the SA has molested and has never admitted molesting, though the child may have repeatedly accused the SA of sexual abuse.

The basis for working the Ninth Step is the foundation created by the first eight. SAs cannot be truly sorry and humble if underneath their apologies they are still waiting for eventual victory or if they continue to harbor contempt for their victims. In working this step, a goal is that rigorous self-examination and making amends will vindicate a patient rather than expose him/her. This step diminishes the patient's use of projection onto others and helps him/her accept responsibility for many past and present aspects of his/her life. This, in turn, facilitates insight in psychotherapy, as well as the ability to make meaningful behavioral changes.

C H A P T E R 7

Phase 3 of Treatment: Advanced Recovery (Intimacy and Autonomy)

Advanced recovery usually involves more traditional, in-depth psychotherapy that has shifted from supportive and cognitive-behavioral techniques to personality reconstruction. The major objective in Phase 3 of treatment is to help the recovering individual achieve intimate relationships, yet function in an independent manner. As long as there is a continuing emphasis on maintaining a sober core, any method of uncovering psychotherapy may be used at this time: psychodynamic, psychoanalytic, reconstructive, intersubjective, or a personalized integration of these techniques. Success in vocational, academic, and recreational pursuits is also developed further in this phase. However, the best therapeutic approaches are still more directive, interactive, and interpersonal than the traditional "neutral screen" of psychoanalysis.

The therapist may even demarcate the transition into this phase by explaining to the patient that there will be changes in the therapist's behavior and expectations of the patient. Explaining that the therapist will be less directive and more explorative will help prepare the patient for these changes. The therapist will also interpret transference more, structure the therapy around psychodynamic themes to a greater extent, and examine dreams in more detail and depth. Other issues that will be worked on include the role of unconscious conflict, including the origins of narcissistic rage (Dodes & Khantzian, 1991). The roles played by substance use in the recovering patient's emotional life, including the substitution of chemicals for soothing object relations, are interpreted, and more adaptive solutions continue to be developed.

It is often very difficult, if not impossible, for the therapist who has been involved with the patient in a variety of directive roles— ranging from confronter to supporter and teacher—to make the shift necessary to perform relatively nondirective, psychoanalytically oriented psychotherapy in this phase. Another reason why the shift is difficult is that the therapist who has "rescued" the patient from a painful "bottom" is often overidealized to such an extent that a shift to analyzing the transference and to more nondirective therapy is impossible. The deprivation of contact and gratification inherent in such a shift can not be tolerated, and overidealization leaves the negative transference unavailable for exploration. Thus a number of alternatives should be explored. The patient may need to shift to a new therapist who can assume this role more readily, as long as both patient and therapist keep in mind the continuing importance of sobriety. Some patients may be able to sustain a high level of intimacy without reconstructive psychotherapy. These patients can use the honesty and self-scrutiny they have gained from Twelve-Step work, together with more directive psychotherapy, to achieve intimacy and a high level of emotional autonomy in most psychosocial spheres. Many patients with 2 to 6 or more years of sobriety will enter treatment for the first time and will be able to work in psychoanalytic psychotherapy.

Once a patient's core identity as a recovering SA is in place, the patient can shift from external behavioral control to internalization of control through identification, expansion of focus, and the use of uncovering psychotherapy (Brown, 1985). Brown acknowledges that this is a difficult time for most patients, since they must simultaneously maintain an identity as SAs and apply cognitive-behavioral controls over substance abuse, while exploring underlying issues contributing to the substance abuse or hindering a satisfying sobriety. Both therapist and patient must risk a heightened but manageable anxiety in order for greater insight to occur. Wallace (1985b) states that after an SA is taught to use preferred defenses to achieve and maintain sobriety in the early stages of treatment, addressing these defenses directly to achieve real changes in personality is a task of later therapy after years of abstinence. He further states that to establish secure and comfortable sobriety, the SA must gradually exchange the learned defensive coping strategies for nondefensive authentic relationships. Zimberg (1985) concurs that a more traditional psychotherapeutic approach can occur only after sobriety is established and maintained.

Intense anxiety or anger can develop when defenses are lowered and uncovering psychotherapy is attempted. The patient's identification as an SA must be solid in order for him/her to tolerate the anxiety necessary for insight. Controls on substance abuse must be intact and ready for reimplementation as needed. During all phases of therapy, the patient and therapist must be constantly aware of the centrality of drugs and/or alcohol. Even in this final phase, specific triggers for relapse are identified and explored, particularly when painful affects emerge. Desires to use substances may be warning signals to stop uncovering, or, when interpreted as such, may permit the reconstructive psychotherapy to continue. Slips and relapse will certainly be repeated threats and may sometimes occur, even in this phase. These slips or near-slips provide opportunities for a microdissection of the feelings, relationships, and events that preceded them. When the patient is able to connect these stressors with cravings, there is a sense of great relief, as passivity is turned into activity (Dodes & Khantzian, 1991).

PSYCHODYNAMIC THEMES IN PHASE 3

Once again, the need for an individualized approach must be emphasized. Each patient will require a focus on different sets of psychodynamic themes. As noted above, one universal theme will be the meaning and role of substance abuse for each patient, although the cluster of unconscious meanings will vary in each individual (see Chapters 1 and 2). Other themes that will be worked on in this phase include (1) grief centering around the loss of drugs/alcohol and the associated life style, as well as other losses, (2) childhood molestations, abuse, separations, and other severe traumas which will require abreaction and letting go; (3) transference and countertransference issues; (4) the need to become aware of narcissistic vulnerabilities, and to relinquish narcissistic entitlement, rage, and other related characterological behaviors; (5) residual dysfunctional affects such as severe anxiety and depression, for which psychotherapy and pharmacotherapy may be needed (of course, potentially addicting chemicals of all kinds are strongly discouraged for pharmacological relief); (6) the continuing need for healthy self-care and maintenance of a sober core; and (7) the achievement of intimacy. In addition to these themes, relapse prevention training is continually practiced.

Grief and Loss

Even though most individuals in Phase 3 of therapy have been sober for several years, there is still considerable mourning for drugs/alcohol and for associated friends and behaviors. Dreams about drugs and alcohol continue, though in this phase they generally represent warning signs more than a working through of loss. Grief work in this phase may also arise from long-repressed feelings about early parental or sibling losses through death, divorce, or abandonment, as well as lost decades of relationships with family members. The latter often include the addict's children from prior as well as present relationships.

Therapists need to be particularly empathic and understanding as recovering SAs struggle with their grief, since the SAs are generally quite vulnerable in this area. I often remind those SAs who have been isolated from their feelings for decades that their painful state is better than the void of no feelings at all, and that in opening the door to their pain they will also open themselves up to experience more joyful feelings.

Letting Go of Early Traumas

With an intact sober core, many early traumas such as physical, emotional, and sexual abuse can be worked with in Phase 3. Some patients will have attended specific self-help groups for these issues (e.g., groups for incest survivors). I usually advocate that patients not attend these types of groups until they have at least 1 year of stable sobriety. These painful experiences are then often well dealt with in group settings that include similar victims, be they therapist-led or self-help. Dealing with these traumas requires that a therapist be even more empathic than in working with grief and loss. I will sometimes meet with a patient who has been sexually abused and the perpetrator of the abuse to discuss the molestation incident(s). This needs to be done with empathy toward the offender as well as the victim, and perpetrator "bashing" needs to be kept to a bare minimum. If this is not done, the result may be retaliatory sadism directed toward the patient, or total emotional devastation of the perpetrator and secondary severe guilt by the patient.

Transference and Countertransference Issues

Countertransference is described in detail in Chapter 8. As therapy intensifies in this phase, the patient may develop intense transference feelings. These can be worked with as long as they do not threaten to overwhelm the patient's autonomy and sobriety. Both negative and positive transferences can be facilitated and eventually analyzed in Phase 3, though successful therapy will often be met with eternal (unanalyzed) gratitude.

Relinquishing Narcissistic Behaviors

By this stage, patients will have given up many of their narcissistic, selfish behaviors as a result of their Twelve-Step work, but others will remain. In my experience, patients with solid sobriety can handle confrontation of the narcissistic aspects of their personalities more effectively than most persons who have never been addicted, because their Twelve-Step program has well prepared them for these confrontations. Emotionally, they are as taken aback and anxious as other individuals, but in this phase of therapy they expect to be confronted about and to relinquish their narcissistic behaviors. They may also increase their meeting attendance, time with their sponsors, and Twelve-Step work to help provide balm for their wounds as each set of narcissistic behaviors is confronted.

Residual Dysfunctional Affects

Many patients continue to experience a great deal of depression and anxiety (including panic disorder), even after years of appropriate working of the Twelve Steps. Some of these patients, with primary affective and anxiety disorders, have self-medicated for years and cannot recover without appropriate medication. In any case, residual anxiety and depression may benefit from appropriate anxiolytics or antidepressants — preferably those that are nonsedating, as these drugs can be abused. Benzodiazepines and other more addicting sedatives should be avoided at all costs, particularly on any long-term basis; these drugs are so cross-tolerant with and psychopharmacologically similar to alcohol that they induce strong cravings for the latter or for a bigger or better "high" with stronger illicit drugs. They also lower inhibitions which can lead directly to substance abuse as well as other relapse prone behaviors.

Traditional psychotherapy that focuses on what causes the painful affects, either in the patient's present life or in the transference, can be quite helpful. Just releasing the affects in a sober, nurturing, "holding" therapeutic environment may be sufficient to moderate these painful feelings. In this phase, painful affects from recollection of childhood traumas and their unconscious meanings in dreams and fantasies can be readily worked with as long as the sober core is maintained. The maladaptive aspects of unconscious fantasies and wishes are interpreted and replaced with more realistic wishes and wants.

Healthy Self-Care

In Phase 3, the external self-care function of the therapist has been generally eliminated, except when it is reactivated by the patient's danger signals and overt cries for help. Patients who are SAs have been relatively deprived of adequate caring and protection from their parents, but by this phase they have internalized ample aspects of these qualities through their psychotherapy and Twelve-Step work. Taking self-care to a higher plane is another aspect of this phase (Khantzian & Mack, 1983). The patient is helped to recognize, utilize, and tolerate anticipatory affects such as embarrassment, shame, guilt, fear, worry, and anxiety, so as to avoid or escape from dangerous and self-punitive situations and relationships. Other components for self-care include the ego-executive functions for self-preservation. These include reality testing, judgment, self-control, and the ability to make cause–consequence connections. Thus, in this phase the patient is further developing the ability to plan actions to anticipate harm and danger; this is based on the patient's now developed capacity for self-comforting, self-valuing, and self-care (Khantzian & Mack, 1983). It is made possible by the patient's increased awareness through giving up primitive defenses and substituting more mature ones. At the same time as there is improved self-care, there is the development of altruism that is not compromised by self-destructive and martyred behaviors.

Achieving Intimacy

The attainment of a high level of intimacy with a significant other is the *sine qua non* of Phase 3 of treatment. An integrally related goal is intimacy with one's own parents, siblings, children, and close friends. It is assumed that the intimate relationship with the significant other is sexual while the others are not. An intimate relationship has certain qualities, although no human interaction can reach perfection even in any single aspect of intimacy. These attributes include the following, according to Coleman (1987):

1. The partners in an intimate relationship are able to express positive and negative thoughts and feelings in a meaningful and constructive manner — one that is mutually acceptable and respectful, and that leads to the psychological well-being of the individuals involved. The most difficult aspect of this is the ability to tolerate and process anger.

2. The partners are able to use this communication to define the boundaries of the relationship; to express caring, concern, and commitment; to negotiate rules and roles; and to resolve conflicts.

3. Sexual experience, which is often considered as synonymous with intimacy, is only one aspect of its expression. In the intimate relationship with the significant other, the sexual act is an important final common pathway and marker of overall intimacy. A definition of satisfying sexuality in such a relationship would include tenderness, nur-

turing, and affection in foreplay and afterplay, as well as a mutually satisfying orgasmic response. A healthy sexual experience also includes the following (Coleman, 1987):

 a. Relative freedom from shame and guilt.
 b. Spontaneity, creativity, and playfulness.
 c. Comfort with each other's boundaries, preferences, and taboos.
 d. The ability to negotiate and compromise, so that the needs of both individuals are met.
 e. A balanced perspective in which sex neither becomes too important nor is neglected.
 f. A balance among sexual, romantic, and working love.*

In dealing with any of the psychodynamic themes discussed above, dreams may often help bring unconscious conflicts to the surface. In Phase 3 dreams are worked with quite actively, as the next section illustrates.

CASE VIGNETTE: THE USE OF DREAMS IN BOB'S ADVANCED RECOVERY

In his eighth month of psychotherapy, Bob reported his first dream: "I lost a dog. The dog was the only thing I had in the world. I lost the dog. I was going around this dark, murky city, desperately trying to retrace my steps. I never found the dog." In working with this dream, I first asked myself, and then asked Bob, a series of questions. The answers helped Bob to use the dream properly, at a level commensurate with his ability to deal with the material at that time in his therapy. The questions and answers were as follows:

 1. What material was spontaneously discussed just prior to and after Bob's account of the dream? What were the current themes in therapy? How was this material relevant? In this case, Bob's fears of getting close and admitting that he wanted intimacy were being discussed.
 2. What was the day residue? Bob said, "I was talking about being truthful and Carla leaving me. It's the fear of not being liked. There is something fundamentally wrong with me, so if I'm open and honest people will see what's wrong. So I hide. Something is wrong with me; I don't know if it's good or evil."

---

*A love that has the positive characteristics of intimacy as described above.

3. What were the feelings in the dream? "A sense of panic, a frantic search. I felt alone, not emotionally connected to anything. It felt weird."

4. What were the defenses against the feelings in the dream? "I felt this before. Not me. I don't want to feel like this again."

5. What did that feeling remind Bob of in the past? "I'm not sure. Not being loved. I can't get in touch with it."

6. What came to Bob's mind when he thought of the specific elements in the dream? "First the dog. Our family had one. I remember, a small collie which always got into trouble when I wasn't there. My father said he found her a home where she'd be looked after. I suspected he put her away."

7. How could Bob use this material to change his behavior? As this material evolved, I stated that Bob feared he would lose his wife if he asserted or revealed himself with her—that he mistrusted loving her as he mistrusted his childhood experience of loving a dog (i.e., if he loved something, he would lose it). I also pointed out that his fear of losing Carla put him in touch with very early feelings of being abandoned or betrayed that were no longer realistic in an adult. With this knowledge in hand, Bob was encouraged to risk more openness and assertiveness with Carla. He responded, "In the dream, I felt more childlike."

Bob ended the session by stating, "It's a lot of work to love. It's harder when you're aware of your capacity to love. You get hurt even more."

CASE VIGNETTE: OTHER FEATURES OF BOB'S ADVANCED RECOVERY

Because of his difficulties with control and perfectionism, Bob took longer to obtain a sponsor than any patient I have ever worked with who utilized AA. He obtained his sponsor after over a year of sobriety, instead of in Phase 1 or early Phase 2 of therapy, as do most patients. Even after choosing a sponsor, he proceeded gradually, requiring 6 weeks to ask a man with solid sobriety (who was also a friend of Bob and Carla) to be his sponsor. He had also learned in advance that this man would "be delighted to sponsor me," Bob said. "I feel a sponsor is there to give me guidance and direction about the right program to serenity. He will help with the steps to put the demons behind. For the first time, I see it as a help. I don't have the same sense of giving up control because I don't consider it a control issue. Its time has come. I have a sense of accepting or anticipating. It's going to be different."

Bob also showed more self-acceptance: "You said I'm too hard on myself. Maybe I am a better person than I give myself credit for. I'm trying to help people at work. Am I being too hard on myself? Maybe I can like and accept myself more." Moreover, he began to look critically and realistically at some of his own projections—for example, that he was not worth my concern or the concern of a sponsor, and that a sponsor would only want to work with him to gratify his own need to control Bob. I supported him for being critical of his own projections and for checking them out rather than holding on to them.

Even after 2 years of psychotherapy, Bob still required a great deal of structure and support to relieve his anxiety in sessions and to stabilize him in his daily activities with his family and at work, as well as to continue his explorative psychotherapy. Nevertheless, he continued to build more intimate relationships with his wife and children.

By the middle of his third year of psychotherapy, Bob began to diminish the frequency of his sessions with me. He now needed the therapy less to maintain his sobriety, but more to facilitate his personal growth and intimacy with significant others, as well as to come to terms with his past. In particular, he was working on taking a stand with his mother and ex-wife. He was able to tell his mother that he would no longer communicate with her if she continued to be hurtful to him. He also wrote his ex-wife that he expected her to take some financial responsibility for herself, and that he wanted to have more responsibility for their children (including, if possible, their moving into his home in the United States). He stated, "I want out of the guilt with both my mother and my ex-wife. I want to ask for what I want, instead of saying I don't deserve anything." I supported Bob for his gains and encouraged him to recognize how self-generated they were, as they had come during the time he had cut down on his therapy. He replied, "It's kinda nice to do it with you as well as to do it without you."

I dealt with his having cut down to one AA meeting a week by telling him about Arlene, another patient of mine. I stated that I do not usually talk about other patients, but this narrative made such an important point that I wanted him to hear it, and I had obtained her permission to tell it. The story was as follows: "Arlene had 10 years of very successful sobriety, in which she was in psychotherapy and very active in AA. For the next 6 years she continued not to drink, but stopped going to AA. Then she relapsed for 6 months and was hospitalized in my chemical dependence program. She was quite resistant to every aspect of her recovery this time, and relapsed again 1 month after her discharge. She again returned to the hospital, but this time she rededicated herself to sobriety, including working the Twelve Steps and maintaining close contact with a sponsor. She now was truly sober again and seemed quite happy for the first time in over a year. I added to Bob, "You're growing wonderfully, but it would be easier to continue if you had a strong sober core right now." Bob responded, "I honestly know I'd be better off if I worked a more active program." Shortly after this session, he returned to his regular meetings.

By the end of his third year of therapy, we were more open with each other as Bob continued to grow. He stated that recently he had been withdrawing a bit from Carla, particularly when stressed by work. I asked him what he needed to do to change this.

BOB: Recognize that that is what I'm doing. Realize that I do best when I'm open to help from others.

DR. KAUFMAN: And fight it like hell [emphasizing the need to continue working on it consciously].

BOB: I'm not comfortable enough with it. I used to think my job was to solve it all myself. Now I know I do better when I don't consciously push it.

DR. KAUFMAN: It's about surrender and a balance between changing through hard work and through surrender.

BOB: I can do it in some parts of my life, not all. Yet I see how much fuller life can be if I go down that path. I know more about myself and my own potential. The question is how to convert the potential into reality. Did you see *What about Bob?* Maybe I can "baby-step" my way to my potential.

DR. KAUFMAN: What is your potential?

BOB: It's so very different from where I've come. It's the difference between feeling that what goes wrong is my fault and I'm under immense pressure to solve my problems, and "Gee, shit happens." I'm not bad, I'm good. I'm giving up living my life as "It must be my fault. I can't handle this or I can't face this."

DR. KAUFMAN: You're moving back and forth between the two, but you're moving more in the direction of "Shit happens" and "It's not my fault."

BOB: It's getting too abstract.

DR. KAUFMAN: How would you put this into effect with Carla tonight?

BOB: I'm afraid she'll judge me. I project into her the personification of what's holding me back—that everything is my fault.

DR. KAUFMAN: That's a very important idea.

BOB: When I feel really good about myself, I can be more open with her. When I'm not, she becomes my inhibiting committee [punitive superego]. Then I associate her with my mother. This is weird and Freudian.

At this point, I supportively taught him about the universality of selfobjects and how common they were between men and their wives and mothers. Bob took it back on himself: "It's my creation, my projection onto her. I don't have to make her my mother. I change over time. If we're both committed it will work." He then sensed that I was involved in my inner thoughts and asked what I was thinking. I shared my fantasy accurately because I thought it would be helpful to him now.

DR. KAUFMAN: I'm thinking about my wife's birthday party tomorrow and what kind of a speech I'll make in her honor.

BOB: Two years ago I wouldn't have asked because I didn't feel I had the right to ask. Not to know but to ask. Now it's okay to ask.

DR. KAUFMAN: Why is it okay now?

BOB: Because I like you and I was curious, and it's okay to be curious.

DR. KAUFMAN: [I was now feeling warmly encouraging and close.] Before we end therapy, I'd like to see you take a cake for your third birthday [in AA].

BOB: I was thinking about that too today. It's only three months away.

DR. KAUFMAN: You have more self-acceptance and self-worth now, so that you should be able to handle it.

BOB: I feel much more accepting of myself.

At this point I realized that I was indirectly offering to attend Bob's AA birthday celebration, but that we would have to work on his feelings stirred by this subject before the event transpired. Bob continued to work on his fears of openness with his wife, and noted how sharing at AA meetings was correlated with being more open with her.

After this, Bob took a few months' break from therapy, in part because of professional commitments and in part because of resistance based on wanting to do it on his own. He appeared at our next session wearing a beard for the first time (I have had a beard for years), but he was casual about why he had grown it. The identification with me was obvious, as was his resistance to looking at it, so I bypassed this issue. He shifted to informing me that he had just had his third AA birthday, and that for the first time, he had taken a cake at a meeting. He stated, "I felt really good, really supported by the people there. For the first time, it was okay to be an alcoholic. I finally gave up and said that I truly need help. A lot of people offered it and gave it. It's easier to tell people about myself now. The cake was a celebration of what is. It's wrong to pretend that it's not that way."

I supported him for taking the cake and asked whether he had remembered my offer to attend the ceremony. He replied, "I forgot. I'm sorry. It was selfish of me." As he explored his forgetting, he was able to say, "I wanted it to be something I could do on my own." As Bob spoke further, he became able to accept that I could have been there to support him without taking it away from him: "I see it's not binary, not either–or. Thank you." I segued from this to the issue of termination.

DR. KAUFMAN: What are your thoughts about continuing here versus being on your own?

BOB: Uncertainty, fear, a sense of missing you. I have made a powerful journey and you have helped significantly. I have a fear I will regress without you, yet I feel on a solid footing, so I can do it myself. I also like seeing you. You guide me through self-discovery. I don't know when or how people stop coming to see you. I'm a little confused. Part of me says that I should continue with you, and part says that maybe I could do it myself. Maybe the confusion is okay.

DR. KAUFMAN: It would be most helpful if you would make a clear decision about stopping therapy now and working with me for a few sessions on that process, or continuing and setting specific goals, rather than staying in therapy without coming regularly.

BOB: Working on closing would bring a completeness to this. It seems natural. Then I wouldn't be left hanging. You say it with confidence and calmness. It's reassuring. Summarize or say goodbye. Either are viable, and it's up to me to choose. I see that you're open to both. I'll let you know.

Bob waited several months before he returned for his final session. He stated that he was feeling better because he now realized that there was not much in life he could control, particularly "other beings."

DR. KAUFMAN: Sounds like it is working for you.

BOB: The more I let go, the happier I am.

DR. KAUFMAN: How's Carla reacting to this change?

BOB: She'd be happier if I explained more about how I see things and asked for more of her help. I'm still too solitary to have a strong, open relationship.

DR. KAUFMAN: You've done the same thing with me. You avoided dealing directly with the issue of whether to stop therapy or not by not calling me for several months.

BOB: I'm sorry, and could have done differently but would I have meant it?

DR. KAUFMAN: I don't need an apology. The issue is running rather than dealing directly.

BOB: "Running" is a term that I bristle at and am sensitive to. If I avoid conflict, it lowers my self-confidence.

DR. KAUFMAN: What are your thoughts about not making a conscious decision about how to stop therapy?

BOB: You'll say, "That's not right"—that fear disturbs me because you're supportive of whatever I choose. Yet I had a concern that you'd disapprove of my decision. I still have an overriding urge about wrong decisions. I can't afford them. Somebody else telling me I do the wrong thing.

DR. KAUFMAN: Besides who? Your mother, Carla?

BOB: Maybe. Maybe also my father. When I went through this discovery process—sensing what it was like when I was small—there was my mother saying, "Neh, Neh, Neh, Neh," and my father saying I couldn't match up to him, but in a more distant voice. [Bob's associations then shifted to his competence, which was now individuating him from his father.] I am more self-confident now, and I can use external feedback to reinforce my positive image of myself. I'm starting to make friends even at work. These people like to see me come in. I'm not the same ogre. I have a solid self-image now unlike when I was small. What's entering my memory was that the put-down came from more than my mother, and my father wasn't totally on my side against her. . . . This therapy led me to increase communication with my ex-wife, which reinforced how badly I feel about not communicating with you. I looked away from you just then because I'm projecting my own self-disapproval onto you.

DR. KAUFMAN: It's growth that you understand that you've made a lot of positive changes. We should stop now until you want to grow some more—or are in more pain again. [Bob was silent for a while, so I asked him what his thoughts and feelings were.]

BOB: My initial reaction was "Damn you."

DR. KAUFMAN: Why?

BOB: So you don't want to help me any more. But I'm not coming, so someone else has made the decision for me. Yet that's okay. Stopping is—let's see if I can explore things myself. If I need help in the future, you'll be there for me. Damn you, you made the decision I should have made 2 months ago.

DR. KAUFMAN: You feel I've taken control and kicked you out?

BOB: I rationalize. I didn't make the decision, and therefore if it's wrong, I didn't make a mistake.

DR. KAUFMAN: If you don't ask, then nobody says "No" to you.

BOB: I should make the decision and stick with it. You didn't make the decision to stop. I actually did months ago, though not directly. [In a few moments of parting intimacy, Bob asked several questions about me in relation to him.] You always call me Bob and I call you Dr. Kaufman. Do you ever refer to patients as Mr. or Mrs.?

DR. KAUFMAN: It must feel one-sided to you. I'm just not comfortable calling people Mr. or Mrs., and I encourage them to call me whatever name they like, such as Ed or Kaufman or Dr. K.

BOB: I keep you at a distance by calling you Dr. Kaufman.

DR. KAUFMAN: Which you need to be comfortable.

BOB: Or I wouldn't do it. Did you finish the book?

DR. KAUFMAN: Almost. Are you anxious about the section that discusses your therapy?

BOB: Yes, I am now. I'd like to read it. I feel it will provide me more insights. [When I asked Bob about including him in my book several years before, he had clearly stated that he did not want to read anything about him that I had written, because it would be too frightening to him. Thus, his request was another example of his enhanced self-esteem and confidence, as well as an indirect way of holding on to me.] It was hard to say that.

DR. KAUFMAN: Some time on your own will help you grow without the mantle of therapy hovering over you.

BOB: Goodbye. I know I'll see you again. [We shook hands in farewell, as at the end of all of our sessions.]

Bob's termination was quite far from the active working-through process suggested in this book, let alone more psychoanalytic approaches. Yet many feelings of fondness, gratitude, and anger were expressed, as well as substantial insight and newfound strength and self-confidence. In view of the sparseness of our visits the last 4 or 5 months of therapy (two, to be exact) it was certainly time to stop, and my approach was sufficiently directive to initiate the termination. Bob was insightful enough to deal with his passive aggressiveness appropriately; he also felt quite close to me during our parting moments. I agreed with him that we would meet again, and my hunch was that he would be stronger the next time.

This clinical example also demonstrates that phases in psychotherapy are rarely discrete, although they are most helpful in describing a model.

ASPECTS AND FUNCTIONS
OF TWELVE-STEP WORK IN PHASE 3

The Twelve Steps, though often practiced less actively in this Phase 3 of therapy, in and of themselves provide ongoing psychodynamic work through the following principles (Brown, 1985): (1) giving up grandiosity and omnipotence through acceptance of a Higher Power; (2) engaging in critical self-examination; (3) obtaining relief from denial and loneliness; (4) dedicating oneself to a lifetime of openness and honesty; (5) achieving humility; (6) making the past real and assuming responsibility for harm caused; (7) obtaining relief from guilt; (8) accepting responsibility for restitution of harm done; (9) implementing a design for daily living (i.e., strengthening autonomous ego function); and (10) shifting defense mechanisms from those that are limiting (e.g., denial and projection) to healthier altruism and sublimation. Chappel (1992) also emphasizes that making amends in a sensitive and caring way repairs damaged relationships and helps develop skills which lead to intimacy.

Although the Tenth, Eleventh, and Twelfth Steps are emphasized in this phase of psychotherapy, the recovering SA continues to work and live the first nine on a daily basis. The First, Second, and Third Steps are reworked to maintain the sober core. The Fourth through Seventh Steps are part of the continuing personal inventory described in the Tenth Step; the Eighth and Ninth Steps are also utilized as part of this self-reflection, in order to avoid continued harm to others and, when it occurs, to recognize it and make amends.

The Tenth Step is as follows: "[We] continued to take personal inventory and when we were wrong promptly admitted it." As described above, this personal inventory is achieved through a daily reworking of the Fourth through Ninth Steps, but with an emphasis on the Fourth. As Chappel (1992), has noted, this step is a continuing stimulus to character development and to personal and relational growth. How much greater this universe would be if we all (especially world leaders) could admit promptly to ourselves and others when we were wrong and make an effort to right these wrongs (Chappel, 1992)! Indeed, this step helps our patients work over and work through the intellectual insights they have gained from their psychotherapy, and turn them into genuine or emotional insight and action. Brown (1985) emphasizes that while the first nine steps deal with the wreckage of the past, the last three steps are the "action steps," providing a plan for daily living in the present. Members are reminded that they do not "wipe the slate clean" (Brown, 1985) with the Fourth Step; they are requested to continue lifelong self-examination. Brown (1985) reminds us that regular honest self-examination and continuing restitution are incompatible with drinking and the type of thinking that permits it. In the Tenth Step, self-restraint is practiced, as it promotes slowing down and engaging in self-reflection rather than acting on impulse.

The Eleventh Step is this: "[We] sought through prayer and meditation to improve our conscious contact with God as we understood Him, praying only for knowledge of His will for us and the power to carry that out." Chappel (1992) considers this an advanced spiritual health step, in that it involves a daily reworking of the first three steps with aspects of the Fifth and Seventh Steps. The idea here is that the internal search for knowledge and power leads to a sense of purpose and meaning.

Finally, the Twelfth Step is as follows: "Having had a spiritual awakening as the result of these Steps, [we] tried to carry this message to others, and to practice these principles in all our affairs." Here, the recovering person puts into practice all he/she has learned and, by giving it away to others, gets it back manyfold. The appropriate Twelve-Step adage here is "You can't keep it if you don't give it away." Belonging to the group is enhanced by the idea that every member has something to give to another. Working with newcomers also reminds sober group members of their own vulnerability and of how they themselves, in an AA phrase, "are only one drink away from a drunk." The altruistic act is linked to "enlightened self-interest" (Chappel, 1992). The message that is shared is of the sober members' struggle with alcohol and/or drugs, the strength they have found in working a program, and the hope that newly recovering SAs can find similar relief and healing. Sponsoring new group members not only helps develop altruism, but deepens the sponsors' own growth in the same way that being psychotherapists deepens therapists' understanding of themselves. When a sponsor works the steps with a newer member, it generally deepens the sponsor's own Twelve-Step work.

At a patient's Twelve-Step birthday, someone generally says, "It is a miracle that you are sober." When I hear this, I think often (particularly in the case of a chronic relapser and/or a difficult dually diagnosed person), "I wonder whether that supportive person knows what a miracle really has taken place."

TERMINATION (OR NOT)

The final step in advanced recovery is working through termination. In my own experience, the therapeutic process is rarely finalized with SAs, since the door should always be left open for their return— particularly during severe external crises or at major critical points in the life cycle, such as marriage, childbirth, parents' deaths, or children's entering adolescence. In addition, they are encouraged to continue in Twelve-Step groups at varying levels of intensity as needed for the rest of their lives.

When there is not a crisis, the patient in advanced recovery may require less external Twelve-Step involvement. However, the years of Twelve-Step practice live on in the internalization of healthy ego functioning, including self-scrutiny, self-care, and self-valuing, as well as responsibility for one's own actions and their effects on others. Generally, some external Twelve-Step practice is necessary in order to maintain this internal change, such as attending at least one meeting a week, reading the Big Book, working the Twelve Steps on a daily basis, maintaining weekly contact with one's sponsor, and/or sponsoring others. I disagree with Dodes and Khantzian (1991) that a patient can remain chemical-free without any Twelve-Step contact, and I do not support that position for my patients.

Just as Twelve-Step groups do not encourage termination, the therapist may continue a relationship by exchanging notes or cards or by attending Twelve-Step birthdays. Even though there may be no formal or full termination, there is an ending to the phase of active psychotherapy, which is worked on in the same way that most therapies are terminated. Thus, the patient may exhibit anger at abandonment, depression, threats of relapse, detachment, and finally autonomy. The lack of a complete termination may rob the patient of the feeling of total autonomy, but it is still preferred, because it reminds the recovering person who was truly dependent on drugs and/or alcohol of the need for a lifetime program that enhances abstinence and includes careful self-scrutiny and honesty.

Countertransference and Other Mutually Interactive Aspects of Psychotherapy with Addicted Persons

Until recently, little has been written on therapists' specific countertransference reactions to SAs. Many psychoanalysts have theorized about the psychodynamics of SAs but very few have written about specific countertransferences. Those who have done so have devoted surprisingly little of their effort to it. Fortunately, a recent shift in viewpoint has generated interest in this vital issue. Countertransference has traditionally been considered as a liability (to be overcome immediately by the therapist's own personal psychotherapy), or as unconscious and unavailable. Presently it is more commonly regarded as an extremely valuable tool, as new approaches help therapists access and utilize these feelings to create meaningful change in their patients. In my opinion, current developments in the utilization of countertransference are as exciting and innovative as any recent developments in psychotherapy.

A contemporary concept of countertransference is quite broad. To paraphrase the description by Imhoff (1991), it encompasses the total emotional reaction of the therapist to the patient, including the entire range of conscious, preconscious, and unconscious attitudes; beliefs and feelings; and their verbal and nonverbal behavioral manifestations. This contemporary view acknowledges the importance of reciprocal cycles of interaction between patient and therapist. This concept includes the therapist's tuning into his/her own unconscious feelings and fantasies about the patient, in order to learn aspects of the patient's behavior that are not consciously obvious. The more the therapist is aware of his/her own underlying feelings, the less they will be acted out in a manner that is harmful to the patient. Thus a therapist can learn by tuning into his/her own positive or negative feelings that a patient is evoking feelings such as love or anger. Rather than expressing these feelings directly or indirectly, the therapist should first attempt to understand how the patient is provoking these feelings or tapping the therapist's own issues. Self-knowledge then permits the therapist to understand emotionally what the patient is experiencing.

As therapists learn to tune into their own feeling states, they will identify patients' conflicts and feelings before these become overt. In this way, the therapists can use countertransference as an extremely helpful tool. Moreover, countertransference is now viewed as a critical pathway for significant change, particularly in the therapy of personality disorders, which are generally present in SAs (Craig, 1988).

Sandler (1976) was one of the first analysts to emphasize that a therapist's proclivity to replay the roles of significant figures in a patient's past is a function of countertransference. Acknowledging these projections and projective identifications as they are experienced in the countertransference provides a great deal of important information, as well as a critical vehicle for bringing about change in patients. Sandler (1976) noted that, as in the case of transference, the field has shifted from viewing countertransference as an obstacle to viewing it as a meaningful facilitator of change. Countertransference is another way of "listening with the third ear." Therapists should not be self-critical when they experience countertransference; rather, they should use these feelings to maximize therapeutic effectiveness. This approach is not totally new in concept, although the nomenclature has changed. Alexander and French (1946) did not mention the term "countertransference" in their seminal book *Psychoanalytic Therapy*. Instead, they substituted technical maneuvers in which the therapist changes behaviors to provide a "corrective emotional experience" (Orr, 1954), which is in part a way of utilizing countertransference.

The interactional view of countertransference was well described by Langs (1978). Langs viewed countertransference as a reciprocal process in which the patient provokes and projectively identifies with the therapist, so that the therapist responds with countertransference behaviors, affects, and fantasies. The patient's communications and symptoms then are derived from the therapist's countertransference.

Six contemporary phenomena that are inextricably fused with countertransference are also discussed in this chapter: parallel process;

therapist codependence, denial, enabling, and burnout; and therapist family-of-origin issues. Parallel process (Doehrman & Gross, 1976) is another psychodynamic way of viewing countertransference, and it is described in detail. Therapist codependence, denial, enabling, and burnout are four concepts commonly used to denote aspects of countertransference in the field of substance abuse. I utilize them here as components of the overall working concept of countertransference; each contributes to a fuller understanding of the wide range of therapist reactions to these patients. Finally, the therapist's own unresolved family issues — often regarded as totally separate from countertransference by family systems theorists, can also be used to further the understanding of the therapist's unconscious reactions to patients. These six countertransference-related phenomena are discussed following the detailed discussion of different views and types or aspects of countertransference. Some of these different ways of looking at countertransference may seem redundant or repetitive, and indeed almost any single countertransference reaction of the therapist can be viewed in each of these contexts. Nevertheless, each contributes to a full understanding of patient–therapist interactions and how to use them in psychotherapy.

TRADITIONAL VERSUS CONTEMPORARY VIEWS OF COUNTERTRANSFERENCE

The Classic Psychoanalytic View

Much of the information we have on countertransference comes from the psychoanalytic literature and has been only minimally applied to SAs. An excellent introductory work from the substance abuse literature is an article by Imhoff et al. (1983). Kernberg's (1984) psychoanalytic writings on the subject focus on patients with BPD (see Chapter 4). However, his observations are applicable to most SAs, since substance abuse and BPD have many aspects in common and are frequently found in the same patients. Countertransference reactions can be seen in a progressively widening framework, ranging from narrow or classical to totalistic (Kernberg, 1984). Even in its classical definition, "countertransference" has several connotations. These include the therapist's (1) unconscious reactions or own transference to a patient's transference, (2) unconscious reactions to the patient as a whole, and (3) blind spots in understanding because of unresolved neurotic conflicts. An integral part of the early, classical view was that countertransference is infantile and undesirable (Freud, 1910/1957) and should be resolved through further personal analysis. Freud's view of countertransference is most applicable to our reactions to relatively highly integrated or neurotic patients (Hedges, 1983) than it is to most SAs.

A Totalistic View

A broader, totalistic view (Kernberg, 1965) is far more helpful to a contemporary therapist working with SAs. The totalistic approach emphasizes the reciprocity in patient–therapist interaction (Langs, 1978; Hedges, 1983), as well as the diagnostic and therapeutic utility of countertransference. Therapists are reminded that either overt or covert expressions have a great deal of impact and should be kept to a discreet minimum (Langs, 1978). Overt expressions should be carefully planned and timed according to a well-defined treatment plan; these are described later in this chapter.

This approach emphasizes concentric circles of progressively deeper and more focused meaning. The first definition or outermost circle, as suggested at the beginning of this chapter, is the total emotional reaction of the therapist to a patient, including conscious and unconscious responses to a patient's reality as well as the transference. This layer also involves the therapist's own real and neurotic needs (Kernberg, 1965). Included here are both appropriate and inappropriate emotional responses to the patient's past life, present life, material, content, affect, attitude, personality, defensive style, and diagnosis. Each of these nine issues or any combination of them can evoke powerful countertransferences in the treatment of SAs. In addition, many therapists have difficulties with patients who demonstrate behaviors or characteristics common in SAs, such as child molestation, wife beating, competitiveness, hostility, obsequiousness, severe depression, poor hygiene/cleanliness, a diagnosis of HIV/AIDS, self-destructiveness, borderline personality traits, and so on.

This broad definition of countertransference includes several more general therapist responses. One's attitude toward being a therapist *vis-a-vis* being a patient is of particular importance, especially if it involves the feeling that being a therapist is superior to being a patient. This problem could manifest itself in untherapeutic superiority, condescension, or pity. Other therapist responses based on being a therapist include the "variety of controlling, competitive, voyeuristic, sadistic, exhibitionistic, or nurturing impulses gratified in the therapist by virtue of playing a central role in someone else's life" (Wallerstein, 1990, p. 338). Therapist omnipotence often promises a rapid cure, which in turn helps to bring about an overidealized transference. When magical promises are not fulfilled, the patient may rapidly switch into extreme hostility or run from therapy. Other maladaptive therapist responses involve certain therapist personality traits, including specific defenses and adaptive responses. These traits are accentuated by any stressor that leads to therapist anxiety, but particularly by powerful transferences, which are experienced as "onslaughts." Therapists may lack empathy in general or may have difficulties in empathizing with certain types of patients.

Within a totalistic view, several types of aspects of countertransference may be thought of as linear, in that they may reach from the outermost circle through each layer into one's core issues. These include objective versus subjective countertransference; positive and negative countertransference; empathy; idealization; gender-related aspects; projective counteridentification; and other interactive issues. These are discussed next.

TYPES OR ASPECTS OF COUNTERTRANSFERENCE

Objective versus Subjective Countertransference

MacKinnon and Michels (1971) suggest that some of the therapist's "objective" emotional responses to patients should not be considered countertransference. These are reactions to a patient "as he actually is" or reactions "that the patient would elicit in most people" (p. 28). I would challenge that view, as tempting as it often is; reactions such as liking, sympathizing, or feeling antagonistic are highly subjective. Still, some people do consistently evoke such negative emotions in most of the people they meet. It is helpful for therapists to realize that these emotions may be those that patients frequently evoke in others, rather than countertransference per se. However, it would be most untherapeutic if therapists were merely to dismiss their reactions with the rationale that anyone would feel that way toward this type of patient. Rather, these patients' pattern of provoking these feelings in most people they encounter needs to be understood and is best explained within their interactions with their therapist.

Giovacchini (1987) terms such universal reactions "homogeneous" countertransference, and cautions that even these feelings, though expected in most experienced therapists, have infantile elements. He contrasts this with "idiosyncratic" responses generated by the therapist's own psychic imbalance.

Vannicelli (1989) has applied psychoanalytic theories of countertransference to group therapy with adult children of alcoholics. The principles which she emphasizes are most appropriate to work with SAs themselves (about 50% of adult children of alcoholism, in my experience, are themselves SAs). Following Winnicott (1949), Vannicelli separates countertransference reactions into "subjective" and "objective." Subjective reactions are those that relate to the therapist's own past and personal idiosyncrasies. Horney (1949) described an objective countertransference, in which the therapist's love or hate is an objective reaction to the actual personality and behavior of the patient. However, in both cases the therapist's countertransference is a result of the interaction between himself/herself and the patient. Since no one has ever fully resolved all of his/her conflicts, therapists should strive to be aware of the possibility of subjective or idiosyncratic countertranferences. They should therefore attempt to be aware of the types of situations, feelings, and patients that provoke these responses, so that they can understand these feelings in themselves and put them into appropriate context. These feelings can tell a therapist a great deal about what is going on under the surface of a patient *if the therapist can separate his/her own contribution from the patients.* When this is accomplished, the therapist will learn a great deal about the patient from countertransference feelings, be they subjective or objective (Vannicelli, 1989).

Positive Countertransference

Unrecognized positive countertransference feelings may be as destructive to therapy as negative feelings. Patients experiencing loving behaviors from their therapist may feel overwhelmed in a number of ways. They may feel seduced, sexualized, swallowed up, merged with, or quite guilty. They may feel that the therapists are offering gratifications that can never be fulfilled, and this will inevitably lead to their feeling betrayed and quite angry. Positive countertransference feelings occur frequently toward patients who were caretakers in their families of origin. In therapy, such patients are exquisitely sensitive to the therapists' own needs, innately knowing just what to say and do to help the therapists feel great. Their altruism also makes these patients likable, even when it verges on masochism. If not confronted, they will be unable to learn to meet their own needs.

Therapists may also become aware of their defenses against countertransference reactions before the emotions are experienced. Thus they should tune into being overly nice or indulgent to their patients as a defense against anger or rejection (Vannicelli, 1989). Whenever a therapist feels that he/she has been manipulated into giving a patient some indulgence he/she does not ordinarily give, there is countertransference for having given it, and secondary dislike and/or anger toward the patient for having been successfully manipulative. Common indulgences include excessive support, activity, or feedback; overt or covert gifts; extending sessions; giving out home telephone numbers; and/or prescribing abusable medications (particularly when any of these behaviors is unusual in the therapist).

Negative Countertransference

When therapists are angry and on the verge of rejecting their patients, it often helps to understand why the patients are so provocative and manipulative. Some SAs may feel a compulsion to repeat the seduction or rejection they experienced in their own families. Some may have lost all coping mechanisms except for those used to obtain drugs or to manipulate others to continue their dependent, passive aggressive, pseudoindividuated life style. No matter how clearly these factors are understood, such patients' manipulations often anger therapists.

Imhoff et al. (1983, p. 501) suggest that an SA may see his/her therapist as a "paragon of virtue" who embodies everything the patient is not. This seeming dichotomy provokes the patient's desire to even the score. The patient tries to "cajole, humiliate and deceive the therapist"—to bring him/her down to the patient's own level. By tuning into his/her countertransference, the therapist becomes aware of the pull toward retaliating or being sucked in. He/she can step back and point out the patient's manipulation, revealing his/her own emotional responses when necessary to facilitate the patient's insight into the manipulative behaviors.

Winnicott (1949) emphasizes that therapists typically feel hate toward psychotic and antisocial patients. Furthermore, these patients expect a mixture of love and hate in their interactions with all significant persons. Winnicot suggests that therapists share their hate judiciously, as not to do so would be experienced by the patients as unreal. This sharing is most appropriate later in therapy, when the patients can properly accept it, and should follow the constraints on therapists' sharing that are described later (see "Other Interactive Issues," below). At times, no matter how well a therapist understands his/her countertransference, he/she will dislike a patient.

Therapists can learn to feel more positive toward "unlikable" patients by looking into themselves for similar qualities, by emphasizing the patients' good traits, by understanding the evolution of the patients' personality and behavior, and/or by discovering that they have been genuinely helpful to the patients. Nevertheless, a therapist should not treat too many patients that he/she dislikes, as this often leads to burnout. Poor therapist–patient fits do exist and a change in therapist may be helpful to both parties.

SAs' primitive use of denial may elicit anger, frustration, and withdrawal on the part of many therapists who feel the patient is perfectly capable of accepting that which they are denying.

Other patients may be manipulative, but SAs' manipulations are particularly powerful and threatening, perhaps because their oral needs feel so insatiable and their aggression so primitive and overwhelming. Also, SAs are quite skilled at manipulations because they have relied on such techniques rather than on more normative coping mechanisms. Many therapists reject substance-abusing patients because of their poor prognosis, or because prior apparent successes have often soured. Phase-related therapy as described in this book, as well as by other authors (Brown, 1985; Khantzian et al., 1990), is one way to avoid such repeated disappointments and burnout.

Countertransference and Empathy

I have discussed the many ways in which tuning into countertransference feelings can enhance therapists' empathy as well as understanding. Unfortunately, countertransference problems can also block therapist empathy just as readily. Almost any aspect of countertransference difficulties discussed in this chapter can lead to impairment of empathy. In fact, empathy is probably one of the first therapist qualities to be damaged whenever there is negative countertransference or general burnout. However, several issues are specific to blockage of empathy. A major obstacle to empathy is self-absorption, which is in turn related to the therapist's own unresolved narcissistic needs. The therapist's tendency to experience others as selfobjects may preclude the recognition of their individual personalities and points of view (Chessick, 1985). Therapist inflexibility is another common source of lack of empathy, which results in a focus on skills and techniques to such an extent that relationships with patients become dehumanized (Chessick, 1985). In this context, gestures of empathy are made, but they are stale and lack freshness and individual specificity.

Countertransference and Idealization

"Idealization" refers to the conscious or unconscious process in which the therapist (or other significant person) is given undue value as a result of emotional overestimation, exaltation, or aggrandizement (Kohut, 1971). In most patients, the idealization does not lose touch with the reality of their therapists' assets and limitations (Chessick, 1985). However, in many formerly addicted patients, particularly those with strong narcissistic features, idealization may take on such powerful exaltation that it may elicit negative countertransference responses of embarrassment and distancing in many therapists. Other therapists may become accustomed to a certain level of idealization and may find that they dislike or distance themselves from patients who do not offer this. In such cases, some degree of idealization may be essential to forming a therapeutic alliance, and the absence of idealization may be quite crippling to an essential working alliance.

Therapists may themselves idealize certain aspects of substance-abusing patients and/or their recovery. Too much therapeutic idealization will obviously lead to blind spots. Therapists may also idealize the recovery movement, particularly the fellowship, camaraderie, care and support network it provides, as well as the honesty and self-scrutiny displayed by those who practice the Twelve-Steps. Although the pitfalls of excessive idealization are evident, it should be noted that the inability to idealize patients, their recovery, and their progress in therapy may lead to lack of therapeutic interest, empathy, zeal, and involvement.

Gender-Related Aspects of Countertransference

Most male and female therapists have unavoidably been socialized according to stereotyped gender views. Thus most female therapists are comfortable with pre-Oedipal nurturing transferences, and may tolerate or even encourage these needs, wishes, and fantasies in their patients. Male therapists often have difficulty recognizing and tolerating patients' wishes for primitive touching, rocking, and sucking and may often react with repulsion or denigration.

Female therapists generally have more difficulty with erotic, sexualized (Oedipal) transferences because they feel guilty about their own presumed seductiveness or urges. Male therapists are much more often quite content with their female patients' sexual longings and may even revel in them. On the other hand, homophobic male therapists may be repulsed by their male patients' wishes for either early, tender gratification or developmentally later, sexualized gratification (Wrye & Wells, 1989).

Projective Counteridentification

A form of countertransference first described by Melanie Klein (1946/1984) is projective counteridentification. "Projective counteridentification" is the therapist's response to the patient's projective identification. The latter describes the process by which a patient projects his/her inner destructive forces into the therapist, who responds by acting in accord with the patients's unconscious wishes and repeating the behavior of parental figures in the patient's past. Projective identifications are also seen in other dyadic relationships outside of therapy, particularly when relationships are close or loving. The therapist will inevitably first receive this projective identification without being aware of its contents, meanings, and affects. He/she *unconsciously* reprojects its pathological contents back into the patient, in a nondetached form. The more aware the therapist is of the process and his/her own reactions, the less projective counteridentification there will be, and the more the projective identification will be detoxified and made more benign for the patient's reidentification.

Countertransference and projective identification are inextricably woven together, and it is often difficult for a therapist to distinguish whether he/she is dealing specifically with one or the other. Projective identification differs from projection in that it relies on the other person's (the therapist's) participation in the process. It is interactional and dyadic, whereas projection only requires one person, the projector, for it to take place (Vannicelli, 1989). In the aware therapist, the disruptive impact of these projected forces is neutralized as they are understood and introjected, and subsequently reinternalized by the patient. Projective identification is a primitive form of projection that begins when the patient projects behavior or affect into the therapist. According to Grinberg (1962), the therapist is a *passive* recipient of these patient projections. The therapist's conflicts or anxiety may be activated or intensified by the content of the patient's material, or as a reaction to powerful projections (Grinberg, 1962). The therapist's own ego strength always plays a role in the process and determines the intensity of his/her response. In one of the most extreme forms of productive counteridentification, a therapist may feel a loss of self as the patient's projections threaten to transform him/her into the object the patient unconsciously desires. In a still more extreme form, this phenomenon can explain the sexual seduction of the therapist by the patient (or, carried further, the patient by the therapist).

When therapists listen closely to their patients, respond *calmly* to their affects, and find meaning in their distress, they provide what is termed a "holding" (Modell, 1976) or "containing" (Bion, 1962) function (Hamilton, 1988). Holding helps to detoxify the patient's projective identifications, which are so powerful that many therapists feel overwhelmed or confused by them. The more primitive or pathologic the introject, the more powerful and frightening the introject's effect will be (Hamilton, 1988).

Many therapists react to these projective identifications by being inattentive, feeling bored, imposing overly punitive restrictions, or engaging in other distancing behaviors. Hedges (1983) describes a type of projective identification in which the patient externalizes the child's role into the therapist and identifies with his/her own parents ("active replication"). This is in contrast to the more common "passive replication," in which the patient assumes the child's role and projects his/her parents' role onto the therapist.

"Detoxified reprojection" sounds almost mystical. In fact, it is accomplished through well-defined steps over an extended period of time. It occurs as the therapist becomes aware of the projection and actively helps a patient to realize its conscious and unconscious implications, symbolism, defenses, and underlying pathological introjects. Insight into projective identification does not generally occur until the later stages of therapy. A therapist's ability to identify with a patient's painful emotions and vulnerability often begins with a powerful countertransference, which then becomes a building block for empathy. Thus contemporary therapists have shifted their attitudes 180 degrees—from viewing countertransference as a foreign object to be immediately extruded, to viewing it as a potential first step toward increasing their own empathy as well as promoting personality change in their patients.

Other Interactive Issues

Many other aspects of therapist personality and behavior are integrated with countertransference. These include self-disclosure, therapist errors, and active versus passive posture and personality style (Khantzian et al., 1990).

Self-disclosure should be guided by a simple rule of thumb: The therapist should always share personal information for the good of the patient, and not to relieve or gratify himself/herself. Because of their frequent early deprivations, SAs need a greater degree of genuineness and openness than the majority of other patients. This need should be balanced against not overburdening the psychotherapy with responses that lead to an inappropriate focus on the therapist and his/her own life issues or needs (Khantzian et al., 1990). Many substance-abusing patients' questions are part of their need to know their therapists better, so as to identify with therapists as role models and/or healthy egos (Khantzian et al., 1990). Other questions are part of the normative, warm interactions that go on between an SA and a therapist; not to answer them, particularly in the early stages of therapy, can lead to irreparable narcissistic wounds. On the other hand, many questions asked by an SA may be attempts to divert the emphasis of the therapy away from the patient, to test the therapist's love, to provoke or distance the therapist, or to place the therapist in impossible double binds. In such cases, it is often best to back away from content and focus on the interactive process that is taking place.

The issue of how to deal with the patient's catching the therapist in a countertransference error is complicated. It is often best to admit such mistakes openly, yet therapists should avoid turning therapy sessions into their own confessionals. When a therapist has substantially provoked a reaction, it creates a double-bind situation for the patient, who will then feel quite responsible for something he/she did not cause. The patient's confusion and anxiety are greatly relieved when the therapist acknowledges responsibility. Once the therapist has admitted his/her own role, he/she should nevertheless not hesitate to use the provoked material if it can be helpful to the patient. Thus, therapist errors can often be meaningful grist for the therapeutic mill. Sharing of the therapist's own misfortunes may be empathic or may be evidence of negative countertransference or of parallel process (see below).

The therapist should be aware of his/her own innate tendencies to be active or passive, and to realize that active therapists tend to do better with SAs than therapists who function passively (Okpaku, 1986). Khantzian et al. (1990) state that it is not the activity or passivity of the therapist that is important, but the therapist's awareness of his/her stance, the ways in which it affects others, and its possibilities for bringing about change. Nevertheless, Khantzian et al. (1990) emphasize that these patients need therapists who can actively and empathically engage them around their vulnerabilities. These authors further cite the need for the therapist to be "flexible enough to fill and model a range of roles" (p. 163), from "firm and directive" to "yielding." The need for a "supportive posture in which the therapist communicates respect, admiration, empathy and real concern for distress" is critical (p. 163). It is also suggested that the patient be encouraged to act as a collaborator with the therapist in self-understanding and growth, rather than to conform to the model of active therapist and passive patient (or vice versa).

A TREATMENT-PHASE-RELATED VIEW
OF COUNTERTRANSFERENCE

This present phase-related method of psychotherapy with SAs requires the therapist to make major attitudinal shifts that vary in each phase.

Countertransference in Phases 1 and 2 of Psychotherapy

In the process of establishing abstinence (Phase 1), the therapist may often need to be quite confrontational. Once the patient is detoxified, the therapist shifts first to the role of an educator (or utilizes others to play this role). In early recovery (Phase 2), the therapist develops the educator role by teaching new coping skills, relapse prevention, and more adaptive utilization of defense mechanisms.

Most therapists who follow this model will have patients who are involved (often quite deeply) with AA or other Twelve-Step groups. A patient's sponsor will become a very important person at this point, and this can easily arouse countertransference reactions. Many therapists are quite threatened by the role and importance of sponsors and may become quite competitive with them. A simple technique that I often use is to meet with the sponsor and patient together, in order to develop and review mutual goals and how best to achieve them. This helps the sponsor to be part of the therapeutic team rather than a competitive adversary. In this phase, the therapist should be comfortable in shifting among various roles—those of an educator, of a person who helps the patient maintain his/her sober identity, of a cognitive-behavioral therapist, and of a psychodynamic therapist—as prescribed by the patient's needs.

Although SAs elicit powerful therapist emotions throughout the course of therapy, how therapists deal with these countertransferences will vary with each stage of the therapy. Early on, a therapist should move rapidly to resolve, dissolve, or diffuse intense patient–therapist interactive responses, rather than analyze or share them. SAs often stimulate intensely positive or negative emotions in their therapists quite early in treatment, as they manipulate, seduce, provoke, test, fuse with, and/or reject the therapist.

Positive feelings are aroused by patients who tap therapist omnipotence, narcissism, or rescue fantasies. Patients send messages that evoke positive countertransferences such as the following quite early in therapy:

> "You're the first therapist who ever understood me" (Levine & Stephens, 1972).
> "You're the first therapist I've ever met who knows how to work with addicts/alcoholics/teenagers/women/a real man."
> "You really know how to work with my dreams."
> "You know just how much medication I need for sleep/pain, detox."
> "You're so sensitive that you know how terrible my life is."
> "I've never told anyone else this."
> "Let's you and I as the only knowledgeable people in the program [world] put one over on them" (Levine & Stephens, 1972).
> "Forget about this transference bull; you really are a sexy guy/woman."

"I'm too sick/helpless to be responsible. (So you take care of me.)"
"Your clothes are so hip/elegant/casual/coordinated."
"Your interpretation of that dream/my transference really turned
    my life around."

A naive, narcissistic, or grandiose therapist may be all too ready to
believe these patient remarks. With this kind of boost to the ego, such
a therapist may continue treatment as if it were a wonderful honeymoon, denying how impaired the patient continues to be. Many therapists may also experience negative countertransferences to the seductive
aspects of these remarks.

Alternatively, in early treatment, SAs can also manipulate their
therapists with hostile behavior and remarks such as these:

"You can't understand me; you're not an idealist/you're too con-
    servative/you're too square."
"You can't understand me; you're Hispanic/black and I'm
    white/Oriental or vice versa" (Levine & Stephens, 1972).

Patients use these statements in an attempt to manipulate their therapists into giving more gratification than is helpful. Patient negativity
may also take the form of aggressive remarks, which can either manipulate or distance a therapist:

"Discharge me, or my mob/gang/brother will get you."
"Write a letter that my treatment is complete, if you know what's
    good for you."
"Keep me in the hospital or I won't pay you."
"You're like a cop, not a therapist."
"Give me more medication or I'll leave you for another doctor."
"You don't trust me to go to parties where there's booze/to make
    it without AA/to go back to my cocaine addict husband/to go
    off my Antabuse/enough to show you really understand me."
"By asking me to go to AA/NA/CA, you're setting me up so you
    can reject me."
"Your limits remind me of my father at his worst."
"Don't tell my mother I overdosed. It will kill her."

A therapist may often feel forced into the role of an authoritarian
limit setter with such a patient, in order to require that the patient
follow certain essential guidelines and adhere to the treatment contract. Here the therapist should point out how the patient provokes
this posture, and as soon as possible should remove himself/herself

from this authoritative role (Kernberg et al., 1989). At times, the limit-setting role is so counterproductive to the therapeutic alliance that it is helpful to have two therapists, with one serving mainly as an administrative limit setter. A licensing board or parole officer may serve this function well if such an agency or individual is a part of the treatment network. Often a single therapist can maintain both roles, particularly if he/she can overcome common countertransference issues pertaining to limit setting, such as fears of patient rage and devaluation and desires for idealization (Kernberg et al., 1989).

It is not at all unusual for a therapist to be seduced or coerced by patients who display these manipulative attitudes. To feel positive delight in a recovering patient, or an urge to reject a hostile patient, is normal. The knowledgeable therapist tunes into these feelings, gathering valuable information, but *does not act* on them. The major exception is a calculated (but spontaneously delivered) sharing of therapist feelings in order to provide a patient breakthrough. In the early phases of therapy, neutral or positive countertransferences are more readily shared with patients than are negative ones. Strong therapist anger or dislike is just too overwhelming at this point. Warm, loving, or nurturing therapist emotions are more readily accepted, although these too can be quite threatening, particularly if they are experienced as seductive or invasive. The therapist must strike a balance in order not to gratify the patient's dependent, aggressive, and sexual needs within the transference, and yet to permit his/her humanity, warmth, and concern to come through (Kernberg et al., 1988).

Countertransference in Phase 3 of Psychotherapy

Powerful countertransferences may be evoked in any stage of psychotherapy with SAs, and therapists should be aware of them from the onset. However, they will become more amenable to intervention later in treatment, and therapists are more likely to explore them in depth at that time. In advanced recovery (Phase 3), a major issue is achieving intimacy. The extended period of time that a patient usually spends in therapy prior to reaching this phase lends itself to an intimate relationship with the therapist. Often this intimacy can readily be transferred to an external love object if the therapist is able to let go of his/her own attachment to the patient. This may be difficult because the long-term therapy of an SA is often characterized by dramatic life changes, stimulating the therapist's Pygmalion fantasies. The therapist's ability to let go will also facilitate termination. Although the patient is in analytic psychotherapy in this phase, it is often quite helpful to meet with the patient and his/her new partner together, to educate the couple about support and communication and to resolve mutual transferences. In this phase, another difficult shift in therapist attitude is required—namely, to the role of a more nondirective yet probing therapist who respects the need for the patient's readiness to return to a core identity as a recovering SA (Brown, 1985).

One example of a countertransference reaction that is dealt with more extensively later in therapy is projective counteridentification, defined above and illustrated in the case example provided later in the chapter. Early in therapy, projective identifications are avoided where possible through early interpretation, encouragement of repression, and an emphasis on sobriety through working the Twelve Steps. In later phases, when sobriety is intact, the full process can be permitted to transpire, but it must always be monitored carefully. Still, projective identifications may flourish at any point in the therapy, and it is critical that the therapist be aware of them so that affects can be detoxified, rather than experienced as overwhelming by either therapist or patient.

COUNTERTRANSFERENCE-RELATED PHENOMENA

Parallel Process

A very important set of therapist countertransference reactions can be considered as part of "parallel process." Parallel process occurs when a therapist, in his/her life outside the therapy, experiences a powerful situation that is very similar to the patient's situation (Doehrman & Gross, 1976). This leads the therapist to place undue emphasis on issues, attitudes, or transferences from his/her own past or present life or therapy with the patient. It is no accident that therapists often find their patients to be working on the same issues that therapists are addressing in their own therapy. Commonly, too, therapists find that patients are working on themes espoused by the therapists' mentors or by the authors of articles they are currently reading. A variation of this occurs when a therapist's behavior to a patient is motivated by competition with a colleague who previously treated the patient or who has written of successes with similar patients. This phenomenon arises as well in group supervision, or in instances when a therapist is called upon to present a case to colleagues and feels judged or evaluated by them or has a need to impress them.

Parallel process also takes place when the therapist acts toward a supervisor as a patient has acted toward the therapist, or when the therapist acts toward a patient as a supervisor or another therapist has acted toward the therapist. For example, a patient of mine became anxious and confused when I shook his hand at the end of the session—a new interaction for us. When I presented this case to my supervisor, he extended the supervision time by 30 minutes, leaving me confused by his need to indulge me.

Perhaps the most powerful instances of parallel process occur when a patient's real-life experiences mirror those of a therapist (e.g., divorce, difficulties with supervisors, existential crises, or the death of a parent, child, or other loved one). Similar events in a therapist's past or present life may have caused him/her difficulties. This overidentification can be used to facilitate empathy, but it can backfire into pity or can cause the therapist to overlook core aspects of the patient's contribution to his/her own difficulties. Therapists' reactions to patients on the basis of their own prejudices about abortion, religion, contraception, and politics are further examples of parallel process.

Therapist Denial, Enabling, Codependence, and Burnout

Therapist "denial," "enabling," "codependence," and "burnout" are terms used in the chemical dependence field to describe phenomena related to countertransference. All four may occur during any phase of therapy. Therapists, particularly those who do not work primarily with SAs, will often deny that their patients are abusing or dependent on drugs and/or alcohol. They may be aware of their patients' substance use, but may not treat it as a serious problem because of their fallacious belief that the use of chemicals is secondary to the underlying psychological problem, and that when the latter is unearthed the substance abuse will go away. Commonly, therapists compare their own use of drugs and alcohol to their patients'; using that standard, they often deny their patients' use as well as their own.

Therapists may deny substance use or relapse because of their need to see their patients as improving. They may also deny the consequences of use, particularly if they overidentify with patients in their struggle with society or their families. Therapists who maintain contact with family members, employee assistance counselors, or probation departments have the advantage of tracking the effects of substance use, but this must be balanced with maintaining patients' trust and confidentiality. Therapist "enabling" and "codependence" are terms that are frequently used interchangeably. I believe that they reflect different aspects of the same phenomenon of therapist overinvolvement. Thus, codependence occurs when patients and/or their outcomes become overly important to therapists' own psychological well-being. Enabling occurs specifically when a therapist either continues to treat someone in psychotherapy who is actively dependent on drugs or alcohol, or protects a patient from the consequences of his/her actions. As a result of the therapist's behavior, the patient is then enabled to continue drug and alcohol abuse.

Therapists who are not familiar with the concept of codependence would still recognize all of the characteristics attributed to that entity as problematic countertransference if they observed other therapists relating to their patients in that manner. Therapists do not have to have had parents, siblings or spouses who were themselves SAs to manifest codependent behaviors. They may behave codependently if, in their own moods and sense of self as they grew up, they were particularly sensitive to the pain or lack of well-being in others. Most therapists learn very early in their training not to accept the degree of responsibility for healing others that codependent persons accept.

Treating patients while they continue to abuse drug/alcohol gives them the illusion that they are doing something about their problems when in fact they are not. Writing letters to get chemically dependent individuals off from work or out of jail is enabling them by reinforcing that they are immune from the consequences of their actions. It may also prevent them from hitting the level of "bottom" necessary to make them truly sincere in seeking help. The most overt enabling behavior occurs when doctors continue to prescribe habituating medications to patients who are abusing them. Most substance-dependent patients are extremely skillful in these manipulations, and physicians may not be aware that they are being manipulated.

If therapists are overinvolved with their patients to a point of accepting excessive responsibility for their welfare or failures, they are more likely to experience burnout. Therapists are also vulnerable to burnout if they treat more than a few patients who are continuing to drink or use drugs. Burnout can result when therapists are exhausted from trying too hard or doing too much of the work, or when the ratio of successes to failures is lower than they can tolerate. It can also occur simply if therapists work too hard and have no means to recuperate. Burnout is often manifested as physical and mental exhaustion, a negative self-concept, poor attitude about the job, and loss of concern and feeling for clients (Stillson & Katz, 1985). Therapists can prevent burnout by attention to self-preservation through nurturing themselves, and thinking of themselves as valuable and treasured resources. This self-nurturing stance is in contrast to narcissistic distancing, which separates a therapist from patients during sessions. The necessary self-repair occurs primarily through nurturing intimate relationships outside of therapy, as well as through living a well-rounded life with proper attention to diet, health, exercise, spirituality, recreation, family, and socialization (Imhoff et al., 1983).

Therapists may feel a sense of success rather than failure when patients relapse and then ask for help, particularly early in the relapse process. This is because the patients are actively seeking help and struggling to return to abstinence. Some patients have to be detoxified 10 or 15 times before they finally become sufficiently motivated to accept the help they need. Therapists should view slips, particularly if they lead to greater self-knowledge and resumption of a therapeutic program, as aspects of the process of recovery rather than indications of failure. (Of course, too kind a view of slips is enabling behavior.) Therapists can also redefine what they consider "success." Certainly, substantially longer periods of abstinence after treatment than before, or shorter, less severe relapses and generally better functioning, should not be denigrated as goals (Stillson & Katz, 1985).

In giving workshops around the United States, I have been struck with the amount of burnout that exists and the extent to which it has grown in the last 10 years. Part of this may be a result of changing social conditions, such as shrinking resources allocated to the poor and homeless, which have left therapists who work with these patients very frustrated by their inability to help motivated clients. Stillson and Katz (1985) point out that other sources of burnout are countertransference feelings that involve taking on the characteristics of patients. Thus therapists may feel hopeless or passive, and may even drink or use drugs. Therapists may also respond to the impulsiveness of patients' needs and try to meet them immediately—a good source of burnout, as well as a poor model for teaching necessary postponement of gratification. Stillson & Katz (1985) point out that therapists' understanding and using the feelings that patients create in them (i.e., a knowledge of countertransference) will help them to feel competent and avoid burnout.

Therapist Family-of-Origin Issues

Still another way to view a therapist's out-of-control responses to a patient is from a family systems point of view, in which the therapist replays unresolved issues from his/her own family of origin with the patient and the patient's family. The converse of this is frequently true when the patient is dealing with more than one therapeutic person at the same time, as in hospital or clinic settings. In this situation, the patient will frequently play one therapist off against the other in much the same way as the patient formerly manipulated his/her parents or was manipulated by them. A therapist's ability to avoid being drawn into recreating this system depends on knowledge of his/her own family and development, as well as of coping mechanisms for not being drawn into such "splitting" and manipulative behaviors. Therapists may also react inappropriately to other aspects of patients because of similarities to their own families of origin or procreation.

RECOGNITION OF COUNTERTRANSFERENCE

Although countertransference reactions are as varied and multitudinous as human personality quirks, there are ways in which therapists can tune into their behaviors so as to detect that they are experiencing countertransference. Some of these have been mentioned throughout this chapter, but they are summarized here. Overt behaviors that signal countertransference are obvious; yet therapists may easily deny these signs, attributing them to realities such as busy schedules or the like. The overt behaviors include (Vannicelli, 1989) lateness, changing or cutting short appointments, not returning phone calls, not holding a patient to his/her therapeutic contract, changing appointment times, drowsiness, and falling asleep. (Despite therapists who feel that falling asleep is an appropriate confrontation of a patient's boring qualities, I am of the opinion that falling asleep by the therapist is always inappropriate and invariably damages the therapeutic alliance.)

Somewhat less overt manifestations of countertransference include rapid shifts in therapist behavior, particularly in areas such as these: being more solicitous or hostile; being more self-serving; making more interpretations that are premature and unnecessary; decreasing verbal productions (Imhoff et al., 1983); and experiencing inappropriate or unusual affective responses, or stereotyped or repetitive responses, to the patient (Vannicelli, 1989).

Covert signs include shifts in attitude that are unexpected or capricious; preoccupation with thoughts, dreams, and/or fantasies (particularly regressive, dependent, or sexual ones); feeling stuck; wanting to miss a session (Vannicelli, 1989); or wishing the patient would cancel. Some of these signs may not be expressions of personalized countertransference, but may indicate life style problems. They may occur when therapists are so busy in their personal or professional lives that they have too many obligations to meet in one lifetime. Therapists who are too overworked to meet their patients' appropriate needs will by definition have countertransference problems with most if not all of their patients.

Vannicelli (1989) proposes that a therapist can recognize countertransference issues by taking a structured, self-reflective stance in which the therapist tunes into basic aspects of the therapy, such as what the basic ground rules are, how they are communicated, and how the therapist handles modifications initiated by himself/herself or by the patient. When the ground rules are not explicit, or when either patient or therapist consistently violates them, countertransference is in evidence.

Therapist behaviors toward SAs may be characterized by disengagement as well as overinvolvement, just as SAs' extratherapeutic relationships may be. An SA's behavior either sucks others into enmeshment or drives them away. Thus therapists should carefully examine evidence for extreme behavior in either direction, particularly nonverbal. Enmeshed touching behaviors include hugging, stroking, kissing, sitting very closely, or even engaging in prolonged handshakes. Other nonverbal seductive therapist behaviors include revealing dress, posturing, or lingering eye contact. I prefer a Twelve-Step type of confirming hug at the end of a session when touch is indicated, as other types of more intimate touching are generally inappropriate. (See Chapter 9 for further discussion of "Twelve-Step hugs.") More primitive touching, such as rocking or rubbing, is also almost always inappropriate and counterproductive with these patients. Although touching should be spontaneous and natural, it should be weighed carefully and often be discussed before and/or after the actual touching takes place.

Nonverbal distancing behaviors include sitting at a greater distance; cessation of prior appropriate/social touching; not giving eye contact; shifting to silence; and withholding of interpretation, suggestion, direction, or other direct gratification that was previously given. Therapists who are feeling distant can confirm this feeling by tuning into their own restlessness, fidgeting, consumption of liquids, smoking, glancing at their watches, intense wishes to have sessions end, or hopes that their patients will not show up.

Still other signs of countertransference include having dreams or experiencing anxiety or preoccupation about a patient or group of patients; feeling deprived of being a human being with a patient; losing one's basic therapeutic abilities; or feeling helpless. Therapists' tuning into thoughts that cross their minds when they are with patients, or thoughts about the patients when they are not present, can also provide indications of countertransference.

A CASE HISTORY

A patient came immediately to mind as I was writing this chapter. Anita* was a 35-year-old, single attorney who had been unable to work

---

*A pseudonym has been used; certain identifying facts have been changed to insure confidentiality.

at her chosen profession for 3 years because of "depression." She intermittently treated her depression and food cravings with intranasal cocaine. She was referred to me by her East Coast psychiatrist, who did not know me; the referral was based solely on my dual membership in the American Psychoanalytic Association and the American Society for Addiction Medicine. The psychiatrist stated that he felt these dual credentials were necessary to treat someone like Anita.

I initially changed Anita's antidepressant drug to one with less uncomfortable side effects, and she responded with rapid improvement, immediately overidealizing me and her new medication. She revealed a history of repeated abusive relationships with men, in which she described herself as a helpless victim. She was abused in every imaginable way as an adult, including rape, unpaid loans, theft, unkept promises, and numerous bruises from severe beatings. She recalled no physical abuse during her childhood. Her mother was a recovering alcoholic, with 5 years of sobriety through a rehabilitation program and AA after a lifetime of alcoholism. The mother was the overidealized object; the father was viewed as rejecting, demanding of perfection, and unaware of who Anita was as a real person. At times the parental roles of good and bad object were reversed.

I continued to be Anita's overidealized savior as long as the medication worked and she did not use cocaine. When she again began to use cocaine, she called repeatedly in a total state of panic. She became furious at me when I did not agree that her paranoid perceptions were real and did not agree to fix her problem instantly. After several nights of hourly phone calls, my limit setting became progressively harsh and rejecting. After the second of these paranoid episodes, she responded to my interdiction and began to attend CA meetings regularly. She rapidly found a home base where several meetings were held daily, but did not select a sponsor. A man with 2 years of cocaine sobriety befriended her, and she rapidly became sexually involved with him. Shortly thereafter, she claimed that he had borrowed money from her and refused to pay it back, and that he was insulting her to the other CA members. She dropped out of CA, stating that the men there were no better than her ex-con boyfriends.

After a short period of sobriety, she began to attribute some of her many somatic complaints to the antidepressant I had prescribed, and chastised me severely for not knowing that the drug could cause these effects and not immediately stopping the drug. I found myself forgetting to call-forward my telephone calls to my secretary during her sessions, changing the times of her sessions, and starting late. She was unable to confront me, but told her litany of complaints about me to everyone around us. She became sexually involved with her former cocaine pusher and again started using coke. Early in her "slip" she was able to confront me about my rejection, but I was unable to see my own participation in the process. Finally, she came early to a rescheduled session to see my car pull away. She stormed into my secretary's office and angrily told her that she was leaving. When I arrived back a few minutes later at our appointed time, I was told that she had left very angrily. This caused a serious rift in our working alliance, to which I had certainly contributed. I too had responded to her hostile dependence by rejecting her, as had her father and every other male in her life. I called and apologized for not waiting for her. We resumed treatment, and I started Anita on a new antidepressant, to which she initially responded very positively. However, I made the mistake of not addressing my own projective counteridentification at that time, even though I was becoming aware of it. In retrospect, this was because of my own guilt about rejecting her as everyone else had.

After 14 months of treatment, Anita had her most disturbed, paranoid cocaine psychosis to date, and was hospitalized involuntarily as "gravely disabled" (unable to care for herself). She was too disturbed to be housed in the hospital's open chemical dependence unit, so she was first placed in the locked psychiatric building. After a premature discharge at her insistence, she immediately had another brief cocaine binge and was rehospitalized on the chemical dependence unit. She completed 2 weeks of inpatient treatment and 2 weeks more in a 5-hour daily partial hospital program. Shortly before her discharge from the latter program, she appeared far better integrated than I had ever seen her, looking every bit the competent professional woman that her past work record proclaimed.

At this point I realized that Anita, through projective identification, had produced in me rejecting behaviors similar to those that she reported in her father (and denied in her mother), as well as in every significant heterosexual relationship in her adult life. Then I shared my feelings with her, and owned that they were my responsibility and were antitherapeutic; I also compared what was going on between us with her relationships outside of the therapy. In response to my intervention and attitudinal shift, her projective identification diminished greatly, as did my own projective counteridentification. In the hospital, she was able to see the many ways that she provoked people to treat her like a victim, as well as her splitting people into good and bad objects and playing them against each other. This was accomplished by the treatment team's multiple, loving confrontations of her behavior. As she faced her last days in the partial hospital program, she began to deal directly with the many stresses she was facing, particularly a new career training program. At this point, I found myself being much more supportive and empathic with her. Still, she focused on the side effects of the new antidepressant, discontinuing it and chastising me for not "hearing" her complaints. I pointed out to her that she not only alternated between praising and denigrating the significant people in her life; she treated her medications in the same way. Three years after her hospitalization, she was still sober and had completed her career retraining program successfully. She was most recently involved in the "best relationship of her life" for 12 months with a man who did not abuse her and was quite supportive, although their relationship was not sexual. However, he drank heavily on a daily basis (but, according to Anita, never showed signs of intoxication). They were able to end their relationship without any mutually destructive behavior and out of a clear understanding of the ways in which it was destructive for both of them. Perhaps this man represented her soothing, drunken mother of childhood.

Patients' slips into substance use and abuse, like those of Anita, always evoke some measure of countertransference, because these slips put everyone close to the patient into a no-win double bind. The proper therapeutic stance is to be neither too rejecting nor too accepting. The therapist who demands too rapid a commitment to too many measures for total sobriety, and offers immediate cessation of treatment if the measures are not followed, will invariably be replaying the role of hostile, rejecting parent. The therapist who accepts slips with unconditional love, and requires no constraints toward a commitment to sobriety, will not only be an enabler; he/she will also be fulfilling the role of the overprotective parent who perpetuates helplessness and chemical dependence. A flexible middle ground, uncomplicated by unresolved countertransference, is the most helpful approach.

MANAGEMENT OF COUNTERTRANSFERENCE REACTIONS THAT INTERFERE WITH PSYCHOTHERAPY

1. The first step is the recognition of antitherapeutic countertransference feelings (i.e., feelings that are out of control to such an extent that a therapist is unable to utilize them to be helpful). The signs of countertransference have been described above. The most direct signs of countertransference that can interfere with therapy include the therapist's feeling stuck, anxious, furious, rejecting, incompetent, trapped, manipulated, or preoccupied with a patient.

2. The next step, according to Kernberg et al. (1989), is to identify the source of the countertransference. These authors suggest that the therapist first look for obvious provocations (e.g., acting out) that

directly threaten or endanger the therapist. The therapist next should note the uniqueness of his/her reaction to a given patient as another clue to countertransference.

3. Next, the therapist examines carefully "who's doing what to whom" and what early experiences are being duplicated, maintaining empathy with the patient's dominant state as well as with his/her projections (Kernberg et al., 1988). The ability to perform these steps while maintaining a carefully delineated therapeutic role permits the therapist to utilize primitive wishes and fears in order to understand the patient (Kernberg et al., 1989).

4. Following recognition and understanding of the source, the therapist must actively intervene to change the situation if he/she is unable to resolve uncontrollable countertransferences.

5. This is generally done either by consultating with a trusted colleague or supervisor, returning to therapy, or rereading a helpful text (Vannicelli, 1989). Finally, with an understanding of the problem and how to deal with it, the therapist must put a solution into practice.

6. Once the therapist has achieved this state of readiness, the patient is usually remarkably cooperative in again bringing up the issue, re-experiencing the affect, or reproducing the scenario that elicited the countertransference response. The therapist, armed with understanding and a "bag of solutions," not only will have insight but will exude a calming presence, which also aids in resolution of the countertransference or in detoxification and "holding" of the projective identification.

7. The experience of intensive personal psychotherapy with transference resolution is very helpful in dealing with powerful countertransferences. The second essential ingredient is to have worked with these therapist reactions under the guidance of a capable and trusted supervisor. Under the spell of powerful, uncontrollable countertransferences, the therapist should first turn to consultation; if that is not sufficient, he/she should consider a return to psychotherapy.

A further utilization of the countertransference as a therapeutic tool has been proposed by Hedges (1992), and is very appropriate in Phase 3 of psychotherapy with SAs. He suggests that the transference–countertransference engagement replicates the seduction or abuse that the patient experienced in childhood. Here the therapist may assume the role of either abused or abuser. Hedges (1992) suggests that the interpretation of countertransference be accomplished through 10 basic therapeutic strategies: (1) a focusing on the symbiotic character structure by tuning into images and metaphors that go beyond empathic attunement to the therapist's primary identification with the patient's parent or infant self; (2) creating an atmosphere in which the therapist can present the material playfully, freely, tentatively, creatively, and spontaneously; (3) avoiding therapist ventilation, discharge, or confession; (4) aborting any sense of blaming or accusing the patient for the therapist's reaction; (5) being wary of the patient's agreeing out of false-self conformity; (6) prefacing the interpretation with the patient's anticipated negative reaction; (7) avoiding the error of not making the interpretation for fear that the feeling belongs only to the therapist; (8) being cautious about feeling that the therapist can always be totally correct; (9) timing the interpretation when there is an appropriate bridge of mutual understanding; and (10) retaining a measure of uncertainty about "how much is one's (i.e., the therapist's] own."

The work of Hedges has evolved out of the intersubjective view of therapist–patient interactions, as presented by Stolorow et al. (1987) and others. This view represents a move away from content to deeper "corrective emotional process" interpretations. It can be utilized to achieve the last pieces of work with addicts and alcoholics—again, when their sobriety is sufficiently stabilized. However, this type of countertransference interpretation, when made according to the 10 guidelines listed above, is much easier for patients to tolerate than unexplained or unintroduced impulsive displays of therapist affect. Still, even the latter may be useful if the therapist recognizes and, when appropriate, shares their origins within the the interactional context.

CONCLUDING COMMENT

The field of psychoanalysis has made great contributions to therapists' understanding and use in treatment of their own reactions to patients, whether these are referred to as "countertransference" or called by some other name. This chapter has attempted to make these concepts available and understandable to therapists from all backgrounds and levels of experience.

CHAPTER 9

The Integration
of Individual
and Group Therapy

Substance abuse is a severe illness that pervades every aspect of an individual's existence. It is rare that so extensive an illness can be reversed by individual therapy alone. Thus I espouse an integration of individual therapy, Twelve-Step work, group therapy, and family treatment, with specific combinations of treatments tailored to each individual's needs.

GROUP THERAPY
WITH SUBSTANCE ABUSERS THEMSELVES

Group therapy has frequently been designated as the treatment of choice with SAs (Cahn, 1970; Hoffman et al., 1976; Khantzian et al., 1990, Vannicelli, 1992). As I see it, group therapy is an essential component of the integrated, individualized approach to addicts and alcoholics. The advantages of group therapy for SAs, as suggested by Vannicelli (1992), are as follows:

1. Groups reduce SAs' sense of isolation through the recognition that they are not alone and that they can be understood. This leads to instant, early bonding, with ties that develop increasing depth as a group becomes more cohesive over time. In the later stages, sobriety rather than the disease becomes the glue that holds the group together.
2. Groups provide ongoing support, safety, and containment.

3 . Groups instill hope by providing new members with access to longer-term members who are successful.
4. Groups permit members to learn from watching others. Many conflicts are more easily resolved by first watching and helping others work through them, then applying what is thereby learned to oneself.
5. Groups provide members with information about coping and relapse prevention strategies, community resources, and support groups.
6. Groups permit members to model ways of communicating and interacting.
7. Groups provide a laboratory for the study of the members' actual here-and-now interactions, as well as a variety of transference reactions particularly those related to siblings.

Another important advantage of group therapy is the dilution of powerful dependent, aggressive transferences, which can overwhelm a patient and lead to relapse. Groups can gratify dependent needs without overwhelming patients or therapists.

As I also discuss in regard to family therapy in Chapter 10, there are advantages and disadvantages in utilizing a therapist for the group who is not the members' individual therapist. Personally, I prefer to act as both the individual and the group therapist. However, I often utilize cotherapists for groups, particularly a recovering addict/alcoholic and/or a female (the latter provides a ready opportunity to work out maternal transferences). All patients in my own long-term groups start out in individual therapy with me. I also conduct my own weekly inpatient group, in addition to the three or four groups that are held daily by the hospital program.

Although I have conducted my own long-term outpatient group for SAs for most of my professional career, at the present time I employ a master's-level therapist with over 15 years of sobriety to conduct these groups with my outpatients. In general, it is preferable to have all patients who are in group therapy have the same status in regard to individual therapy with the primary group therapist; that is, either all receive it or none do. If the leader sees some group members individually and not others, then those who are seen individually are felt to have special status with the group leader (Vannicelli, 1992).

Group therapy varies with each of the three phases in the individual psychotherapy of these patients. Many of the basic principles of group therapy with SAs are similar to those described in connection with individual psychotherapy (see Chapters 5–7) and family therapy (see Chapter 10), and are not repeated here.

Phase 1 of Treatment

In the first phase of psychotherapy, the type of group utilized will depend on the treatment setting—hospital, residential, intensive outpatient (also termed partial hospitalization), or limited outpatient.

In hospital settings, educational groups are an essential part of the early treatment process, and the subjects covered in these groups are quite similar to those in educational family groups, which are described in the following chapter. The major differing emphasis in patient educational groups is on the physiological aspects and risk factors of drugs of abuse and alcohol. Other important issues covered didactically in these groups are as follows: (1) assertion training; (2) other compulsive behaviors, such as sexuality, eating, working, and gambling; (3) relapse prevention; (4) the prolonged abstinence syndrome; (5) leisure skills; and (6) cross-addiction. All educational groups include appropriate coping strategies, some of which are developed from the experiences of recovering members.

One advantage of 28-day residential programs (now more often 7- to 21-day programs, followed by intensive 6-hour-a-day outpatient treatment) is that group therapy can be started immediately after drinking or drug use stops. In their first few sober days, SAs are so needy that their resistance to groups is low. After a few days of sobriety, defenses resolidify, and therapy is often resisted. Without alcohol or drugs to relieve life's problems, SAs are depressed and frightened. They feel they have nothing to contribute to society or to a group, yet they desperately need support. At this stage, the therapists and the group should show newly sober SAs how to borrow the confidence that life without alcohol or drugs is possible and better than life with it. This hope is best offered by a therapist or cotherapist who is a recovering SA with solid sobriety. Therapeutic groups in these settings will also deal with appropriate expressions of feelings, relationships with significant others, childhood molestations and abuse, self-esteem building, and development of strategies for self-care.

A critical aspect of group therapy here is for SAs to experience the sharing of a group of individuals struggling against their addiction. This helps to overcome feelings of isolation and shame, which are so common in these patients. The formation of a helping sober peer group that provides support for a lifetime, in and out of Twelve-Step groups and formal psychotherapy sessions, is very helpful and dramatic when it occurs.

In residential settings, particularly therapeutic communities such as Phoenix House or Daytop, recovering SAs are used as primary therapists in the first phases of the program. The techniques that they utilize include identification, love and concern, confrontation, responsibility, acting "as-if," reward and punishment, stratified groups, and emphasis on the present (Kaufman, 1972).

In outpatient programs, there is less of an opportunity to perform uncovering therapy in the early phases. The more infrequent the therapeutic contact, the lesser the ability to deal with underlying conflicts. Also, there is less protection and less of a holding environment than in residential settings.

Voluntary group therapy is often difficult to establish in methadone maintenance programs. However, mandatory groups may be effective with SAs. I have utilized several principles in setting up voluntary groups in methadone programs (Kaufman, 1978):

1. Select as group leaders persons with high status in the program, such as program directors, respected psychiatrists or psychologists, or other therapists.
2. Time groups to coincide with methadone dispensing. (Most patients are not motivated to return a second time in a day, or on a day they do not receive methadone.)
3. Use the patients' negative feelings as an impetus to start groups. Thus, groups can be started with patients who complain about conditions or who "hang out" around the program.
4. Have counselors draw their groups from patients in their own caseload, so that there is an established therapeutic alliance.
5. Begin some task-oriented groups (e.g., groups centering around women's issues, patient government, socialization, health and sex education, detoxification, or discussion).
6. Group leaders should be consistent and hold groups if even only one member appears. A cotherapist should direct the group if the primary leader is absent for any reason. (This is particularly important in the early phases of such groups.)
7. The milieu of the clinic must shift so that patients are not motivated to get methadone for as little effort as possible, but rather to participate in a maximum number of helping activities. (This principle has been developed in the course of the recent defending of therapeutic services for methadone patients.)
8. Avoid placing patients in the same group who have severe conflicts with each other outside of the program.
9. Use pretreatment group experiences or a didactic group to prepare patients for the working group (e.g., to develop communication skills, explore fears, develop trust in leaders and other patients, and provide support and reassurance).

Others, particularly Woody et al. (1986), have developed detailed group therapy techniques for methadone patients. In addition, Brown and Yalom (1977) and Vannicelli (1992), working with alcoholics, and Khantzian et al. (1990), working with cocaine addicts, have adapted psychodynamic techniques for group work with these patients.

Ex-addicts and recovering alcoholics are valuable as cotherapists, particularly in the early stages of groups (they may even serve as primary or sole therapists at this stage). Commonality of experience with clients, by itself, does not qualify an individual to be a therapist. Recovering persons should have at least 2 years of sobriety before they are permitted to function as group therapists. The techniques that help SAs become experienced therapists are best learned gradually and under close supervision, preferably by both experienced paraprofessionals and professionals. As noted earlier, another helpful pairing in cotherapy is male–female pairing, which provides a balance of male and female role models and transferences.

During the early sessions of group therapy with SAs, the focus is on the shared problem of substance abuse and its meaning to each individual. The therapist should be more active in this phase, which should be instructional and informative as well as therapeutic (Fox, 1962). SAs tend toward confessionals and monologues about prior drinking/drug use. These can be politely interrupted or minimized by a ground rule of "no drunkalogues/drugalogues." Romanticizing past use of drugs or alcohol is strongly discouraged.

The desire to drink/use drugs and the fear of slipping are pervasive early concerns in these groups. The patients' attitude is one of resistance and caution, combined with fear of open exploration. Members are encouraged to participate in AA or other Twelve-Step groups; yet the high-support, low-conflict, inspirational style of such groups may inhibit attempts at uncovering, interactional therapy. There may be a conspiracy of silence about material that members fear could cause discomfort or lead to drugs or drinking. The therapists can point out to the members that they choose to remain static and within comfortable defenses, rather than expose themselves to the discomfort associated with change. Patients usually drop out early if they are still committed to using drugs or drinking. Other patients who drop out at this stage do so because they grow increasingly alarmed as they become aware of the degree of discomfort that any significant change requires.

Therapists should not be overly protective and prematurely relieve the group members' anxiety, since this fosters denial of emotions. On the other hand, the members' recognition of emotions and responsibility must proceed slowly, since both are particularly threatening to SAs. Patients at this stage are superficially friendly, but do not show real warmth or tenderness; "Twelve-Step hugs" (see below) are an easy way to begin to show physical support. Group members are also afraid to express anger or to assert themselves. However, sudden irritation, antipathy, and anger toward the leaders and other members inevitably begin to appear as the group progresses. Gradually, tentative overtures of friendship and understanding are manifested.

Phase 2 of Treatment

In the second phase of treatment, the emphasis in group therapy is quite similar to that in individual therapy. Therapists should continue to focus on cognitive-behavioral techniques to maintain sobriety. Intensive affects are abreacted toward significant persons outside of the group, but are minimized and modulated between group members. In this stage there evolves a beginning awareness of the role of personality and social interactions in the use of drugs and alcohol. SAs are ambivalent about positive feedback. They beg for it, yet reject it when it is given. They repeatedly ask for physical reassurance such as a warm hug, but may panic when they receive it because of fear of intimacy and a re-experiencing of their unmet past needs. A "Twelve-Step hug"* is comforting but less threatening and is appropriate between patients. Therapists should be relatively discreet about giving even Twelve-Step hugs to patients, but hugging is more appropriate in group settings, where it is less potentially seductive and more of a group norm.

There is a fear of success and a dread of competing in life, as well as in the group. Success means destroying the other group members (siblings) and loss of the therapists (parents). Rigidity and denial are greater in groups of SAs than in any other groups I have worked with except those of chronic schizophrenics. They are afraid to talk about unpleasant experiences because they fear they will be overwhelmed by their previous pain. They are reluctant to explore fantasies, since the thought makes them feel as guilty as the act. They view emotions as black or white. This makes them withhold critical comments because they fear their criticism will provoke chaos and substance use in other members. This withholding may be on a conscious or unconscious level. They are frequently overly conscientious. Those who were older siblings or were raised by substance-abusing parents have often felt that they had to be the responsible members of their families even when they were children. Thus they assume blame and guilt for the emo-

---

*A "Twelve-Step hug" is generally an inverted V, with the tops of shoulders touching and mutual back patting. It is warm but without intimacy or sexuality.

tional pain of other group members. Rage has been expressed either explosively or not at all. Its expression in Phase 2 of group therapy should be encouraged, but gradually and under slowly releasing controls.

The other crucial affect that must be dealt with is depression. Initially, a severe depression occurs immediately after detoxification. This appears vegetative in its severity but usually remits rapidly, leaving SAs with a chronic low-grade depression, which is frequently expressed by silence, lack of energy, and vegetative signs. These patients should be drawn out slowly and patiently. Ultimately, they are encouraged to cry or mourn. A distinction is made between helping these patients deal with despair and rushing to take it away from them.

Role playing or doubling may facilitate expression of anger. In "doubling," a therapist or another group member will sit behind a patient and express feelings that seem obvious yet are dammed up. When the patient finally expresses anger, he/she should be cheered and rewarded by the group. Assertiveness training may increase the ability to express anger and to accept it.

The success of Phase 2 of group therapy with SAs depends on the therapists' and the group members' ability to relieve anxiety through support, insight, and the use of more adaptive and concrete strategies for dealing with it. Alcohol and drugs must become unacceptable solutions to anxiety. In this vein, it is important not to end a session with members in a state of grossly unresolved conflict. This can be avoided by closure when excessively troubling issues are raised. Closure can be achieved by the group's concrete suggestions for problem solution. When this is not possible, group support, including contact between members outside of group sessions, can be offered. Brown and Yalom (1977) utilize a summary of the content of each group, which is mailed to members between sessions and helps provide closure and synthesis.

Phase 3 of Treatment

In the final phase of treatment, SAs in group therapy will express and work through feelings, responsibility for behavior, interpersonal interactions, and the functions and secondary gain of drugs and alcohol. In this phase, reconstructive group techniques as practiced by well-trained professionals are extremely helpful; indeed, they are essential if significant shifts in ego strength are to be accomplished. Here, the SAs will become able to analyze defenses, resistance, and transference. The multiple transferences that develop in the group are recognized as "old tapes" that are not relevant to the present. Problems of

sibling rivalry, competition with authority, and separation anxiety become manifest in the group, and their transference aspects are developed and interpreted. Conflicts are analyzed on both the intrapsychic
and interpersonal levels. Ventilation and catharsis take place and may
be enhanced by group support. Excessive reliance on fantasy is abandoned (Fox, 1962).

A study of alcoholics found that those who survived a high initial
dropout rate stayed in groups longer than neurotic patients (Yalom
et al., 1978); thus, it seems that a substantial number of SAs in Phase
2 should reach this final phase. By the time SAs have reached Phase
3, they act like patients in high-functioning neurotic groups. They have
accepted sobriety without resentment and can work to free themselves
from unnecessary neurotic and character problems (Fox, 1962). They
have developed a healthy self-concept, combined with empathy for
others, and have scaled down their inordinate demands of others for
superego reassurance. They have also become effectively assertive rather
than destructively aggressive and have developed a reasonable sense
of values. More fulfilling relationships with spouses, children, and
friends can be achieved (Fox, 1962).

When one or more members leave the group, the decision to leave
should be discussed for several weeks before a final date is set. This
permits the group to mourn the lost member(s) and vice versa. This
is true regardless of the stage of the group, but the most intense work
is done when termination occurs in Phase 3. In open-ended groups,
the leadership qualities of the graduating member(s) are then taken
over by others, who then may apply these qualities to life outside the
group.

GROUP THERAPY INVOLVING FAMILY MEMBERS

Other forms of group treatment, such as multiple-family group treatment and couples groups, combine the principles of group and family
work.

Multiple-Family Group Treatment

Multiple-family group treatment is a technique that can be used in any
treatment setting for SAs, but is most successful in hospital and residential settings, where family members are usually more readily available.
In a residential setting, the group may be composed of all of the families, or the community may be separated into several groups of three
or four closely matched families (Kaufman, 1982). Most multiple-family

groups now include the entire community, because this provides a sense of the entire patient group as a supportive family. In residential settings, these groups meet weekly for 2–3 hours. In hospitals, a family week or weekend is often offered as an alternative or adjunct to a weekly group.

There are often as many as 10 to 15 families and 40 to 50 individuals in multiple-family groups. Families should be oriented and interviewed prior to their entering in the group. The group includes identified patients and their immediate families, as well as any relatives with significant impact on the family. Friends and lovers are included if they are an important part of the SAs' network and are drug-free. If they abuse drugs or alcohol, they are excluded from the group until they control this symptom; otherwise, they are often quite disruptive or destructive in the group. However, there are no rigid guidelines about excluding family members or friends, since meaningful material and a true picture of a family may come from anyone who knows a patient.

In a multiple-family group, an experienced family therapist often works with program counselors as cotherapists. In addition, group members frequently function as adjunctive family therapists. Usually family members take their cues from primary therapists and will be appropriately confronting, reassuring, and supportive. Didactic sessions for family members are often held to teach the difference between appropriate support and enabling. At times the needs of a particular family's members prevent this, and their anger at their alcoholic/addicted relative will spill over onto other identified patients in the group. At other times, a family's protective and possessive qualities may be inappropriately directed toward group members. Families also share experiences and offer help by acting as extended families to one another and to the residents outside the actual therapy hours.

Early in treatment, family members support one another by sharing the pain they have experienced as a result of having SAs in their families. Each family's sense of loneliness and isolation, in dealing with this major crisis, is attenuated by sharing the burden with other families. The ways in which the SAs have manipulated them are quite similar; when these are revealed, they help these families to form a common bond. Group members commiserate over each family's suffering. Each family is encouraged to break the pattern of perpetuating substance abuse through overprotection. The family learns to see the hostile aspects of this, rather than its benevolence. Many patients who have difficulty with the demands of residential treatment will try to convince their families to take them home and "protect" them. Intervening in this system helps prevent early treatment termination.

As therapy progresses, the role of the families in producing and perpetuating substance abuse is identified. Patterns of mutual manipulation, extraction, and coercion are identified. The family members' need to perpetuate the patients' dependent behavior through scapegoating, distancing, protection, or infantilization is discouraged, and new methods of relating are taught and practiced. Family members tend to feel guilty when the SAs confront them with their role in the addiction cycle. Similar confrontations have occurred in families' homes and recur in the early phases of multiple-family therapy. If a therapist does not intervene, a family may retaliate with anger, guilt induction, or undermining of growth, and/or enter a coalition with the SA that permits him/her to leave treatment.

Parents of SAs, in particular, must be given a great deal of support in family sessions because of their own guilt and the tendency of the identified patients as they feel empowered in early recovery to attack them. For some parents, even the public admission that there are any family problems leads to shame and reactive hostility. Such parents may require individual family therapy sessions and individual support. When they can overcome their embarrassment about expressing feelings in the "public" group, they have made a valuable step toward more open and honest expression of feelings in general.

Multiple-family therapy groups help patients achieve and put into practice insights about their families that are achieved in other settings. Family sessions are often a true test of whether or not SAs have really changed and can put their insights into practice. Many families learn to express love and anger directly and appropriately, for the first time, in these groups.

Later in multiple-family group treatment, families may express intense repressed mourning, which enhances a healthier family adaptation. Mourning is readily expressed about siblings who have died from an overdose; in still later phases, abandoning or deceased parents may be mourned. Families and individuals also mourn lost opportunities and relationships of all kinds. When the anxiety stirred up by early shifts has been resolved, more advanced tasks can be assigned. Family secrets and myths are also revealed in later multiple-family treatment. In the final phase, each family and identified patient separate from the group. However, family members are free to return to handle slips even if the identified patient does not participate (Kaufman & Kaufmann, 1992).

Couples Groups

There are two types of couples groups—one for the parents of youthful SAs, and another for SAs and their spouses.

After couples of both types have been part of a multiple-family group for several months, they usually request couples sessions. The frequently stated rationale is that there are problems that relate only to a couple that cannot be resolved with the children present. Couples often have difficulty dealing with their own dysfunction or other issues in family or multiple-family therapy with the children present (Kaufman & Kaufmann, 1992). This boundary is generally appropriate, and thus ongoing couples groups should be an integral part of any family-based treatment program.

When the presenting problem of substance abuse is resolved, content shifts to marital problems. It is often at this point that parents want to leave a multiple-family therapy group and attend a couples group. In the couples group, the multiple-family group's procedures are reversed: Partners should not speak about their children, but rather focus on the relationship between themselves. If material is brought up about a child or children, it is allowed only if it is relevant to problems that the partners have. Invariably, five issues are emphasized: communication, control, money, sex, and intimacy (Kaufman & Kaufmann, 1992).

Partners must support each other while learning the basic tools of communication. When one partner gives up substance misuse, this is a critical period; the nonusing partner must adjust the way in which he/she relates to the using partner. There are totally new expectations and demands. Sex may have been used for exploitation and pacification so often that both partners have given up hope about resuming sexual relations and have stopped making serious efforts toward mutual satisfaction. In addition, drugs and alcohol have often physiologically diminished the SA's sex drive. Sexual communication must be slowly redeveloped. Difficulties may arise because the recovering SA has given up the most precious thing in his/her life (drugs or alcohol) and often expects immediate rewards. The SA's spouse, in turn, has been "burned" too many times and may be unwilling to continue to provide rewards, even when sobriety stabilizes the SA. Both the SA and the spouse in such a situation are asked to re-evaluate their expectations for trust. Couples groups in a program for either adult or adolescent SAs provide a natural means for strengthening intimacy.

It is critical that shifting a couple to a couples group not be done simply because such groups exist, but with the full knowledge that the group will support and strengthen the couples bond and weaken the individual parent–child relationships. If this is kept in mind, the specialized couples group can be extremely helpful and, in some cases, essential.

Spouses and parents of SAs are encouraged to attend Al-Anon, Nar-Anon, Co-Anon, or Coda (Codependents Anonymous), as appropriate, to help diminish their reactivity and enhance their coping and self-esteem. Such groups also facilitate an attitude of loving, detached acceptance. Ablon (1974) states that the chief dynamic of the group process of Al-Anon is the learning experience that results from a candid exchange and sharing of reactions and strategies for behavior related to living in a household with an alcoholic or problem drinker. The experience of others provides a basis for a comparison and a stimulation of self-examination, leading to new insight in all areas of life experiences. However, Al-Anon or a similar group is frequently not enough for a spouse, perhaps because the approach is not individualized. Hence, separate groups for spouses may be an essential additional resource.

Other Types of Groups

Another type of group that may be used is a significant-others group. This group may include parents, lovers, employers, close friends, and other important members of the SAs' network. In addition, separate groups for adolescent and younger children of SAs offer support and an opportunity to discuss their special problems.

Research Support for Family Involvement

Many studies have demonstrated that spousal involvement facilitates alcoholics' participation in treatment and aftercare (see Cadogan, 1973). In addition, it increases the incidence of sobriety and enhanced functioning after treatment. Furthermore, the greater the involvement of spouses in different group modalities (Al-Anon, spouse groups, etc.), the better the prognosis for treatment of alcoholics (Wright & Scott, 1978). My own work with Pauline Kaufmann demonstrated that involvement of the families of adolescent drug abusers in multiple-family group treatment and couples groups cut recidivism from over 50% in families without family group treatment to 20% when families participated (Kaufman & Kaufmann, 1992). There is thus considerable research support for the efficacy of family involvement in group treatment of SAs.

The Integration
of Individual
and Family Therapy

I was fortunate in that Nathan Ackerman, considered by many the father of family therapy, was one of the primary teachers in my psychoanalytic training. As early as the 1960s, Ackerman espoused an integration of family therapy and psychoanalytic techniques, which has continued to influence my work to the present time. The need for integration is relatively clear in the early phases of therapy. Dealing with the family is one more aspect of involvement with the patient's ecosystem, which includes working with the treatment team, Twelve-Step groups, sponsors, employers, employee assistance counselors, managed-care workers, parole officers, and other members of the legal system. It is generally true that upon entering treatment, the family is the most critical part of this ecosystem.

In Chapter 5, the importance of the family in the initial assessment phase has been discussed. With patients in their teens and 20s, there is a focus on working with the patients in their families of origin. Stanton et al. (1982) strongly suggest that family therapy not begin with a marital dyad until work with an addict and his/her parents has freed the addict from an enmeshed triangle with his/her parents. I agree with this in principle only. Many addicts enter therapy in highly dysfunctional relationships with spouses or significant others; these must be dealt with early in therapy, as these dyadic difficulties are often primary causes of relapse. On the other hand, as the case history later in this chapter demonstrates, I commonly do begin with the patients and their families of origin, and shift the emphasis in the later phases of therapy toward achieving or sustaining intimacy with a significant other. This, of course, varies with the age of a patient and his/her involvement with each subsystem.

Many heavily emotionally laden family issues can be dealt with during early inpatient or residential treatment. The protectiveness of this setting permits powerful family issues and secrets to be worked on, such as sexual and physical abuse, enmeshment, coalitions, scapegoating, and other severe emotional abuse. After discharge from the protected residential environment, many of these issues cannot be dealt with again in any depth until sobriety is stable for a year or two.

There are inherent problems with one person's functioning as both individual therapist and family therapist, particularly as long-term therapy deepens the bond between the individual therapist and the patient. This alliance may be so strong as to preclude a meaningful alliance between the therapist and other family members. On the other hand, if the therapist bonds well with other members of the family, the identified patient may experience intense jealousy or feel that the special patient–therapist relationship is threatened.

Family therapy often calls for greater self-revelation by the therapist (see "Joining," below), which may be incompatible with deeper, nondirective individual therapy. A patient may have extreme difficulty with the required changes in personal style, affect, and interaction when the therapist shifts from individual to family work. Moreover, a therapist may have difficulty in making these changes. All of these issues can be worked through and are excellent grist for the therapeutic mill, if there is a meaningful therapeutic alliance. Nevertheless, a patient may simply be unable to tolerate the shifting role and attitude of the therapist from the individual to the family mode of therapy, and may require referral to a different family therapist. Many therapists are also, understandably, unable to maintain both roles.

My approach to family therapy utilizes a synthesis of several different (even seemingly contradictory) treatment systems. The use of varying techniques depends on the unique needs of each family and stems from a commitment to individualized treatment plans. My approach to individual therapy has been greatly influenced by family therapy, particularly family therapy with only one individual present. My family approach incorporates psychodynamic techniques as well as strategic, structural, communications, systems, and behavioral methods. An important influence on my approach has been prolonged and deep exposure to the complicated and unique characteristics of SAs and their families, and to their needs for certain specific treatment principles, as well as for a wide variety of change techniques (Kaufman, 1985).

Feldman (1992) emphasizes the synergism between individual and family therapy. He states that individually oriented techniques are the most effective means of achieving intrapsychic changes, whereas family therapy is the best way to promote interpersonal changes. Efforts to change dysfunctional family interactions often lead to the recognition of intrapsychic problems, which provide critical material for individual psychotherapy. In addition, intrapsychic individual change may often be blocked by family dysfunction. When the latter is corrected, insights by the individual are more readily translated into meaningful behavioral change, either within or outside of the family. Family sessions are also effective in determining whether the insights of individual therapy have been translated into behavioral change.

Some therapists may find it difficult to integrate psychodynamic approaches with the more directive restructuring techniques. Liddle (1985) has noted that model integration is a complicated, sophisticated, and challenging task.

I term my system of family therapy "structural–dynamic," because it is a fusion of structural–strategic techniques with psychodynamic methods. Within this system, the therapist is seen as an active, dynamic participant rather than a passive, neutral screen. My method of family therapy consists of (1) family diagnosis, (2) family contracting, (3) family education, (4) joining, (5) restructuring, (6) utilization of psychodynamic constructs, and (7) communications therapy.

FAMILY DIAGNOSIS

In family diagnosis, the therapist looks at family interactional and communication patterns and relationships. As noted above, I prefer a family systems approach that utilizes structural concepts, but also considers a psychodynamic understanding of the personality of each individual. However, a difference from most psychoanalytic approaches is that the therapist is urged to become a part of the family and actively to shift his/her own alliances within the family system. Using the structural model, I examine the family's rules, roles, boundaries, and flexibilities. I look for coalitions (particularly transgenerational ones), shifting alliances, splits, cutoffs, and triangulation. I observe communication patterns, confirmation and disconfirmation, unclear messages, and conflict resolution. I also note the family's stage in the family life cycle. Finally, I note mind reading (predicting reactions and reacting to them before they happen, or knowing what someone thinks or wants), double binds, and fighting styles.

During the first visit, I rarely use an extended genogram (which includes all aunts, uncles, and cousins), but I always obtain an abbreviated three-generational genogram that focuses on the identified patient, his/her parents, and any progeny; if the patient is part of a couple, it should also include the partner's parents, as well as any prior marriages on either side. In addition, I include other members of the household and any other significant relatives with whom there is regular or important current contact. In stepfamilies, the initial genogram must include the noncustodial parent(s) and the geographical location and family situation of all children from prior marriages, as these may be extremely significant. As therapy progresses, and other important family members from the past and present are discussed, a full but informal family genogram is gradually developed (Kaufman, 1985).

In assessing a family and its members, it is critical to assess their strengths as well as their weaknesses. The use of combined individual, subsystem, and total family assessments has been termed "integrative multilevel assessment" by Feldman (1992). This type of evaluation produces a more comprehensive evaluation than any single focus. It provides consensual clarification and validation of self-reported behaviors and sequences, as well as evidence that alleged changes can be translated into action, particularly in the most difficult battlefields of the families of origin and procreation.

FAMILY CONTRACTING

The contract is an agreement to work on mutually agreed-upon, workable issues. The contract should always promise help with the identified patient's problems before it is expanded to include other issues. Goals should be mutual. If there is disagreement about them, then work on resolving disagreements should be made a part of the contract.

The preliminary contract is drafted with the family at the end of the first interview. In subsequent sessions, the concept of a contract is maintained, so that family assignments and tasks are agreed upon and their implementation is contracted by the family. The likelihood that the family will return after the first session is greatly enhanced by a contract that develops measures for problem resolution. Initial contracts should include the length of therapy; duration of sessions; cost; and which members will attend and in what combinations. The therapist may also choose to include his/her own style, techniques, and expectations of the family. Everyone in the household, and all other involved family members (such as grandparents and siblings away at college), should be invited and urged to attend sessions. The greater the number of family members involved, the more thoroughly the family is understood. When working with a family system that appears limited to an enmeshed mother–SA dyad, it is particularly important to involve at least one other family member to provide sufficient leverage for structural change.

The length of therapy may be flexibly renegotiated at the end of the initial time period, particularly if family members feel they have made noticeable gains. Whereas the initial contract should provide for some relief of the symptoms of the identified patient, subsequent contracts, if agreed to, can focus on other family members.

There are many specific modifications of the contract with SAs. The family chooses a system to achieve abstinence and agrees to pursue that system after it has been negotiated as part of the initial evaluation. In addition, family members other than the identified patient should agree to attend a type of support group (see Chapter 5 and 9), and should specify the location and number of meetings they will attend. Involving all siblings and both parents in treatment, in the case of a youthful SA, is an important aspect of the contract. In order to do this, it is essential that the therapist be sufficiently flexible to be available at times when all family members can be present, or to make home visits when necessary.

The family should be provided with the beginnings of a method of diminishing overreactivity to substance abuse in the initial contract. They may be coached to disengage from the identified patient, using strength gained from support groups and the therapist. At times, this disengagement can only be accomplished by powerful restructuring or paradoxical interventions (see below).

FAMILY EDUCATION

A substantial amount of family education is generally very helpful in the early stages of the family's involvement in therapy. In many inpatient addiction treatment programs, the family spends several days or more receiving appropriate education. If this is not available, then I will try to duplicate many aspects of this education process in early sessions. When the SA is male, I often provide a book I have written that covers much of this material—*Help at Last: A Complete Guide to Coping with Chemically Dependent Men* (Kaufman, 1991).

Some of the issues covered in the education process are as follows: (1) the physiological and psychological effects of drugs and alcohol; (2) the disease concept; (3) the principle of cross-addiction (which helps families learn that a recovering cocaine addict should not drink, or that a recovering alcoholic should not use cocaine or other drugs of abuse); (4) common family systems concepts that emphasize the family's roles in addiction and recovery, including enabling, scapegoating, and codependence; (5) the phases of treatment, with an emphasis on the deceptiveness of the "honeymoon" period in early recovery; (6) the importance of Twelve-Step groups for the family (Al-Anon, Co-Anon, Alateen, etc.), and ways to utilize support groups.

JOINING

In "joining," the therapist adjusts himself/herself in a number of different ways in order to affiliate with the family system. Joining enhances the therapist's leverage to change the system. The therapist alternates between joining that supports the family system and its members, and joining that achieves growth by challenge. The therapist's verbal and nonverbal behavior demonstrates to the family that he/she understands them, values them, and is committed to (as well as capable of) helping them change (Feldman, 1992).

In joining with the family, the therapist alternates between existential engagement and disengaged expertise. The therapist must be capable of joining each subsystem, including that of siblings. Each family member must be able to feel the therapist's firm commitment to healing. The therapist must make contact with all family members, so that they will follow the therapist even when they believe that he/she is being unfair. With the families of SAs, the therapist must join with them by respecting and not challenging their initial defensiveness (Kaufman, 1985).

Minuchin has categorized joining according to two different systems: techniques (Minuchin, 1974) and degree of proximity (Minuchin & Fishman, 1981).

Techniques of Joining

There are three types of joining techniques: "maintenance," "tracking," and "mimesis."

Maintenance

Maintenance requires supporting the family structures and behaving according to the family rules. The therapist may initially speak to the family through the family spokesperson or "switchboard." When a family is being pushed beyond its ability to tolerate stress, maintenance techniques can be used to lower stress. Maintenance operations include supporting areas of family strength, rewarding, affiliating with a family member, complimenting/supporting a threatened member, and explaining a problem. The therapist uses the family's own metaphors, expressions, and language.

Joining with every member of the family is part of the art of family therapy. A thorough knowledge of various aspects of adolescent culture (e.g., music) is helpful with young SAs. A knowledge of the drug culture and vocabulary is helpful with addicts. With recovering alcoholics or addicts of any age, a basic knowledge of the Twelve Steps of AA, NA, or CA is important.

Tracking

In tracking, the therapist follows the content of the family's interactions by listening carefully to what everyone has to say, and by providing comments and expressions that help each family member know he/she has been heard and understood.

Mimesis

Mimesis involves the therapist's adopting the family's style and affect as reflected by the members' action and needs. If a family uses humor, so should the therapist, but without double binds. If a family communicates through touching, then the therapist may also touch if he/she is comfortable doing so.

Mimesis is frequently done unconsciously, but it may be consciously used in family systems therapy; by contrast, in individual psychoanalytic psychotherapy it is generally contraindicated, as are most overt joining techniques.

The most significant joining occurs when the therapist communicates to the family that he/she understands them and is working with and for them. Thus, paradoxically, the most profound joining comes when the therapist challenges the family's dysfunctional maneuvers in ways that give them hope that the therapist can make them better.

Joining with all family members may be too difficult for one therapist, particularly in a family with an adolescent identified patient. I have often found it necessary to utilize a cotherapist who takes the position of advocate for the adolescent in the family sessions. This enables me to join more effectively with the parents and facilitate their limit setting. In other cases, the adolescent is begging for limits underneath his/her bravado, and a single therapist can easily join with the adolescent as well as the parental system. After long-term individual therapy has progressed for several years, it may be helpful to refer an SA and his/her family to, or conduct family sessions jointly with, a neutral family therapist.

Joining Classified by Degree of Proximity

In joining a family from a close proximity, the therapist may feel emotionally drawn in, as if he/she were a member of the family. The therapist in this position should push himself/herself to find positive aspects in all family members, particularly ones who are disliked (Minuchin & Fishman, 1981). In joining from a middle position, the therapist gathers important information by observing his/her own ways of interacting with the family, without being incorporated into the family system. Here it is often important to shift emphasis by tracking from content to process. In joining from a disengaged position, the therapist may have the role of an expert or director. Family recognition of the therapist as expert provides substantial leverage for change to the therapist. Perhaps even more than most techniques, joining becomes much more spontaneous and less deliberate as therapy progresses.

RESTRUCTURING

Unlike joining, "restructuring" involves a challenge to the family's homeostasis and takes place through changing the family affiliations and interactional patterns. In restructuring, the therapist uses expertise in social manipulation, with the word "manipulation" being used in a positive rather than a pejorative sense. Techniques used for change include actualizing transactional patterns, marking boundaries, assigning tasks, reframing, utilizing paradox, balancing and unbalancing, and creating intensity. Joining is necessary as a prerequisite and facilitator for change production, and the therapist frequently alternates between joining and restructuring.

Actualizing Family Transactional Patterns

Family members usually direct their communications to the therapist; they should be reminded to talk to each other rather than to the therapist. They should also be asked to enact transactional patterns instead of describing them. Manipulating space is a powerful tool for generating actualization. Changing seating may create or strengthen boundaries. Asking two members who have been chronically disengaged and/or communicating through a third party to sit next to and face each other can actualize strong conflicts and emotions.

Families in which there is substance abuse frequently gravitate to a rehash of past fights, hoping to entrap the therapist into deciding who started the fight, who is wrong and right, and what the proper decision is. It is critical not to be triangulated into such a position, but rather to have the family choose an unresolved conflict and actualize their problem-solving methods or lack of them in the session. If a family arrives with a member who has been using drugs and/or alcohol, the family should not be dismissed; the members' interactions should be observed, as this will demonstrate how they interact during a good portion of their time together. Of course, if drinking/drug use is a repeated problem, then the family must develop a system to end the substance abuse before therapy can continue.

Most families will enter therapy trying to look as good as possible. Actualizations unleash sequences that are beyond a family's control and permit the therapist to see the family as it really is. They may be staged by the therapist to reveal or change dysfunction, or they may be spontaneous and permitted to evolve or guided in a therapeutic direction.

Marking Boundaries

Basic ground rules are established that protect individual boundaries. Each person should be spoken to, not about; and no one should talk, feel, think, answer, or act for anyone else. Each family member is encouraged to tell his/her own story, and to listen to and acknowledge the communications of others. Nonverbal checking and blocking of communications should also be observed and, when it is appropriate to do so, should be pointed out and halted. "Mind reading" is very common but is strongly discouraged, because even if the mind reader is correct it almost always starts an argument. (Issues related to communication are discussed more fully in "Communications Therapy," below.)

Symbolic boundaries are established in the session by the therapist's placing his/her body, an arm, or a piece of furniture between family members; rearranging members' seating; or having members make or avoid eye contact. These boundaries are supported and strengthened by tasks outside of the session. The most important boundary shifts are weakening the ties between an overinvolved parent and child, and strengthening the boundary that protects spouses or partners from in-laws, affairs, and the rest of the world external to the nuclear family. Then direct work can more easily be done to support the spousal bond.

If a role or tie is removed from a family member, this relationship should be replaced by building ties with other family members or people outside the family.

Assigning Tasks

Tasks are perhaps the most important technique in family therapy, representing the major road to change in much the same way transference does in individual psychoanalytic psychotherapy. There are four major purposes of tasks (Haley, 1977): to gather information through tasks that probe and actualize; to intensify the relationship with the therapist; to continue the therapeutic change process outside of the session; and to enable people to behave differently.

There are many ways to motivate families to perform tasks, some of which flow from other aspects of the principles of family therapy (Haley, 1977). The therapist should (1) join the family first, using family language and metaphors to frame the tasks; (2) choose tasks in the framework of family goals, particularly those that are directed towards correcting the symptoms of the identified patient; (3) choose tasks that bring gains to each member of the family, particularly if there is conflict about doing the tasks; (4) have the family members accomplish a task in session before they are given one for homework; (5) if family members are improving, use their progress to prescribe further change so that they can improve even more; (6) use his/her position as an expert to emphasize the need to perform the tasks; (7) cut off disagreement about doing the tasks and tell the family members to "do it anyway"; and (8) provide the general framework of the tasks, and then work with the family to develop the specifics.

Haley (1977) has also made a number of suggestions for how to give tasks properly so that they will be successfully accomplished. I have also integrated these into my work as rules of thumb with substance-abusing families. The therapist should (1) be specific; (2) give the tasks clearly, concisely, and firmly; (3) formulate the tasks throughout the session (highlighting important areas), but be certain to emphasize all specific tasks at the end of the session; (4) be as repetitious as necessary to have the family remember the tasks; (5) involve everyone in the household (one person may perform the task, another help, and another supervise, plan, or check on it); (6) review how each family member may avoid performing his/her role or prevent completion of the task; (7) make the task part of contracting at the end of each session; (8) review the task at the beginning of the next session; (9) use failures as learning experiences to reveal the dysfunctional aspects of the family or the poor timing of the task; (10) support the family members in what they have learned from not doing the task; (11) remember that negotiations about the task may be more important than the actual task; (12) avoid letting the family members off easily, particularly if they forget the task; (13) explore why they let themselves down; (14) build incrementally from easy to more difficult tasks; and (15) use tasks used to achieve structural change.

Reframing

In "reframing" (Minuchin & Fishman, 1981), the therapist shifts the conceptual framework of information received from the family, transforming it into a form that will be most helpful to changing the family. Reframing begins at the start of the first session as the therapist receives information from the family, molding it so that the family members feel that their problems are clear and solvable. Reframing is achieved by focusing material as it is received, selecting the elements that will facilitate change, and organizing the information in such a way as to give it new meaning. Perhaps the most common use of reframing is broadening the symptoms of an identified patient to include the reactivity of the entire family system. Positive reframing is often used to shift from hopelessness to an understanding of the helpful and protective aspects of family interactions.

Utilizing Paradox

Paradoxical techniques work best with chronic, rigid, repetitive, circular, highly resistant family systems, particularly ones that have had many prior therapeutic failures (Papp, 1981). Paradox is not utilized when family motivation is high, resistance is low, or the family responds readily to direct interventions (Papp, 1981). It is also not used in crisis situations (e.g., violence, suicide, incest, or child abuse); here the therapist needs to provide structure and control. Paradox is likewise avoided with paranoid identified patients and with families exhibiting widespread mistrust. Paradox is used to slow progress so that a family will be chafing at the bit to move faster.

When an individual's behavior is prescribed, it is related to its function in the family system. The symptom should only be prescribed if its function in the system is understood and if it can be prescribed in a way that changes the functioning of the system. At times, it seems that paradox is a way of making a psychodynamic or system interpretation that motivates the family to change behavior in a way that classical interpretations do not—for example, encouraging an adolescent SA to continue to act out because his/her parents need the behavior to argue about, in order to avoid feeling close enough to have a sexual relationship.

Balancing and Unbalancing

The therapist moves back and forth between "balancing" and "unbalancing." Balancing techniques tend to support a family, and unbalancing tends to stress the family system.

Balancing is similar to Minuchin and Fishman's (1981) "complementarity." It challenges the family's views of symptoms as part of a linear hierarchy and emphasizes the reciprocal involvement of symptom formation, while supporting the family. Mutual responsibility should be emphasized, and tasks that involve change in all parties should be given. The therapist must be aware that an individual's view of his/her responsibility for a symptom may be so skewed that what the therapist feels is perfectly balanced may feel very unbalanced and unfair to that person.

Unbalancing involves changing or stressing the existing hierarchy in a family and should only be attempted after the therapist has achieved a great deal of power through joining.

Creating Intensity

Techniques that create intensity (Minuchin & Fishman, 1981) enable the family to hear and incorporate the messages sent by the therapist. One simple way to be heard is to repeat the same phrase or use different phrases that convey the same concept. Another way of creating intensity, "isomorphic transactions," uses many different interventions to attack the same underlying dysfunctional pattern. The amount of time a family spends on a transaction can be increased or decreased, as can the proximity of members during an interaction.

UTILIZATION OF PSYCHODYNAMIC CONCEPTS AND TECHNIQUES

There are two cornerstones for the implementation of psychodynamic family techniques: the therapist's self-knowledge and a detailed family history. The better therapists understand their own roles in their own families, the better they are able to understand their representations to the families they treat. Every family member will internalize a therapist's good qualities, such as helpfulness, warmth, trust, trustworthiness, assertion, empathy, and understanding. Likewise, they may incorporate a therapist's less desirable qualities, such as rage, despair, and emotional distancing. Thus therapists need to understand how and when these qualities are being identified with by their patients.

The more a therapist understands about a family's history and prior patterns, the better he/she will be able to help that family not to repeat dysfunctional transactions or personalized transference reactions. When a couple is stuck, I frequently use individual sessions for both partners or conduct family-of-origin-oriented therapy for one partner (with the other partner present). These sessions are used to understand and shift patterns that have been repeated unchanged over several generations.

The psychodynamic concepts discussed here are countertransference, interpretation, resistance, working through, and projective identification.

The Use of Countertransference

The use of countertransference has been discussed in detail in Chapter 8 of this book. A fundamental difference in work with families is that the therapist may have a countertransference problem toward the entire family system or style, or toward any individual subsystem or member of the family. The therapist may particularly rally to the defense of the identified patient against "oppressive" family members, which can set up power struggles between the therapist and family.

Judicious expression of countertransference feelings may at times be helpful in breaking fixed family patterns. For example, sharing children's anger at a controlling parent may give the children enough support to express their anger at this parent in a manner that finally makes an impact.

The Role of Interpretation

Interpretations can be extremely helpful if they are made in a reciprocal way, without blaming, inducting guilt, or dwelling on the hopelessness of long-standing, fixed patterns. The goal is always to change the present. Repetitive patterns and their maladaptive aspects to each family member can be pointed out, and tasks can be given to help them change these patterns. Some families need interpretations before they can fulfill tasks. An emphasis on mutual responsibility when making any interpretation is an example of the helpful fusion of structural and psychodynamic therapy.

Overcoming Resistance

"Resistance" is defined as any behaviors, feelings, patterns, or styles that prevent involvement in therapy or that delay or prevent change

(Anderson & Stewart, 1983). In a substance-abusing family, key resistant behaviors that must be dealt with involve the failure to perform functions that enable the SA to stay "clean." It is important to understand resistance and to have methods for overcoming it. The greater the resistance by the family, the greater the demand on the therapist's energy and creativity. Resistance may be conscious or unconscious, purposeful or accidental; it may emanate from one family member or from the entire system (Anderson & Stewart, 1983).

Some forms of resistance, such as the defense mechanisms of denial, rationalization, somatization, intellectualization, displacement, and acting out (see Chapter 3), occur in all types of therapy. Other forms of resistance—collusions, myths, family secrets, scapegoat maintenance, pseudomutuality, and pseudohostility—are specific to family therapy (Anderson & Stewart, 1983). Every family has characteristic patterns of resistant behavior, in addition to isolated resistances. The family "style" may contribute significantly to resistance: Some families may need to deny all conflict and emotion and may be almost totally unable to tolerate any displays of anger or sadness, while others may overreact to the slightest disagreement. It is important to recognize, emphasize, and interpret the circumstances that arouse resistance patterns (Anderson & Stewart, 1983).

In individual psychodynamic psychotherapy, the concept of resistance is integral and essential to the overall change process. In family therapy, resistance is more often viewed as an obstacle to be overcome. Nevertheless, overcoming family resistance may lead to a great deal of positive family change in and of itself.

Working Through

The important concept of "working through," derived from psychoanalysis, is quite similar to the structural concept of isomorphic transactions. It underscores the need to work for an extended time on many different overt issues, all of which stem from the same dysfunctional core. Thus, in order to have real change, a family must deal with a problem over and over until it has been worked through. In psychoanalysis this is termed "the transition from intellectual to genuine or emotional insight" (Fenichel, 1945). This process is ususally much quicker in family than in individual therapy, because when an appropriate intervention is made, the entire family system may reinforce the consequent positive change. If the homeostatic system pulls the family's behavior back to old maladaptive ways, then it will become necessary to work the conflicts through in many different transactions until more stable change takes place.

Projective Identification

It is important to realize that projective identification is much more common than is generally realized, and that it is often an integral part of relationships that are considered "normal." This defense is not used solely to rid oneself of primitive rage and aggression, but also of wishes to devaluate, dominate, and control, which are based on primitive envy and the wish to cling parasitically to the significant other (Horowitz, 1983). Projective identification is particularly relevant to couples work, because it involves both an intrapsychic defense mechanism and an interpersonal transaction — for example, the significant other undergoes an identification or fusion with the projected content, and thus has the experience of being manipulated into a particular role (Horowitz, 1983). This process of being manipulated is also quite confusing and anxiety-provoking to the significant other.

Some time ago, Dicks (1967) wrote that projective identification not only is the cement that binds marital partners in their love–hate interactions, but provides the material for most of their disagreements and tensions. Thus, identifying projective identification in marital and total family therapy, as well as its affect-laden roots in each member's family of origin, can be extremely helpful in resolving conflict, particularly between partners who battle constantly. (See the case history in Chapter 3 for an extensive example of projective identification in a couple as well as in the couple's environment.)

COMMUNICATIONS THERAPY

Yet another family approach to SAs and their significant others is communications therapy. Again, this is particularly useful in dyadic couples work. The proponents of this system include Haley (1977), Watzlawick et al. (1974), Satir (1972), and Bateson et al. (1956). However, pointing out and working with problems in communication are important aspects of all family therapies.

As its name implies, the goal of communications therapy is to correct discrepancies in communication. This is achieved by having participants state their messages clearly, by clarifying meanings and assumptions, and by permitting feedback to clarify unclear messages (Bateson et al., 1956). The therapist acts as an objective governor of communication who teaches people to speak clearly and directly in a structured, protected experience. This can be facilitated by a simple exercise. One partner speaks for 5 minutes without interruptions, while the other listens with encouragement. Next, the second partner tells what he/she has heard; the first partner then provides helpful feedback.

The following individualized rules of communication were developed with a 24-year-old cocaine addict and his pregnant 22-year-old wife after several enactments were observed in the early phases of their couple's therapy.*

Rules of Communication

1. Finish discussing a subject before you jump to another. Skipping around from one topic to another is poor communication and is usually based on anger and hurt. Thus nothing is resolved and anger escalates.

2. Don't assume that you know what the other person means — if you think someone is cutting you down (or complimenting you), check it out before you react.

3. Listen to the other person without interruption. This goes with number 2 — you won't have a two-way communication unless you really hear what the other person is trying to say.

4. Don't put words in the other person's mouth by answering or talking for [him or her]. This makes the other person angry because [it suggests] that you have no respect for [that person] or [his or her] opinions. [Your partner] will get particularly angry if you're wrong but being right will also incite your partner.

5. Talk to each other instead of through a third person, particularly either of your parents or your children.

6. Don't bring up past or present relationships with others when you're trying to prove a point about the relationship between you two. This only confuses the issue and changes the subject. Generally avoid the past when dealing with present problems.

7. Don't replay old arguments over and over again — this solves nothing, it just brings up old hurts and resentments. After you have repeated an argument, either of you has the right to call a truce.

8. Don't make promises or threats that you don't really mean, particularly about leaving.

9. Don't use words like never, always, or you should. Statements like now, sometimes, and could you are much better ways to communicate. There are always exceptions to never and always. In addition, they make the other person angry because they are judgmental, critical, pessimistic, and patronizing.

10. Don't call the other person names — hanging a label on someone means that he or she will hear only the name and not the point you are trying to make. It will make the other person angry, but it won't help you solve a problem.

11. The louder you shout, the less likely your spouse is to hear the content of what you are saying. [He or she] will hear only the volume and react in kind.

*Rules 1–10 are reprinted from Kaufman & Kaufmann (1992, p. 311). Copyright 1992 by Allyn & Bacon. Reprinted by permission.

A CASE HISTORY

The case history that follows demonstrates the successful integration of individual and family therapy, as written by a patient who experienced these therapies over an 8-year period.* I had met Debby G. during her inpatient stay for cocaine and alcohol dependence, a year prior to her beginning therapy with me. She felt she was not ready for psychotherapy at first, but began later after having a year of solid sobriety. She decided to begin at that time because her anger at her mother felt out of control. In her words:

> We began with private sessions every week and family sessions (my family and me) once every few weeks. I didn't emote very much in the private sessions, but I would leave feeling a little better than when I came in. In the family sessions though, I would begin to cry within the first few minutes. I was filled with a pain I had never felt before — not the empty pain I felt while bottoming out on drugs; no, this pain was full and round and grew inside me. I felt worthless; I thought they felt I was worthless. Worthlessness and feeling judged led to anger, but I didn't know how to express anger, particularly with my parents, and so I turned it back on myself. I would judge myself and believe everything they said; I left these sessions feeling terrible, as if my self-esteem had been smashed. I felt lonely, worthless, afraid, hurt.

Debby required a 2-hour supportive debriefing following each 1-hour family session to rebuild her self-esteem. After over a year of sobriety, her sober core was strong enough to withstand the severe emotional pain of her family therapy.

> I decided I could not participate in family therapy any more. I went to my private session that week and told Ed I couldn't handle another session with my parents; it was undermining my sobriety.
>
> Ed's reply stands out in my mind today as the single most important event in my first year of therapy. He told me I had the mistaken idea that family therapy was a tool only to bring families together. He said in my case we were learning that my family was dysfunctional and that I needed to break away from them. I was amazed and relieved. I knew intellectually that my parents had problems relating to me, but in my heart I thought the problem was me. If only I could change, the problem would be solved; yet, every time I tried to do what they wanted, I invariably felt hurt or angry.

---

*The narrative by Debby G. is reprinted from Kaufman & Kaufmann (1992, pp. 271–286). Copyright 1992 by Allyn & Bacon. Reprinted by permission. Names other than Debby's and my own have been changed to preserve confidentiality, and the material is used with Debby's permission as well.

When Ed planted the "breaking away" message, I knew he wasn't lying. He validated my feelings and, because of that validation, I not only felt better but I also drew closer to him. I trusted him a little bit more than I had before.

His validation gave me a new freedom: I could allow myself to feel real anger toward my parents. I was angry at the way my parents had raised me, and I was furious I had the disease of alcoholism. I blamed them for "giving" me the disease. I realized whatever I had done while drinking and using was my fault, [but] I was not a faulty person. My parents did the best they could, but that wasn't good enough; I wasn't ready to forgive them.

Many family therapists, particularly Haley (1977), state that the best way to help patients individuate from their families is first to bring them together. Debby's case illustrates that mechanism, as well as mobilization of rage as a way to facilitate the identified patient's autonomy. The removal of the intrapersonal defenses of denial and intellectualization was facilitated by the family therapy.

The rest of the first year I stayed angry at my parents. I took baby steps in not seeking their approval, support, and love, and I started to accept that they were going to continue to hurt me every so often. This education took the form of not calling them all the time. They live 50 miles away, but I would turn to them for what I thought was approval or love. Every week Ed would ask if I had called them and I would invariably answer, "Yes," then he would ask me to recount these conversations. After some time, I realized that my parents always hurt my feelings in these discussions. I finally acknowledged that I really called them, or at least my mother, to be abused. I was used to it; I thrived on it. I then worked at putting an end to it.

I slowly began to separate from my parents, most importantly financially. I learned how to turn down what looked like free gifts but were really attempts to control me. I could say, "No, I won't take whatever you have to offer because I think you mean something else by it." In this manner, I communicated openly with them for the first time. When I used open communication, not only would the conversation come to an abrupt halt but there was also no way we could take advantage of each other.

Another major breakthrough of this first year was learning how to say, "You hurt my feelings," or "I am angry with you because. . . . " These two phrases were essential keys to recovery; they were the open and honest forms of communication I had never before practiced. As a feeling stuffer, when I felt angry, hurt, or afraid, instead of expressing my feeling during the moment, I reacted later. With my parents, I usually reacted by being angry with my father. For me, communicating openly not only helped me to relieve whatever feeling I was experiencing at the time but it also forced me to be myself. I stopped acting out my mother's form of expression of feelings, namely anger at my father, and began to learn what was appropriate for me.

The last lesson involves issues I learned about in family therapy. I call these the present issue, the expectation issue, and the showing love issue. The first, the present issue, is my personal favorite. This one depicts my sick family at its best. My mother believes that she and my father must be completely fair about presents they give to my sister and me.

As an adult, almost all of the gifts I have received from my parents have been cultured pearls, even though I hate cultured pearls. In fact, I told them this in family therapy.

However, three years after family therapy, my parents returned from a trip to Thailand and Singapore. Thailand is the ruby capital of the world. Before they left for this trip, I said often, " A ruby ring or little bracelet would really be nice, hint, hint. After all, you'll be back just in time for my birthday." Well, my parents came back from Thailand and Singapore and what did they get me? A cultured pearl pendant!

Commonly, people in AA refer to insanity as doing the same thing over and over and expecting a result different from what has always happened before. In my situation, I expect certain actions and reactions by my parents over and over. I first learned about false expectations in the family therapy. I learned that sometimes my expectations of my parents are unrealistic and vice versa, but I have had to work diligently at keeping that knowledge alive. Often I have seen myself fall into the expectation trap not only with my parents but also with men in relationships, girlfriends, bosses, and all sorts of people with whom I come in contact. My expectations of people can become either unrealistically high or unrealistically low because, I believe, I learned this behavior from my parents. Their expectations of me are either too high or too low.

Here we see how Debby was able to combine the family therapy and AA teachings about false expectations to enhance her awareness of punitive selfobjects and of the ways in which she replayed her childhood disappointments as an adult. She used psychotherapy to free herself from these punitive introjects.

The last item, the expression of love issue, was the easiest problem to resolve. Basically, my father had a great deal of trouble showing love or affection. Ed brought this out openly in family therapy, and I simply asked for more attention. My father immediately thereafter began to express love to me and now hugs and kisses me when he sees me; occasionally, he will even hold my hand if we are walking together. This has helped our relationship immensely and he has, to some extent, helped me to express my feelings.

I believe that I too had trouble expressing love, particularly to my female friends. I was not conscious of it before, but I think my father's attempts at correcting something he felt uncomfortable about helped me to do the same. I can now say, "I love you," to my friends on the phone, something I always shuddered at before (giving up the defense of isolation).

Debby's father was able to open up warmly to her for the first time in years as a result of the family therapy. This occurred after Debby asked directly for affection and her father was able to give it, because in dyadic sessions with Debby he learned to do so without retaliation from his wife. He was able to continue to be demonstrative outside of the therapy. Debby felt that her shift in expressing love to friends came as a result of her identification with her father's new expressiveness. I am certain that the underlying warmth that I consistently expressed to her also helped her own expression of positive feelings.

> On a deeper level, I think my going through therapy has enabled my father to express his feelings more openly in a number of ways. During my first and second years of therapy, I was asked to speak at several different types of AA and CA meetings and panels. On one of these occasions, I thought it would be nice to invite my parents, Ed, and my sponsor and her husband to hear me speak. I consider it an honor to be asked to tell my story, and I wanted to share this occasion with some of the people I felt close to. I had no idea the experience would be so enlightening.
>
> On the day I was supposed to speak, my mother got sick with a cold, and my father drove from Los Angeles to Orange County (50 miles in rush hour traffic) without her. At the meeting my father sat near Ed and my sponsor and her husband.
>
> I omitted almost my entire "drugalogue" and focused my sharing on my feelings as a child and an adult, the numbing chill I felt as a practicing addict, and my feelings, experiences, and hopes in sobriety. During my talk I also mentioned that my father was sitting in the room. When I finished speaking, as many people came up to my father as they did to me. So many recovering addicts wanted to tell him how great they thought it was that he came to hear his daughter. When we walked outside my father made some comment about what an inspiration I must be to "those" people. Inside I laughed as I said, "They keep me sober, dad." He was a little taken aback.
>
> Weeks later, though, it was my sister who relayed to me that dad had told the cousins in Canada how proud he was of me. I was amazed; I never thought my parents were proud of me for anything. I instantly felt closer to my father and happy that I could make him feel proud. I also knew that even though he couldn't share his pride with me, he was beginning to share it with others.

Attending a patient's AA birthday or speaking engagement is an important parameter in the treatment of any patient with long-term sobriety. It generally communicates the therapist's full support and recognition of the patient's achievements, without any significant difficulties in violating patient—therapist boundaries. In this case, it also helped Debby to focus on certain aspects of family dysfunctions, as follows:

> The speaking engagement had other repercussions for my family, though. I did not doubt that my mother was psychosomatically ill, but I didn't want

to accept that fact. However, when she called me to tell me how proud she was of herself because she had been sick and had stayed home, I wanted to scream at her over the phone. When I went to see Ed, he began the session by reinforcing my good feelings about speaking. He told me I was great. Then he asked what my parents had said. I told him I thought my father was proud of me and I told him what my mother had said. He commented that it sounded right to him and I asked him why. His reply helped me to learn what my dysfunctional family was all about.

My mother vies with my sister and me for my father's attention. She cannot handle him giving us more attention than her, so she got sick in order to turn the family attention back to herself. That day I not only learned that my father was capable of feeling pride for his children but that my mother felt so ignored that she needed to have the family's attention on her constantly.

I don't remember much else about this first year of therapy, except for Ed trying to bring up my relationship with Bob, my boyfriend (whom I had been seeing for 2½ years), which I would always try to dismiss. Finally, when I was forced to look at my relationship with Bob, I found it more painful than I could have thought in my wildest dreams. Bob and I had a history together — a mentally abusive history for me. Like my mother, Bob criticized me constantly, and I interpreted criticism as love. Although I had stopped calling my mother for criticism, I had not stopped calling Bob. In addition, Bob had seen me through the worst of my drug abuse and now saw the changes occurring in me because of AA and therapy. As I became more whole, the less we got along. He started to lose control over me, both emotionally and sexually.

Debby broke up with Bob in part through a new relationship, which she also terminated in 3 months.

Again, she used an insight she obtained in family therapy to shift a relationship with adult significant others:

For the first time in a long time I was alone — completely alone. There was no one to fall back on, no one to call for abusive criticism, no readily available warmth or sex. I became depressed. I slept a lot and I cried. I had nothing positive to say in AA meetings. I would just go and dump my feelings and leave. I hated work, but at least it was a brief respite every day from my own head. I even cried in Ed's office, which was rare for me in private sessions. I was so out of it I had to ask him what was wrong. He was the one who told me I was depressed. It was this depression, though, that really brought about some major changes for me.

First, Ed was the only person I felt I could turn to who wouldn't tell me just to work the AA steps. I was working the steps, but I was still depressed. He seemed to understand that. I placed full trust in him.

During that period I slept around quite a bit, as men had always been a "quick fix" for me. But I did learn to build my self-esteem in other ways. I became friendly with a woman in CA. With her, I began to learn what intimacy was with other women. We helped each other out, and I felt better about myself. I also started to work out at the gym. This really improved my self-esteem and I began to get the glimmer that maybe I was attractive. I also left my job as a secretary and became an editor.

I recognize now that Ed gave me the encouragement I needed. I was very insecure about interviewing for an editing position, and my parents were anything but supportive. Ed gave me the extra ounce of confidence I needed. He was positive and kind. When I got the job, he congratulated me, implying "You did it!" My mother commented on how nice it was for my old boss to get me the job. The difference two years of therapy made was incredible. I didn't respond when she said it; I just smiled to myself and knew that she would always see it in the negative way she chose to see it.

I visualize the second year of therapy as the emergence of my new self, though I am not sure exactly how this happened. When I asked Ed, all he said was that he reparented me without criticism. He let me be myself. That is not to say I didn't do any work. I believe I did a lot of work, mostly conscious thought and action. I looked at my motives, actions, and reactions, pointed out my behavior patterns to myself and in a safe place learned how to [change them], and made a continual effort to change them.

The third year of therapy was a blossoming for me. After clearing away the most glaring destructive patterns, working through a depression, and building a little self-esteem, I forged ahead to work on the more subtle problems.

I developed intimate and rewarding relationships with some very special female friends. I got sober with six of these women in AA and CA. We formed a group and meet once a month for dinner and a meeting. I now love these women as sisters. I learned through them how to communicate joy and sorrow to a friend and how to say, "You hurt my feelings" and move on. I feel committed to my relationships with them and so I am willing to change my behavior to help our friendships. These are new feelings for me. I was never accustomed to risking or being vulnerable with anyone, least of all another woman. Today I have trust and faith. I know if there are confrontations, they will not end the friendship.

The third year of therapy I came to accept myself—my good traits and my bad traits. I no longer feel at odds with myself because at times I can be very aggressive, loud, and self-obsessed. I know that I am a good person with a lot to give but, like anyone, sometimes my less attractive traits get in the way of that. Today, I am comfortable with who I am.

When Ed announced my therapy would end soon, I was both excited and fearful. I asked him if people got depressed when their therapy ended and he replied they did. What he didn't tell me was that I would revert to whatever old negative behavior patterns would marginally work and that I might even acquire some new ones.

Even on the last day of therapy Ed wanted to talk about my feelings on ending therapy, but I could not get the words out in his office. Just the words, "I'll miss you," were difficult to say. Of course, the minute I got into my car and began to drive out [of] the parking lot, I started to cry.

Before therapy ended, Ed mentioned that I may need to come back for psychotherapy when I get into a relationship. Now I see that he may be right.

Other than missing therapy occasionally, I feel good about having finished it. There are few activities in my life that I consider accomplishments, things that I actually saw through to completion; therapy is definitely one of them. I feel that I swallowed some big truths about myself and changed many of my negatives into positives. I feel proud.

It didn't happen in one room, for one hour of the week. It was a process of living as a trial ground for a new person. It was really a process for which AA has coined the perfect phrase: uncover, discover, and discard. In therapy I did one more thing: build. Not only did I rid myself of the unnecessary baggage I was carrying around but I added a wealth of knowledge and happiness to my life.

Shortly after leaving therapy, I told my parents that I could no longer participate in their dysfunction. I told them this in the most loving way I could, but I was also firm with them. I explained the various roles we played on our family stage and tried to let them know that my part was over.

A few months later I had to make two decisions; the first was to let my parents know I would no longer accept any kind of money from them, the second was not to sleep in their house. The important reason I cannot stay in their home is them. They are very critical and negative, and they know no boundaries. In addition, my mother constantly picks on my father. He shuts off his feelings and it all slides off his back. Frustrated, my mother starts to pick on me.

Debby's two actions here are both examples of working through insights about individuation directly with her parents.

While I do not envision great strides on the horizon, I do see things improving for me and possibly for my family. I certainly feel a strong, loving and supportive bond with my sister and sometimes I feel I am growing closer to my father. I can only hope that my mother is not threatened by these developing relationships, but I am certain she will be.

About a year after writing this postscript, and in her seventh year of sobriety, Debby returned to therapy. Her major issue was a relationship with a man whom she described as the first truly desirable man she had been involved with. She was also concerned about her mother, who was apparently becoming severely depressed and was refusing treatment. Debby mobilized her family and her mother's previous therapist to perform a modified intervention; that succeeded in getting her mother to return to psychotherapy and initiate pharmacotherapy, both of which were somewhat helpful. The problem with her new significant relationship was somewhat more difficult to resolve. This man was just getting out of a bad marriage and wanted time on his own and the opportunity to test other relationships before he made a commitment to monogamy with Debby. She was obsessively preoccupied with his dates, as he was with her sexual relationships prior to him (she had shared these during a long friendship that had preceded their becoming lovers).

In Debby's first session back, she realized that she had let go of her own self-growth program as a result of her preoccupation with this man. She realized it was essential that she resume it; within a week, she was again working out regularly in a gym, socializing with female friends, and going back to her favorite women's AA meeting. She negotiated a reasonable fee so that during this course of therapy she could pay for it entirely on her own (her parents had paid until this time).

Debby began to feel her sense of self-esteem return about 2 months after she returned to therapy. Her new beau joined us for several sessions. He also returned to his individual psychotherapist, who at the same time confronted him about his distancing maneuvers. I pointed out to them that their relationship was maintaining a tenuous balance through their preoccupations with each other's past and present relationships. I stated that they both needed to hold on to their preoccupations in order to maintain distance from each other. They returned again after they had been living together for a month, having handled the transition with surprisingly little conflict. We processed how their romantic love was shifting to a working love while maintaining the former. After a few more individual sessions, Debby terminated again, calling me later to inform me when and where she was celebrating her eighth CA birthday. Shortly before the completion of her ninth year of sobriety, I received a wedding invitation from Debby and her husband-to-be. I had already accepted a prior wedding invitation in another state for that weekend, or I would have gladly attended.

Debby's previous therapy enabled her to work through her current conflicts with her significant other rather rapidly. However, she first had to return to her sober core in order to utilize her self-knowledge and give her the strength to risk the intimacy of a close relationship.

References

Ablon J., Al-Anon family groups. *American Journal of Psychotherapy, 28:* 30–45, 1974.

Abraham, K. The psychological relations between sexuality and alcoholism. In *Selected Papers in Psychoanalysis*. New York: Brunner/Mazel, 1979, pp. 80–90. (Original work published 1908)

Adler, G. *Borderline Psychopathology and Its Treatment.* New York: Jason Aronson, 1985.

Alexander, F., & French, T. *Psychoanalytic Therapy.* New York: Ronald Press, 1946.

American Psychiatric Association. *Diagnostic and Statistical Manual of Mental Disorders* (3rd ed., rev.). Washington, DC: Author, 1987.

American Psychiatric Association. *DSM-IV Options Book: Work in Progress 9/1/91.* Washington, DC: Author, 1991.

Anderson, C. M., & Stewart, S. *Mastering Resistance: A Practical Guide to Family Therapy.* New York: Guilford Press, 1983.

Babor, T. F., Hofman, M., DelBoca, F. K., Hesselbrock, V., Meyer, R., Dolinsky, Z., & Rounsaville, B. Types of alcoholics: I. Evidence for an empirically derived typology based on indicators of vulnerability and severity. *Archives of General Psychiatry, 49:* 599–608, 1992.

Baldinger, R., Goldsmith, B. M., Capel, W. C., & Stewart, G. T. Pot smokers, junkies and squares: A comparative study of female values. *International Journal of the Addictions, 7:* 153–166, 1972.

Banys, P. The clinical use of disulfiram (Antabuse): A review. *Journal of Psychoactive Drugs, 20*(3): 243–261, 1988.

Barnett, M. J., & Trepper, T. S. Treating women abusers who were victims of childhood sexual abuse. In C. Bepko (Ed), *Feminism and Addiction.* New York: Haworth Press, 1991, pp. 127–146.

Bateson, G., Jackson, D. D., Haley, J., & Weakland, J. H. Towards a theory of schizophrenia. *Behavioral Science, 1:* 251–264, 1956.

Bean-Bayog, M. Psychopathology produced by alcoholism. In R. E. Meyer (Ed.), *Psychopathology and Addictive Disorders.* New York: Guilford Press, 1986, pp. 334–345.

Beck, A. T., Freeman, A., & Associates. *Cognitive Therapy of Personality Disorders.* New York: Guilford Press, 1990.

Beckman, L. J. Women alcoholics: A review of social and psychological studies. *Journal of Studies on Alcohol, 36*(7): 797–824, 1975.

Beckman, L. J., Day, T., Bardoley, P., & Seeman, A. The personality characteristics and family backgrounds of women alcoholics. *International Journal of the Addictions, 15:* 147–154, 1980.

Bepko, C., & Krestan, J. *The Responsibility Trap.* New York: Free Press, 1985.

Berenson, D. Powerlessness — liberating or enslaving? Responding to the feminist critique of the Twelve Steps. In C. Bepko (Ed.), *Feminism and Addiction,* New York: Haworth Press, 1991, pp. 67–84.

Binion, V. J. A descriptive comparison of the families of origin of women heroin users and abusers. In *Addicted Women: Family Dynamics, Self-Perceptions and Support Systems* (DHEW Publication No. ADM 80-762). Rockville, MD: National Institute on Drug Abuse, 1980, pp. 77–133.

Bion, W. R. *Learning from Experience.* New York: Basic Books, 1962.

Bollerud, K. A model for the treatment of trauma-related syndromes among chemically dependent inpatient women. *Journal of Substance Abuse Treatment, 7:* 83–87, 1990.

Bond, M. An empirical study of defense styles. In G. E. Vaillant (Ed.), *Empirical Studies of Ego Mechanisms of Defense.* Washington, DC: American Psychiatric Press, 1986, pp. 2–29.

Boothroyd, W. E. Nature and development of alcoholism in women. In O. M. Kalant (Ed.), *Alcohol and Drug Problems in Women.* New York: Plenum Press, 1980, pp. 299–329.

Bowlby, J. Pathological mourning and childhood mourning. *Journal of the American Psychoanalytic Association, 2:* 500–511, 1963.

Bromet, E., & Moos, R. Sex and marital status in relation to the characteristics of alcoholics. *Journal of Studies on Alcohol, 37:* 1302–1312, 1976.

Brook, J. S., Whiteman, M., & Finch, S. Childhood aggression, adolescent delinquency, and drug use: A longitudinal study. *Journal of Genetic Psychology, 153*(4): 369–383, 1992.

Brook, J. S., Whiteman, M., Gordon, A. S., & Cohen, P. Dynamics of childhood and adolescent personality traits, and adolescent drug use. *Developmental Psychology, 22:* 403–414, 1986.

Brown, S. *Treating the Alcoholic: A Developmental Model of Recovery.* New York: Wiley, 1985.

Brown, S., & Yalom, I. D. Interactional group therapy with alcoholics. *Journal of Studies on Alcohol, 38:* 426–456, 1977.

Brownell, K. D., Marlatt, G. A., Lichtenstein, E., & Wilson, G. T. Understanding and preventing relapse. *American Psychologist, 41:* 765–782, 1986.

Burt, M. R., Glynn, T. M., & Sowder, B. J. *Psychosocial Characteristics of Drug-Abusing Women.* Rockville, MD: National Institute on Drug Abuse, 1979.

Cadogan, D. A. Marital group therapy in the treatment of alcoholism. *Quarterly Journal of Studies on Alcohol 34:* 1187–1197, 1973.

Cadoret, R. J., Troughton, E., O'Gorman, T.W., & Heywood, E. An adoption study of genetic and environmental factors in drug abuse. *Archives of General Psychiatry, 43:* 1131–1136, 1986.

Cadoret, R. J., Troughton, E., & Widmer, R. B. Clinical differences between antisocial and primary alcoholics. *Comprehensive Psychiatry, 25:* 1–8, 1984.

Cahn, S. *The Treatment of Alcoholics: An Evaluative Study.* New York: Oxford University Press, 1970.

Carrol, E. N., & Zuckerman, J. Psychopathology and sensation seeking in "downers," "speeders," and "trippers": A study of the relationship between personality and drug choice. *International Journal of the Addictions, 12*(4): 591–601, 1977.

Cashion, B. Female-headed families: Effects on children and clinical implications. In *Journal of Marriage and Family Therapy, 8:* 77–85, 1982.

Chappel, J. Effective use of Alcoholics Anonymous and Narcotics Anonymous in treating patients. *Psychiatric Annals, 22*(8): 409–415, 1992.

Chein, I., et al. *The Road to H.* New York: Basic Books, 1964.

Chessick, R. D. The pharmacogenic orgasm in the drug addict. *Archives of General Psychiatry, 3:* 117–128, 1960.

Chessick, R. D. *Psychology of the Self and the Treatment of Narcissism.* Northvale, NJ: Jason Aronson, 1985.

Cloninger, C. R. A systematic method for clinical description and classification of personality variants. *Archives of General Psychiatry, 45:* 111–119, 1988.

Coleman, E. Chemical dependency and intimacy dysfunction. *Journal of Chemical Dependency Treatment, 1*(1): 13–26, 1987.

Colten, M. E. A descriptive and comparative analysis of self-perceptions and attitudes of heroin addicted women. In *Addicted Women: Family Dynamics, Self-Perceptions and Support Systems.* (DHEW Publication No. ADM 80-762). Rockville, MD: National Institute on Drug Abuse, 1980.

Conley, J. J. Family configuration as an etiological factor in alcoholism. *Journal of Abnormal Psychology, 89*(5): 670–673, 1980.

Corrigan, E. M., *Alcoholic Women in Treatment.* New York: Oxford University Press, 1980.

Craig, R. J. Personality characteristics of heroin addicts: Review of empirical research, 1976–1979. *International Journal of the Addictions, 17*(2), 227–248, 1982.

Craig, R. J. A psychometric study of the prevalence of DSM-III personality disorders among treated opiate addicts. *International Journal of the Addictions, 23*(2): 115–124, 1988.

DeLeon, G. Phoenix house: Psychopathology among male and female drug-free residents. *Addictive Diseases, 1*(2), 135–152, 1974.

DeLeon, G., & Jainchill, N. Female drug users: Sociological and psychological status two years after treatment in a therapeutic community. Presented at the National Alcohol and Drug Conference, Washington, D.C., 1980.

Dicks, H. *Marital Tensions.* London, Tavistock, 1967.

Dodes, L. M., & Khantzian, E. Individual psychodynamic psychotherapy. In R. J. Frances & S. I. Miller (Eds.), *Clinical Textbook of Addictive Disorders.* New York: Guilford Press, 1991, pp. 391–405.

Doehrman, M., & Gross, J. Parallel process in supervision and psychotherapy. *Bulletin of the Menninger Clinic, 40*(1): 1976.

DuPont, R. L. *Getting Tough on Gateway Drugs.* Washington, DC: American Psychiatric Press, 1984.

Ellinwood, E. H., Smith, W. G., & Vaillant, G. E. Narcotic addiction in males and females: A comparison. *International Journal of the Addictions, 1:* 33–45, 1966.

Emrick, C. D., Torrigan, J. S., Montgomery, H., & Little, L. Alcoholics Anonymous: What is currently known? In B. S. McCrady & W. R. Miller (Eds.), *Research on Alcoholics Anonymous.* New Brunswick, NJ: Rutgers Center for Alcohol Studies, 1993, pp. 41–76.

Erikson, E. H. *Childhood and Society.* New York: Norton, 1950.

Esman, A. H. Dependent and passive aggressive personality disorders. In A. M. Cooper, A. J. Frances, & M. H. Sacks (Eds.), *The Personality Disorders and Neuroses.* New York: Basic Books, 1986.

Estep, R. The influence of the family on the use of alcohol and prescription depressants by women. *Journal of Psychoactive Drugs, 19*(2): 171–179, 1987.

Feldman, L. *Integrating Individual and Family Therapy.* New York: Brunner/Mazel, 1992.

Fenichel, O. *The Psychoanalytic Theory of Neurosis.* New York: Norton, 1945.

Forrest, G. C. *Alcoholism and Human Sexuality.* Springfield, IL: Charles C. Thomas, 1982.

Forth-Finegan, J. L. Sugar and spice and everything nice: Gender socialization and women's addiction—a literature review. In C. Bepko (Ed.), *Feminism and Addiction.* New York: Haworth Press, 1991, pp. 19–48.

Fox, R. Group psychotherapy with alcoholics. *International Journal of Group Psychotherapy, 12:* 56–63, 1962.

Fox, R. Group psychotherapy with alcoholics. In M. Rosenbaum & M. M. Berger (Eds.), *Group Psychotherapy and Group Function.* New York: Basic Books, 1975, pp. 521–528.

Freeman, P. S., & Gunderson, J. Treatment of personality disorders. *Psychiatric Annals,*
19(3): 147–153, 1989.

Freud, A. *The Ego and the Mechanisms of Defense.* New York: International Universities
Press, 1966.

Freud, S. *Origins of Psychoanalysis: Letters to Wilhelm Fliess, Drafts and Notes, 1887–1092*
(M. Bonaparte, Ed. and Trans.). New York: Basic Books, 1954.

Freud, S. The future prospects of psycho-analytic therapy. *Standard Edition, 11:* 139–151,
1957. (Original work published 1910)

Freud, S. Beyond the pleasure principle. *Standard Edition, 18:* 3–64, 1955. (Original work
published 1920)

Freud, S. Instincts and their vicissitudes. *Standard Edition, 14:* 109–140, 1957. (Original
work published 1915)

Freud, S. Dostoevsky and parricide. *Standard Edition, 21:* 173–194, 1961. (Original work
published 1928)

Fuller, R. F., & Roth, H. P. Disulfiram for the treatment of alcoholism: An evaluation of
128 men. *Annals of Internal Medicine, 90:* 901–904, 1979.

Galanter, M. Network therapy for addiction. *American Journal of Psychiatry, 150*(1): 28–36,
1993.

Gerstley, L., McLellan, T., Alterman, A. I., Luborsky, L., & Prout, M. Ability to form
an alliance with the therapist: A possible marker of prognosis for patients with antisocial personality disorder. *American Journal of Psychiatry, 146*(4): 508–512, 1989.

Gessner, P. K. Treatment of the alcohol withdrawal syndrome. *Substance Abuse, 1:* 2–5,
1979.

Giovacchini, P. L. *A Narrative Textbook of Psychoanalysis.* Northvale, NJ: Jason Aronson, 1987.

Glatt, M. M. Reflections on the treatment of alcoholism in women. *British Journal on Alcohol and Alcoholism, 14*(2): 77–83, 1979.

Glover, E. On the aetiology of drug abuse. *International Journal of Psycho-Analysis, 1932.*

Glueck, S., & Glueck, E. *Toward a Typology of Juvenile Offenders.* New York: Grune
& Stratton, 1970.

Goldberg, M. Loss and grief: Major dynamics in the treatment of alcoholism. *Psychosocial
Issues in the Treatment of Alcoholism, 2*(1): 37–46, 1985.

Goldsmith, R. J. An integrated psychology for the addictions: Beyond the self medication
hypothesis. *Journal of Addictive Diseases, 12*(3): 139–154, 1993.

Goldsmith, S. J., Jacobsberg, L. B., & Bell, R. Personality disorder assessment. *Psychiatric
Annals, 19:* 139–142, 1989.

Gomberg, E. S. Risk factors related to alcohol problems among women: Proneness and vulnerability. In *Alcoholism and Alcohol Abuse among Women.* Washington, DC: U.S.
Department of Health, Education and Welfare, 1980.

Goodwin, D. W. Genetic componentss of alcoholism. *Annual Review of Medicine, 32:* 93–99,
1981.

Grant, I., & Reed, R. Neuropsychology of alcohol and drug use. In A. I. Alterman (Ed.),
Substance Abuse and Psychopathology. New York: Plenum Press, 1985, pp. 289–341.

Greenblatt, D. J., & Shader, R. I. Treatment of the alcohol withdrawal syndrome. In R.
I. Shader (Ed.), *Manual of Psychiatric Therapeutics.* Boston: Little, Brown, 1975, pp.
211–215.

Griffin, M. C., Weiss, R. D., Mirin, S. M., & Lange, V. A comparison of male and female
cocaine abusers. *Archives of General Psychiatry, 46:* 122–126, 1989.

Grinberg, L. On a specific aspect of countertransference due to the patient's projective identification. *International Journal of Psycho-Analysis, 43,* 436–440, 1962.

Haley, J. *Problem-Solving Therapy.* San Francisco: Jossey-Bass, 1977.

Halikas, J. A., Crosby, R. D., Carlson, G. A., Crea, F., Graves, N. M., & Bowers, L. D. Cocaine reduction in unmotivated crack users using carbamazepine versus placebo in a short-term double-blind crossover design. *Clinical Pharmacology and Therapeutics, 50:* 81–95, 1991.

Hamilton, N. G. *Self and Others: Object Relations Theory in Practice.* Northvale, NJ: Jason Aronson, 1988.

Hare-Mustin, R. T. A feminist approach to family therapy. *Family Process, 17:* 181–194, 1978.

Hart, L. S., & Stueland, D.S. Classifying women alcoholics by Cattell's 16PF. *Journal of Studies on Alcohol, 41:* 911–921, 1980.

Hedges, L.E. *Listening Perspectives in Psychotherapy.* Northvale, NJ: Jason Aronson, 1983.

Hedges, L. E. *Interpreting the Countertransference.* Northvale, NJ: Jason Aronson, 1992.

Helzer, J. E., & Pryzbeck, T. R. The co-occurrence of alcoholism with other psychiatric disorders in the general population and its impact on treatment. *Journal of Studies on Alcohol, 49*(3): 219–224, 1988.

Hendin, H. Psychosocial theory of drug abuse: A psychodynamic approach. In D. J. Lettieri, M. Sayers, & H. W. Pearson (Eds.), *Theories on Drug Abuse: Selected Contemporary Perspectives* (NIDA Research Monograph No. 30). Rockville, MD: National Institute on Drug Abuse, 1980, pp. 195–200.

Hesselbrock, M. N., Meyer, R. E., & Keener, J. J. Psychopathology in hospitalized alcoholics. *Archives of General Psychiatry, 42:* 1050–1055, 1985.

Hill, H. E., Haertzen, C. A., & Davis, H. An MMPI factor analytic study of alcoholics, narcotic addicts and criminals. *Quarterly Journal of Studies on Alcohol, 23:* 411–431, 1962.

Hoffman, H., Noem, A. A., & Petersen, D. Treatment effectiveness as judged by successfully and unsuccesssfully treated alcoholics. *Drug and Alcohol Dependence, 1:* 241–246, 1976.

Hoffman, H., & Welfring, L. R. Sex and age differences in psychiatric symptoms in alcoholics. *Psychological Reports, 30:* 887–889, 1972.

Horney, K. *New Ways in Psychoanalysis.* New York: Norton, 1949.

Horowitz, L. Projective identification in dyads and groups. *International Journal of Group Psychtherapy, 33*(3): 259–279, 1983.

Hurt, S. W., & Clarkin, J. F. Borderline personality disorder: Prototypic typology and the development of therapy manuals. *Psychiatric Annals, 20*(1): 13–18, 1990.

Imhoff, J. E. Countertransference issues in the treatment of drug and alcohol addiction. In N. S. Miller (Ed.), *Comprehensive Handbook of Drug and Alcohol Addiction.* New York: Marcel Dekker, 1991, pp. 931–946.

Imhoff, J., Hirsch, R., & Terenzi, R.E. Countertransferential and attitudinal considerations in the treatment of drug abuse and addiction. *International Journal of the Addictions, 18*(4): 491–510, 1983.

Jaffe, J. H., & Ciraulo, D.A. Drugs used in treatment of alcoholism. In J. H. Mendelson & N. K. Mello (Eds.), *Diagnosis and Treatment of Alcoholism.* New York: McGraw-Hill, 1985.

Johnson, A., & Szurek, S. The genesis of antisocial acting out in children and adults. *Psychoanalytic Quarterly, 21:* 323, 1952.

Johnson, C. W. A descriptive study of 100 convicted female narcotics residents. *Corrective Psychiatry, 14:* 23–26, 1968.

Johnson, V. E. *I'll Quit Tomorrow* (rev. ed.). San Francisco: Harper & Row, 1980.

Kail, B. L., & Lukoff, I. F. Differentials in the treatment of black female heroin addicts. *Drug and Alcohol Dependence, 13:* 55–63, 1984.

Kandel, D. B. Stages in adolescent involvement in drug abuse. *Science, 190:* 912–914, 1975.

Kaplan, H. I., & Sadock, B. J. *Modern Synopsis of Comprehensive Textbook of Psychiatry.* Baltimore: Williams & Wilkins, 1981.

Kasl, C. D. *Many Roads, One Journey: Moving Beyond the 12 Steps.* New York: Harper-Collins, 1992.

Kaufman, E. Group therapy techniques used by the ex-addict therapist. *Group Process, 5:* 3–19, 1972.

Kaufman, E. The psychodynamics of opiate dependence: A new look. *American Journal of Drug and Alcohol Abuse, 1,* 349–370, 1974.

Kaufman, E. The abuse of multiple drugs: I. Definition, classification and extent of problem. *American Journal of Drug and Alcohol Abuse, 16*(1), 106–118, 1976a.

Kaufman, E. The abuse of multiple drugs: II. Psychological hypotheses, treatment considerations. *American Journal of Drug and Alcohol Abuse, 3*(2), 293–301, 1976b.

Kaufman, E. Polydrug abuse or multi-drug misuse: It's here to stay. *British Journal of Addiction, 72:* 339–347, 1977.

Kaufman, E. Individualized group treatment for drug dependent clients. *Group, 2:* 22–30, 1978.

Kaufman, E. Family structures of narcotic addicts. *International Journal of the Addictions, 16*(2): 93–102, 1981.

Kaufman, E. Group therapy for substance abusers. In M. Grotjahn, C. Friedman, & F. Kline (Eds), *A Handbook of Group Therapy.* New York: Van Nostrand Reinhold, 1982, pp. 163–191.

Kaufman, E. *Substance Abuse and Family Therapy.* New York: Grune & Stratton, 1985.

Kaufman, E. *Help at Last: A Complete Guide to Coping with Chemically Dependent Men.* New York: Gardner Press, 1991.

Kaufman, E., & Kaufmann, P. *Family Therapy of Drug and Alcohol Abuse.* New York: Gardner Press, 1979.

Kaufman, E., & Kaufmann, P. *Family Therapy of Drug and Alcohol Abuse* (2nd ed.). Boston: Allyn & Bacon, 1992.

Kaufman, E., & Reoux, J. Guidelines for the successful psychotherapy of substance abusers. *American Journal of Drug and Alcohol Abuse, 14:* 199–209, 1988.

Kendler, K., Heath, A., Neale, M., Kessler, R., & Eaves, L. Alcoholism and major depression in women. *Archives of General Psychiatry, 50*(9): 690–698, 1993.

Kernberg, O. F. The concept of countertransference. *Journal of the American Psychoanalytic Association, 13,* 38–56, 1965.

Kernberg, O. F. Borderline personality organization. *Journal of the American Psychoanalytic Association, 5:* 641–685, 1967.

Kernberg, O. F. Factors in the treatment of narcissistic personality disorder. *Journal of the American Psychoanalytic Association, 18:* 51–85, 1970.

Kernberg, O. F. *Borderline Conditions and Pathological Narcissim.* New York: Jason Aronson, 1975.

Kernberg, O. F. *Severe Personality Disorders: Psychotherapeutic Strategies.* New Haven, CT: Yale University Press, 1984.

Kernberg, O. F. An ego psychology object relations theory of structure and treatment of pathologic narcissism. *Psychiatric Clinics of North America, 12*(3): 723–729, 1989.

Kernberg, O. F., et al. *Psychodynamic Psychotherapy of Borderline Patients.* New York: Basic Books, 1988.

Khantzian, E. Impulse problems and drug addiction. In H. A. Wishnie & J. Nevis-Oelsen (Eds.), *Working with the Impulsive Person.* New York: Plenum Press, 1979.

Khantzian, E. J. An ego–self theory of substance dependence: A contemporary psychoanalytic perspective. In D. J. Lettieri, M. Sayers, & H. W. Pearson (Eds.), *Theories on Drug Abuse: Selected Contemporary Perspectives* (NIDA Research Monograph No. 30). Rockville, MD: National Institute on Drug Abuse Research, 1980, pp. 29–33.

Khantzian, E. J. Psychopathology, psychodynamics and alcoholism. In E. M. Pattison & E. Kaufman (Eds.), *Encyclopedia Handbook of Psychiatry*. New York: Gardner Press, 1982, pp. 581–597.

Khantzian, E. J., Halliday, K. S., & McAuliffe, W. E. *Addiction and the Vulnerable Self*. New York: Guilford Press, 1990.

Khantzian, E. J., & Mack, S. M. Self preservation and the care of the self-ego: Instinct reconsidered. *Psychoanalytic Study of the Child, 38:* 209–232, 1983.

Khantzian, E. J., & Mack, S. M. Alcoholics Anonymous and contemporary psychodynamic theory. In M. Galanter (Ed.), *Recent Developments in Alcoholism* (Vol. 7). New York: Plenum Press, 1989, pp. 67–89.

Khantzian, E. J., & Schneider, R. J. Treatment implications of psychodynamic understanding of opioid addicts. In R. E. Meyer (Ed.), *Psychopathology and Addictive Disorders*. New York: Guilford Press, 1986, pp. 323–333.

Khantzian, E. J., & Treece, C. DSM-III psychiatric diagnosis of narcotic addicts. *Archives of General Psychiatry, 42:* 1067–1071, 1985.

Klein, M. Notes on some schizoid mechanisms. In *Envy and Gratitude and Other Works (1946–1963)* (Vol. 3). New York: Free Press/Macmillan, 1984, 1–24.

Kleinman, P. H., Miller, A. B., & Millman, R. B. Psychopathology among cocaine abusers entering treatment. *Journal of Nervous and Mental Disease, 178:* 442–447, 1990.

Koenigsberg, H. W., Kaplan, R. D., Gilmore, M. M., et al. The relationship between syndrome and personality disorder in DSM-III: Experience with 2,462 patients. *American Journal of Psychiatry, 142:* 207–212, 1985.

Kohut, H. *The Analysis of the Self*. New York: International Universities Press, 1971.

Kohut, H. Thoughts on narcissism and narcissistic rage. *Psychoanalytic Study of the Child, 27:* 360–400, 1972.

Kohut, H. *The Restoration of the Self*. New York: International Universities Press, 1977.

Kosten, T. R. Pharmacotherapeutic interventions for cocaine abuse: Matching patients to treatment. *Journal of Nervous and Mental Disease, 177*(7): 379–389, 1989.

Kosten, T. R., Kleber, H. D., & Morgan, C. Treatment of cocaine abuse with buprenorphine. *Biological Psychiatry, 26:* 170–172, 1989.

Kosten, T. R., & Rounsaville, B. J. Psychopathology in opioid addicts. *Psychiatric Clinics of North America, 9*(3): 515–532, 1986.

Kosten, T. R., Rounsaville, B. J., & Kleber, H. D. DSM-III personality disorders in opiate addicts. *Comprehensive Psychiatry, 23:* 572–591, 1982.

Krystal, H. Trauma and affect. *Psychoanalytic Study of the Child, 36,* 81–116, 1978.

Krystal, H. *Integration and Self Healing: Affect, Trauma, Alexithymia*. Hillsdale, NJ: Analytic Press, 1985.

Krystal, H., & Raskin, H. A. *Drug Dependent: Aspects of Ego Functions*. Detroit: Wayne State University Press, 1970.

Lachar, D., Berman, W., Grisell, J. L., & Schoof, K. A heroin addiction scale for the MMPI: Effectiveness in differential diagnosis in a psychiatric setting. *International Journal of the Addictions, 14:* 135–142, 1979.

Langs, R. *Technique in Transition*. New York: Jason Aronson, 1978.

Lemle, R., & Mishkind, M. E. Alcohol and masculinity. *Journal of Substance Abuse Treatment, 6:* 213–222, 1989.

Levin, J. D. *Treatment of Alcoholism and Other Addictions*. Northvale, NJ: Jason Aronson, 1987.

Levine, S., & Stephens, R. Games addicts play. *Psychiatric Quarterly,* 582–592, 1972.

Levinson, V. R. The compatibility of the disease concept with a psychodynamic approach in the treatment of alcoholism. *Psychosocial Issues in the Treatment of Alcoholism, 2*(1): 7–24, 1985.

Liddle, H. Five factors of failure in structural–strategic family therapy: A contextual construction. In S. Coleman (Ed.), *Failures in Family Therapy.* New York: Guilford Press, 1985.

Liepman, M. R., Nirenberg, T. D., & Begin, A. M. Evaluation of a program designed to help family and significant others to motivate resistant alcoholics into recovery. *American Journal of Drug and Alcohol Abuse, 15*(2): 209–221, 1989.

Lindblad-Goldberg, M. Successful minority single parent families. In L. Combrinck-Graham (Ed.), *Children in Family Contexts: Perspectives on Treatment.* New York: Guilford Press, 1989.

Liskow, V., & Goodwin, D. Pharmacological treatment of alcohol intoxication withdrawal and dependence: A critical review. *Journal of Studies on Alcohol, 48*(4): 356–370, 1987.

Litt, M. D., Babor, T. F., & Del Boca, F. K. Types of alcoholics II: Application of an empirically derived typology to treatment matching. *Archives of General Psychiatry, 49:* 609–614, 1992.

MacAndrew, C. The differentiation of male alcoholic outpatients by means of the MMPI. *Quarterly Journal of Studies on Alcoholism, 26:* 238–246, 1965.

MacKinnon, R. A., & Michels, R. *The Psychiatric Interview in Clinical Practice.* Philadelphia: W. B. Saunders, 1971.

Marsh, J. *Women helping women: The evaluation of an all female methadone maintenance program in detroit.* Paper presented at the National Drug Abuse Conference, Seattle, 1979.

Masterson, J. F. *The Narcissistic and Borderline Disorders.* New York: Brunner/Mazel, 1981.

McAuliffe, W. E., & Albert, J. *Clean Start: An Outpatient Program for Initiating Cocaine Recovery.* New York: Guilford Press, 1992.

McDuff, D. R., & Soulounias, B. Use of brief psychotherapy with substance abusers in early recovery. *Journal of Psychotherapy Practice and Research, 1*(2): 163–170, 1992.

McGlashan, T. H., & Heinssen, R. K. Narcissistic, antisocial and noncomorbid subgroups. *Psychiatric Clinics of North America, 12*(3): 653–670, 1989.

McGuffin, P., & Thapar, A. The genetics of personality disorder. In *Personality Disorder Reviewed,* Royal College of Psychiatrists, pp. 42–63, 1993.

McKenna, T., & Perkins, R. Alcoholic children of alcoholics. *Journal of Studies on Alcohol, 42:* 1021–1029, 1981.

Meller, W. H., Rinehart, R., Cadoret, R. J., & Troughton, E. Specific familial transmission in substance abuse. *International Journal of the Addictions, 23*(10): 1029–1039, 1988.

Merikangas, K. R., Leckman, S. R., Prusoff, B. A., & Weissman, M. M. Familial transmission of depression and alcoholism. *Archives of General Psychiatry, 42:* 367–372, 1985.

Metzger, L. *From Denial to Recovery.* San Francisco: Jossey-Bass, 1988.

Meyer, R. E. How to understand the relationship between psychopathology and addictive disorders. In R. E. Meyer (Ed.), *Psychopathology and Addictive Disorders.* New York: Guilford Press, 1986, pp. 3–16.

Milkman, H., & Frosch, W. On the preferential abuse of heroin and amphetamines. *Journal of Nervous and Mental Disease, 156*(4): 242–248, 1973.

Milkman, H., & Frosch, W. Theory of drug use. In D.J. Lettieri, M. Sayers, & H.W. Pearson (Eds.), *Theories on Drug Abuse: Selected Contemporary Perspectives* (NIDA Research Monograph No. 30). Rockville, MD: National Institute on Drug Abuse, 1980.

Miller, J. S., Sensenig, J., Stocker, R. B., & Campbell, R. Value patterns of drug addicts as a function of race and sex. *International Journal of the Addictions, 8:* 589–598, 1973.

Millon, T. *Disorders of Personality, DSM III.* New York: Wiley, 1981.

Minuchin, S. *Families and Family Therapy.* Cambridge, MA: Harvard University Press, 1974.

Minuchin, S., & Fishman, H. C. *Family Therapy Techniques,* Cambridge, MA: Harvard University Press, 1981.

Modell, A. H. The holding environment and the therapeutic action of psychoanalysis. *Journal of the American Psychoanalytic Association, 24:* 258–308, 1976.

Mogar, R. E., Wilson, W. M., & Helm, S. T. Personality subtypes of male and female alcoholic patients. *International Journal of the Addictions, 5:* 99–113, 1970.

Moise, R. *Three Portraits of Women Entering Drug Abuse Treatment Programs.* Ann Arbor: Women's Drug Research Project, University of Michigan, 1979.

Nace, E. P. Personality disorder in the alcoholic patient. *Psychiatric Annals, 19*(5): 256–260, 1989.

National Client Data System. (1992). [Personal internal memo from the Substance Abuse Mental Health Services Administration] Bethesda, MD: Author.

National Institute of Alcohol Abuse and Alcoholism. *Information and Feature Service,* ADAMHA, December 1, 1982.

New York Times, p. 11, June 20, 1993.

O'Connor, P. G., Waugh, M. E., Schottenfeld, R. S., et al. Ambulatory opiate detoxification and primary care: A role of the primary care physician. *Journal of General Internal Medicine, 7:* 532–534, 1992.

Okpaku, S. O. Psychoanalytically oriented psychotherapy of substance abusers. *Advances in Alcohol and Substance Abuse, 6:* 17–53, 1986.

Oldham, J. M., & Skodol, A. E. Personality disorders in the public sector. *Hospital and Community Psychiatry, 42*(5): 481–387, 1991.

Orr, O. W. Transference and countertransference: A historical survey. *Journal of the American Psychoanalytic Association, 2:* 621–670, 1954.

Papp, P. Paradoxical strategies and countertransference. In A. S. Gurman (Ed.), *Questions and Answers in the Practice of Family Therapy.* New York: Brunner/Mazel, 1981.

Pattison, E. M. Clinical approaches to the alcoholic patient. *Psychosomatics, 27*(11): 762–770, 1986.

Penning, M., & Barnes, G. E. Adolescent marijuana use: A review. *International Journal of the Addictions, 17*(5): 749–791, 1982.

Perry, J. C., & Cooper, S. H. What do cross-sectional measures of defense mechanisms predict? In G. E. Vaillant (Ed.), *Empirical Studies of Ego Mechanisms of Defense.* Washington, DC: American Psychiatric Press, 1986, pp. 32–46.

Perry, J. C., Herman, J. L., van der Kolk, B. A., & Hobe, L. A. Psychotherapy and psychological trauma in borderline personality disorders. *Psychiatric Annals, 20*(1): 33–43, 1990.

Peteet, J. R. A closer look at the role of a spiritual approach in addictions treatment. *Journal of Substance Abuse Treatment, 10*(3): 263–268, 1993.

Rado, S. The psychic effects of intoxicants: An attempt to evolve a psychoanalytic theory of morbid cravings. In S. Rado (Ed.), *Psychoanalysis of Behavior.* New York: Grune & Stratton, 1960, pp. 25–39. (Original work published 1926)

Reed, B. G. Drug misuse and dependency in women: The meaning and implications of being considered a special population or minority group. *International Journal of the Addictions, 20*(1): 13–62, 1985.

Reichman, W. Affecting attitudes and assumptions about women and alcohol problems. *Alcohol Health and Research World, 7*(3): 6–10, 1983.

Rosen, A. C. A comparative study of alcoholics and psychiatric patients with the MMPI. *Quarterly Journal of Studies on Alcohol, 21:* 253–266, 1960.

Rosenbaum, M. *Women on Heroin.* New Brunswick, NJ: Rutgers University Press, 1981.

Rosenbloom, A. Emerging treatment options in the alcohol withdrawal syndrome. *Journal of Clinical Psychiatry, 49*(12): 28–31, 1988.

Rounsaville, B. J., Weissman, M. M., Kleber, H.D., et al. Heterogeneity of psychiatric diagnosis in treated opiate addicts. *Archives of General Psychiatry, 39:* 161–166, 1982.

Ryan, V. S., & Moise, R. *A Comparison of Women and Men Entering Drug Abuse Treat* ment Programs. Ann Arbor: Women's Drug Research Project, University of Michigan, 1979.

Sandler, J. Countertransference and role responsiveness. *International Review of Psycho-Analysis,* 43–47, 1976.

Sandmaier, M. *The Invisible Alcoholics: Women and Alcohol Abuse in America.* New York: McGraw-Hill, 1980.

Satir, V. *People Making.* Palo Alto, CA: Science and Behavior Books, 1972.

Savitt, R. Psychoanalytic studies on addiction: Ego structure in narcotic addiction. *Psychoanalytic Quarterly, 32:* 43–57, 1963.

Schuckit, M. A., Pitts, F. N., Reich, T., King, L. J., & Winokur, G. Alcoholism: I. Two types of alcoholism in women. *Archives of General Psychiatry, 20:* 301–306, 1969.

Schwingel, P., Sperazi, L., & Shelton, D. M. *Major issues in the development of a women's drug treatment program: A case study.* Paper presented at the National Institute on Drug Abuse Conference, San Francisco, 1977.

Shapiro, D. *Psychotherapy of Neurotic Character.* New York: Basic Books, 1989.

Shore, E. R. Drinking patterns and problems among women in paid employment. *Alcohol and Research World,* 16(2): 160–164, 1992.

Spotts, J. V., & Shontz, F. C. A lifetime history of chronic drug abuse. In D. J. Lettieri, M. Sayers, & H. W. Pearson (Eds.), *Theories on Drug Abuse: Selected Contemporary Perspectives* (NIDA Research Monograph No. 30). Rockville, MD: National Institute of Drug Abuse, 1980.

Stanton, M. D. Family treatment approaches to drug abuse problems: A review. *Family Process, 18:* 251–280, 1979a.

Stanton, M. D. Drugs and the family. *Marriage and Family Review,* 2(1): 1–10, 1979b.

Stanton, M. D., Todd, T. C., & Associates. *The Family Therapy of Drug Abuse and Addiction.* New York: Guilford Press, 1982.

Stillson, K., & Katz, C. A supervisory group process approach to address staff burnout and countertransference. *Alcoholism Treatment Quarterly, 2:* 117–134, 1985.

Stolorow, R., Brandshaft, B., & Atwood, G. *Psychoanalytic Treatment: An Intersubjective Approach.* Hillside, NJ: Analytic Press, 1987.

Stone, M. H. *The Borderline Syndrome.* New York: McGraw-Hill, 1980.

Stone, M. H. Long term follow-up of narcissistic/borderline patients. *Psychiatric Clinics of North America,* 12(3): 621–651, 1989.

Stone, M. Borderline personality disorder—contemporary issues in nosology, etiology and treatment. *Psychiatric Annals,* 20(1): 8–10, 1990.

Thomas, A., & Chess, S. *Temperament and Development.* New York: Brunner/Mazel, 1977.

Treece, C., & Khantzian, E. Psychodynamic factors in the development of drug dependence. *Psychiatric Clinics of North America,* 9(3): 209–232, 1986.

Tucker, M. B. A descriptive and comparative analysis of the social support structure of heroin addicted women. In *Addicted Women: Family Dynamics, Self Perceptions and Support Systems* (DHEW Publication No. ADM 80-762). Rockville, MD: National Institute on Drug Abuse, 1980.

Vaillant, G. E. Sociopathy is a human process: A viewpoint. *Archives of General Psychiatry, 32:* 178–188, 1975.

Vaillant, G. E. *Alcoholism and Drug Dependence: Harvard Guide to Modern Psychiatry.* Cambridge, MA: Belknap Press, 1978.

Vaillant, G. E. Introduction. In G. Vaillant (Ed.), *Empirical Studies of Ego Mechanisms of Defense.* Washington, DC: American Psychiatric Press, 1986.

Vannicelli, M. *Group Psychotherapy with Adult Children of Alcoholics.* New York: Guilford Press, 1989.

Vannicelli, M. *Removing the Roadblocks.* New York: Guilford Press, 1992.

Wall, J. H. A study of alcoholism in women. *American Journal of Psychiatry, 93:* 943–955, 1937.

Walker, G., Eric, K., Pironick, A., & Drucker, E. A descriptive outline of a program for cocaine-using mothers and their babies. In E. Bepko (Ed.), *Feminism and Addiction.* New York: Haworth Press, 1991, pp. 7–18.

Wallace, J. Critical issues in alcoholism therapy. In S. Zimberg, J. Wallace, & S. B. Blume (Eds.), *Practical Approaches to Alcoholism Psychotherapy* (2nd ed.). New York: Plenum Press, 1985a.

Wallace, J. Working with the preferred defense structure of the recovering alcoholic. In S. Zimberg, J. Wallace, & S. B. Blume (Eds.), *Practical Approaches to Alcoholism Psychotherapy* (2nd ed.). New York: Plenum Press, 1985b.

Wallace, N. *Support Networks among Drug Addicted Women and Men* (WOMAN Center Evaluation Report). Rockville, MD: National Institute on Drug Abuse. 1976.

Wallerstein, J. S. Transference and countertransference in clinical intervention with divorcing families. *American Journal of Orthopsychiatry, 60*(3): 337–345, 1990.

Washton, A. *Cocaine Addiction: Treatment, Recovery and Relapse Prevention.* New York: Norton, 1989.

Watzlawick, P., Weakland, J. H., & Fisch, R. *Change: Principles of Problem Formulation and Problem Resolution,* New York: Norton, 1974.

Weatherford, V., & Kaufman, E. Adult children of alcoholics: Prevalence of Axis II disorders and dysfunctional family patterns. *Journal of Family Violence, 6*(4): 319–335, 1991.

Weiss, R. D., & Mirin, S. M. Subtypes of cocaine abusers. *Psychiatric Clinics of North America, 9*(3): 491–501, 1986.

Whitehead, P.C. Acupuncture in the treatment of addiction: A review and analysis. *International Journal of the Addictions, 13:* 1–16, 1978.

Whitfield, C. L. Outpatient management of alcoholism. *Psychiatric Annals, 12:* 447, 1982.

Widiger, T., Frances, A., Warner, L., et al. Diagnostic criteria for the borderline and schizotypal personality disorders. *Journal of Abnormal Psychology, 95:* 43–51, 1986.

Widiger, T. A., & Rogers, J. H. Prevalence and comorbidity of personality disorders. *Psychiatric Annals, 19*(3): 132–136, 1989.

Wieder, H., & Kaplan, E. H. Drug use in adolescents: Psychodynamic meaning and pharmacogenic effect. *Psychoanalytic Study of the Child, 24:* 399–431, 1969.

Williams, C. N., & Klerman, L. V. Female alcoholic abuse: Its effects on the family. In S. C. Wilsnack & L. J. Beckman (Eds.), *Alcohol Problems in Women.* New York: Guilford Press, 1984, pp. 280–312.

Wilsnack, R. W., Wilsnack, S. C., & Klassen, A. D. Epidemiological research on women's drinking, 1978–1984. In *Women and Alcohol: Health Related Issues* (National Institute on Alcohol Abuse and Alcoholism Research Monograph No. 16; DHHS Publication No. ADM 86-1139). Washington, DC: U.S. Government Printing Office, 1966, pp. 1–68.

Wilsnack, S. C. The needs of the femal drinker: Dependency, power, or what? In M. E. Chafety (Ed.), *Psychological and Social Factors in Drinking and Treatment Evaluation: Proceedings of the Second Annual Alcoholism Conference of the National Institute on Alcohol Abuse and Alcoholism* (DHEW Publication No. NIH 74-676). Washington, DC: U.S. Government Printing Office, 1973.

Wilsnack, S. C. Alcohol abuse and alcoholism in women. In E. M. Pattison & E. Kaufman (Eds.), *Encyclopedia Handbook of Alcoholism.* New York: Gardner Press, 1982, pp. 718–735.

Winnicott, D. W. Hate in the countertransference. *International Journal of Psycho-Analysis, 30*(2), 69–74, 1949.

Winokur, G., & Clayton, P. J. Family history studies in comparison of male and female alcoholics. *Quarterly Journal of Studies on Alcohol, 29:* 885–891, 1968.

Winokur, G., & Pitts, F. N. Affective disorder: VI. A family history study of prevalences, sex differences and possible genetic factors. *Journal of Psychiatric Research, 3:* 113–123, 1965.

Winokur, G., Reich, T., Rimmer, J., & Pitts, F. N., Alcoholism: III. Diagnosis and familial psychiatric illness in 259 alcoholic probands. *Archives of General Psychiatry, 23:* 104–111, 1970.

Wolper, B., & Scheiner, Z. *Family Therapy Approaches and Drug-Dependent Women* (DHHS Publication No. ADM 81-1177). Rockville, MD: National Institute on Drug Abuse, 1981.

Woody, G. E., McLellan, A. T., Luborsky, L., et al. Sociopathy and psychotherapy outcome. *Archives of General Psychiatry, 42:* 1081–1086, 1984.

Woody, G. E., McLellan, A. T., Luborsky, L., & O'Brien, C. P. Psychotherapy for substance abuse. *Psychiatric Clinics of North America, 9:* 547–562, 1986.

Wright, K. D., & Scott, T. B. The relationship of wives' treatment to the drinking status of alcoholics. *Journal of Studies on Alcohol, 39:* 1577–1581, 1978.

Wurmser, L. Psychoanalytic considerations of the etiology of compulsive drug use. *Journal of the American Psychoanalytic Association, 22:* 820–843, 1974.

Wurmser, L. Flight from conscience: Experience with the psychoanalytic treatment of compulsive drug abusers, II. *Journal of Substance Abuse Treatment, 4:* 169–179, 1987.

Wurmser, L. Denial and split identity: Timely issues in the psychoanalytic psychotherapy of compulsive drug use. *Journal of Substance Abuse Treatment, 2:* 89–96, 1985.

Wrye, H., & Wells, J. K. The maternal erotic transference. *International Journal of Psycho-Analysis, 70:* 673–684, 1989.

Yalom, I. D., Bloch, S., Bond, G., Zimmerman, F., & Qualls, B. Alcoholics in interactional group therapy. *Archives of General Psychiatry, 35:* 419–425, 1978.

Zelen, S. L., Fox, J., Gould, E., & Olson, R. W. Sex contingent differences between male and female alcoholics. *Journal of Clinical Psychology, 22:* 160–165, 1966.

Zimberg, S. Principles of alcoholism psychotherapy. In S. Zimberg, J. Wallace, & S. B. Blume (Eds.), *Practical Approaches to Alcoholism Psychotherapy* (2nd ed.). New York: Plenum Press, 1985.

Index

AUTHOR'S NOTE

In July of 2000, when the first book, *Murder of a Small-Town Honey,* was published in my Scumble River series, it was written in "real time." It was the year 2000 in Skye's life as well as mine, but after several books in a series, time becomes a problem. It takes me from seven months to a year to write a book, and then it is usually another year from the time I turn that book in to my editor until the reader sees it on a bookstore shelf. This can make the time line confusing. Different authors handle this matter in different ways. After a great deal of deliberation, I decided that Skye and her friends and family will age more slowly than those of us who don't live in Scumble River. Although I made this decision while writing the fourth book in the series, *Murder of a Snake in the Grass,* I didn't realize until recently that I needed to share this information with my readers. So, to catch everyone up, the following is when the books take place.

Murder of a Small-Town Honey — August 2000

Murder of a Sweet Old Lady — March 2001

Murder of a Sleeping Beauty — April 2002

Murder of a Snake in the Grass — August 2002

Murder of a Barbie and Ken — November 2002

Murder of a Pink Elephant — February 2003

Murder of a Smart Cookie — June 2003

Murder of a Real Bad Boy — September 2003

Murder of a Botoxed Blonde — November 2003

Murder of a Chocolate-Covered Cherry — April 2004

The Scumble River short story and novella take place:

"Not a Monster of a Chance" — June 2001

"Dead Blondes Tell No Tales" — March 2003

CHAPTER 1
PREHEAT OVEN TO
350°

School psychologist Skye Denison had endured the situation for as long as she could. Improvements on the outside were well and good, but they didn't make her feel any better about the ugliness on the inside. It was time to put an end to her suffering.

She ignored the ringing telephone. There really wasn't anyone she wanted to talk to bad enough to untie the rope, climb down from the ladder, and find the phone in the mess she had created in her dining room. She sighed with relief when the ringing stopped, but let out a small scream of frustration when it started right up again.

Evidently, whoever was calling knew that her answering machine picked up on the fourth ring and was hanging up after the third. This meant it was someone who called her on a regular basis. Skye paused as she tightened the knot. Who would be so determined to reach her that they would keep punching the redial button again and again?

It wasn't her boyfriend, Wally Boyd, chief of the Scumble River Police Department. He had phoned earlier canceling their date for that night with the lame excuse that "something had come up." His call had been the start of her bad day.

Another possibility was her best friend, Trixie Frayne, school librarian and Skye's cosponsor of the school newspaper, but they had already spoken as well. Trixie had called to tell Skye that a cheerleader's parents were threatening to sue the *Scoop* for slander, and Trixie and Skye were scheduled to meet with the district's lawyer at seven a.m. on Monday. Homer Knapik, the high school principal, would have a cow when he heard the news — then make Skye and Trixie shovel the manure.

A quick glance at her watch and Skye knew it couldn't be her brother, Vince. Saturday morning was the busiest time at his hair salon. Skye's godfather and honorary uncle, Charlie Patukas, the owner of the Up A Lazy River Motor Court, wouldn't bother with repeated calls; he'd just jump into his Caddy and come over. After all, few places in Scumble River, Illinois, were more than a five- or ten-minute drive away.

Shoot! That left only one person, and she would never stop dialing until Skye answered. Moaning in surrender, Skye made sure the rope holding the chandelier up out of the way was tied tightly and reluctantly climbed down the ladder, almost tripping on her black cat, Bingo, as she stepped to the floor. He shot her a nasty glare and darted from the room.

She yelled after him, "You know, you could have answered the phone, buddy. You're not earning your keep around here."

The next group of rings helped her locate the handset, and she lifted the edge of the tarp she had placed on the hardwood floor to protect it. Grabbing the receiver, she pushed the ON button and said, "Hello, Mom."

"It's about time you picked up." The voice of May Denison pounded into Skye's ear. "There's a family emergency. Get over here right away."

Skye growled in aggravation as her mother hung up without further explanation. Then her mother's words penetrated the fog of her bad mood. Emergency! Had something happened to Skye's father? Her grandmother? One of her countless aunts, uncles, or cousins?

A busy signal greeted Skye's repeated attempts to call back. No doubt May had taken the phone off the hook to force Skye to come over as ordered, rather than phone and ask questions.

Catching her reflection as she hurried past the foyer mirror, Skye hesitated. Her chestnut curls were scraped back into a bushy ponytail, the only paint on her face was the Tiffany blue she was using on her dining room walls, which did nothing for her green eyes, and the orange sweat suit she had put on to work in made her look like Charlie Brown's Great Pumpkin.

Shaking her head, she decided it would take too much time to transform herself into a presentable human being, and instead grabbed her jacket, purse, and keys from the coat stand. She ran out of the house and leapt into the 1957 Bel Air convertible her father and godfather had restored for her a few years ago, after several unfortunate incidents left her previous cars undrivable.

The Chevy was a boat of a car, which made it hard to lay rubber, but Skye stomped on the accelerator and the Bel Air flew down the blacktop, white vapor pouring from the tailpipe in the below-zero temperature. Seven and a half minutes later, Skye wheeled into her parents' driveway and skidded to a halt on the icy film covering the gravel.

Where were all the vehicles? If there was a family emergency the driveway should be packed with cars and trucks. Did her mom need a ride to the hospital? No, May's white Olds was parked in the garage. What the heck was going on?

Skye flung herself out of the Bel Air and jogged up the sidewalk and across the small patio to the back door. She spared a glance at the concrete goose squatting at the corner. Except for the holidays, when the statue was dressed as anything from a Halloween witch to Uncle Sam, its costume was usually a good barometer of May's mood. Given that it was January 10, too late for New Year's and too early for Valentine's Day, the fact that it was wearing an apron and a tiny chef's hat and had a rolling pin clutched in its wing must mean something, but darned if Skye had a clue as to what.

Shrugging, she continued into the house, calling, "Mom, what's going on? What's the emergency?"

Silence greeted her as she dashed through the utility room's swinging doors and into the kitchen. Still no sign of her mother, but Skye slid to a stop as her gaze swept past the counter peninsula and reached the dinette.

She felt all the blood drain from her head and the room started to sway as she stared at the table. She sank to her knees and closed her eyes, hoping she was dreaming or having a hallucination, but when she opened them again the wedding cake was still there — three layers of pristine white frosting with delicate pink roses and a vine of ivy trailing down its side.

Surely even May, a woman desperate for her daughter to get married and produce grandkids, wouldn't throw an emergency wedding.

Seconds later Skye's mother bustled around the corner from the living room clutching a cordless phone to her right ear. She clicked it off and leaned down. "What are you doing on the floor?" Grabbing Skye's arm, she ordered, "Get up. It's filthy. I haven't had time to mop it yet today."

May was dressed in sharply creased blue jeans, a pale yellow sweatshirt with tiny bluebells embroidered across the chest, and gleaming white Keds. Her short salt-and-pepper hair waved back from her face as if she had just finished combing it, and her mauve lipstick looked freshly applied.

"What's that doing here?" Skye shook off her mother, rose from the light green lino-

16

leum, noting that it looked as immaculate as the day it was laid, and pointed a shaking finger at the offending pastry.

May made a dismissive gesture toward the towering wedding cake. "Oh, that. I was bored last night; your father had a meeting at the Moose, so I decided to practice my recipe."

"Okay." Skye hesitated in asking what her mother was practicing for, afraid the answer would involve Skye, a church, and a long white gown. Instead she demanded, "What is the emergency? Is it Dad, Grandma, Vince?"

"Oh, well . . ." May looked everywhere except at Skye. "I suppose I should have made it clear: Everyone is fine. It's not that kind of emergency." May stepped toward Skye and took her hands. "It's a good emergency. The best. You'll never guess what's happened."

"What?" Skye cringed. Her mother's idea of *good* was often not close to Skye's; heck, a lot of times they weren't even in the same universe.

"I'm a finalist in the Grandma Sal's Soup-to-Nuts Cooking Challenge." Grandma Sal's Fine Foods was one of the area's biggest employers. They operated a huge factory located between Scumble River and

Brooklyn, Illinois, adjacent to the railroad tracks that ran through both towns.

"Wonderful." Skye hugged her mom, happy for May and relieved for herself. A cooking contest would keep May occupied and out of Skye's affairs. "Congratulations."

"Thank you." May took a step back and wrinkled her nose. "You smell funny."

"I was painting my dining room. Remember? I told you I was taking this weekend to finally get some of the downstairs rooms done," Skye reminded her mother, then added, "If you wanted me all clean and pretty, you shouldn't have said it was an emergency."

"But it is an emergency. I needed to explain something to you before you answered your phone again." May took a knife from the drawer by the stove and sliced into the wedding cake.

Skye flinched, still unconvinced that her mother didn't have a groom waiting in the den and a priest stashed in the linen closet. "Explain what?"

"Sit down and I'll tell you." May handed Skye a piece of cake and a fork. "What do you want to drink with that?"

A double martini straight up? Skye settled for a glass of milk.

May finally pulled a stool up to the

counter next to Skye and said, "Now, I want you to promise that you'll let me tell you the whole story before you say anything."

"Okay." Skye frowned; she was a school psychologist, for Pete's sake, a trained counselor. Did her mom really feel it necessary to remind her to be a good listener?

"When I entered Grandma Sal's contest, I couldn't decide which recipe to use. Each entrant was only allowed to send one, but how could I choose between my Two-Hour Decorated Cake and my Chicken Supreme Casserole?"

Skye finished chewing and swallowed. "Well, I think you made the right decision; this cake is scrumptious. I didn't know you knew how to make frosting decorations."

"Maggie taught me the basics."

Maggie was one of May's best friends and the premier fancy-cake baker in Scumble River.

"They're beautiful. You must be a quick learner."

"Thanks." May fiddled with her coffee cup. "Uh, I didn't exactly choose the cake recipe."

"Well, your casserole is great too." Skye forked another bite into her mouth.

"I'm glad you feel that way." May stared out the picture window and kept talking.

19

"Because *you* entered the chicken dish."

"Huh?" Skye choked and had to take a swig of milk in order to speak. "I did what? Why? How?"

"I wasn't sure which recipe would get the judges' attention." May twisted a paper napkin into a raggedy bow. "The cake is more dramatic, but the casserole is more practical, so I wanted to enter both. I just needed another name to use, and I borrowed yours."

"Why me? Why not Aunt Kitty or your friend Hester or Maggie?"

"They were all entering their own recipes. I needed someone who wasn't."

"Then why didn't you tell me?" Skye put down her fork; suddenly the sweet frosting curdled on her tongue.

"Because you would have said no. Then I'd have had to use your father's name, and you know he would have a coronary if I entered him in a cooking contest. He's barely over the fact that I made him wear a pink shirt to the VFW dinner dance."

"Dusty rose," Skye corrected, losing the thread of the argument.

"Pink, red, it doesn't matter what you call it; Jed still finds it hard to accept that dress shirts come in any color but white."

"Uh-huh, let's get back to the contest."

20

Skye tilted her head. There was something her mom was keeping from her. "So you used my name. What does that have to do with me not answering my phone?"

"Because the woman who called to tell me I was a finalist said that they were notifying you next, and I was afraid you'd tell them you hadn't entered and ruin everything."

"I'm a finalist?" Skye took another sip of milk to stop herself from slapping her mother. "Why did she tell you about my entry finaling?"

"While we were chatting she mentioned that more than one entrant with the same last name made the finals. She asked if we were related, and I said yes. I told her that the Chicken Supreme was my daughter."

"Well, they won't let us both compete, so I'll decline when they call." Skye blew out a breath, thankful for her narrow escape.

"No! That's just it. We can both be in the contest. There aren't any rules against it."

"But I don't want to be in it."

"Please. For me?" May's happy expression melted away. "We'll have a great time. We can spend some quality time together."

"I talk to you every day and see you at least twice a week. That's enough quality time for any thirtysomething daughter to spend with her mother." Skye wasn't falling for that old line. The only way May would ever feel she and Skye spent enough time together would be if Skye moved back home. Heck, knowing May, she wouldn't be satisfied unless Skye crawled back into the womb.

"I've been entering this recipe contest for twenty-five years, and I've never made the finals before. I never expected more than one of my recipes to make it this far." May dabbed at a tear with her paper napkin. "This might be my only chance to win. I'm not getting any younger, you know."

"You still have your cake entry." Skye was determined not to let her mother talk her into this. Several of her friends had told her she needed to grow a backbone where her mother was concerned. Of course, they never had to face the heaping helping of guilt May was so good at dishing out to get her own way.

Tears seeped down May's cheeks. "But I want the casserole to have a chance, too. There are four categories: Snacks, Healthy, One-Dish Meals, and Special-Occasion Baking. The winner of each category gets five thousand dollars, and the overall winner gets fifteen thousand. Between us we could win twenty-five thousand dollars. I could finally take your dad on that cruise we've been talking about, and have enough left over to buy him a new used truck. His is running on wire hangers and duct tape."

Skye opened her mouth to say no, but instead asked, "Where and when is this contest? There's no way I can take a lot of time off from work."

"It's at the Grandma Sal's plant, right here in Scumble River." May smiled like a poker player laying down a royal flush. "It starts the first Friday in April and goes through Sunday. Isn't that during your spring break?"

Once again Skye tried to say no, but she couldn't come up with an excuse. Too bad she couldn't claim to be going away for the school vacation, but her mother knew she was spending all her spare cash fixing up the old house she had inherited that past summer.

May was looking at Skye like a puppy asking to be chosen from the animal shelter. How could Skye turn her down? She loved her mother and wanted her to be happy. If that made Skye a weenie, then so be it. There was a difference between having a backbone and being nice to your mom. Heck, there was even a commandment about it.

"I get to keep the cash if I win, right?" Skye teased, knowing her chances of producing a winning dish were slim to none.

"We'll split it," May bargained. "Fifty-fifty — my recipe, your cooking talent."

Skye rolled her eyes. In that case the split should be ninety-ten, in favor of her mother.

After finishing her cake and milk, Skye was on her way out the door when a thought that had been nagging at her subconscious finally surfaced. She stopped and turned to face her mother. "You said there were four categories, right?"

May nodded.

"The cake would be in the Special-Occasion Baking and the casserole in the One-Dish Meals, right?"

May nodded again, this time more slowly.

"So, whose names did you use for the Healthy and Snack divisions?"

"What makes you think I entered those?" May studied her nails intently.

"Let's not do this dance. Just tell me the whole truth. No equivocations."

"What does equivocation mean?" May turned away from Skye and opened the dryer door, taking sheets and towels from its drum.

"Mother!" Skye pulled a towel out of May's hands. "You have three seconds to tell me or I'll drop out of the contest."

May shook out a sheet, remaining silent.

"One."

May picked up two pillowcases and paired them.

"Two."

May closed the dryer door with her knee, her arms full of folded cotton.

"Thr—"

"Uncle Charlie for Snacks and Vince for Healthy."

"Well." Skye had to bite her lip to keep from giggling as she tried to imagine her godfather cooking. "I guess it's a good thing they didn't final."

"Mmm."

"They didn't final, did they?" Skye followed her mother as May walked to the linen closet.

"Yes." May put the clean laundry on the shelf. "Charlie knew I had used his name, and he called just a few minutes ago to say we're in."

"And Vince?" Skye asked. When her brother had become a hairstylist, he'd had a hard time convincing the more narrow-minded townspeople, which included their father, that he was straight. Entering a cooking contest would cause all that talk to flare up again.

"He said it would be a hoot, and he likes the idea of being surrounded by women." May beamed fondly. "He's such a good boy." Vince was thirty-eight, but would forever be a boy to May.

Skye shook her head, hoping neither her mother nor her brother would repeat his statement to Vince's girlfriend, Loretta. Loretta was Skye's sorority sister and sometime attorney. She would not be amused to learn that her boyfriend was one of the only males under seventy among two dozen women.

"It seems wrong for you to have four chances to win, and the others to have only one." Skye wondered how the organizers felt about three finalists coming from the same family — four if you counted Charlie. On the other hand, since the contest had an entry area of only about a forty-five-mile radius, there was bound to be some duplication.

"It's not like I'll be doing the cooking. I just provided the recipes. Sort of like sponsoring a car in a race." May closed the linen closet door. "I checked the rules and there's nothing that says the recipes have to be your own; they just have to be original."

Skye gave up. It wasn't her problem. Her problem was learning how to make Chicken Supreme Casserole without burning down the kitchen. Why did the expanding-bread episode of the old TV show *I Love Lucy* keep running through her mind?

It was the first Thursday in April, April Fools' Day, which was apropos, since Skye had just gotten out of a meeting with the school's attorney regarding the threatened lawsuit against the student newspaper. Due to spring break, there were only one or two people in the school building. Most of the staff was off on vacation, including Trixie, the student newspaper's cosponsor.

The lawyer was confident they'd win the case if it ever went to court, but the stakes were so high Skye was still worried. The superintendent was threatening to do away with the activity if they lost, which would devastate the kids who had worked so hard to make their paper one of the best student-produced newspapers in the state. They had even won a prize for last year's efforts.

Skye cheered herself briefly with the thought that the default mode of school administrators was always no, but they *could* be reprogrammed. Still, why had she ever let Xenia Craughwell write for the *Scoop*?

Granted, Xenia was smart — her IQ was off the charts. She was an excellent writer, and she was seeing an outside therapist, but there was a streak of meanness in the girl that concerned Skye. Xenia just didn't seem to grasp the finer points of right and wrong, which made Skye suspect that it would take more than six months of counseling to make any substantive changes in her.

Xenia had enrolled in Scumble River High in the fall after being kicked out of several other schools, and up until now she had been behaving herself; but Skye should have known from Xenia's record that wherever she went, trouble followed.

Which brought Skye back to the question of why in the world she had allowed Xenia on the newspaper staff to begin with. Skye felt like slapping herself — she had to stop trying to save everyone, and admit that some people were beyond her power to help.

Trying to distract herself from thinking about the lawsuit, she flipped open her appointment book and stared at the pale green index card clipped to Thursday. Her mother's careful printing mocked Skye.

Was she some kind of moron? What in heaven's name was she doing wrong? She'd been practicing the recipe for nearly three months and it still came out a gooey, rubbery mess every time she made it. The only time the dish was edible was when May stood right beside her, guiding her every move.

Poor Wally had dutifully eaten all of Skye's attempts, and gamely lied, claiming to taste improvement each time. Maybe that was why he had broken so many dates lately. At least three or four times since January he had called out of the blue, said something had come up, and had never given her a good explanation for canceling.

He was probably reconsidering his statement that he wasn't looking for a girlfriend who was a good cook. Thank goodness the contest started tomorrow. One more practice casserole and Skye might be minus a boyfriend.

Okay, she didn't want to think about the lawsuit or the recipe. What was more pleasant? *Ah, yes.* She smiled, recalling how excited everyone in town had been about Grandma Sal's Cooking Challenge. In the past, the opening press conference, the welcome luncheon, and the awards ceremony had taken place in Brooklyn, but this year Scumble River's mayor, Dante Leofanti, who was also Skye's uncle, had persuaded the company to move all those events to Scumble River.

Locating accommodations for the three judges, half a dozen contest staff members, and various media personnel covering the three-day extravaganza had been like negotiating a peace treaty, but the mayor had stepped in and gotten everything moving forward.

He had even managed to get the school board to allow him to use the high school gym/auditorium for the contest press conference. As Dante had explained at the town meeting, no way would they let an event that would bring in both positive media coverage and lots of people spending money go back to Brooklyn just to save some scuffing of a hardwood floor.

Skye had watched in awe as her uncle managed to get the townspeople to work together to keep the Challenge in Scumble River. Collaboration was not the strong suit of most of the town's citizens.

Skye tapped the recipe card against her chin, remembering having seen Dante arguing with Uncle Charlie about who got the cottages at his motor court. Charlie would have preferred to give the rooms to the highest bidders, but he and the mayor had agreed to three for the judges, three for out-of-town Grandma Sal's staff, one for Grandma Sal, one for her son and his wife, one for her two grandsons, and two for the media. It was a good thing the cooking challenge was for Stanley County residents only. All the finalists could commute.

Charlie stood firm on the twelfth cabin, explaining that he had a long-term renter and couldn't kick him out. Skye wondered how much the lodger had bribed Uncle Charlie to keep the cabin during the contest.

Overall, the town was ready for the Challenge, even if Skye wasn't. She exhaled noisily. At least, unlike other events Scumble River had hosted, this one was likely to produce nothing worse than burnt chicken. The food might be to die for, but it was unlikely that anyone would be murdered over a recipe.

Chapter 2
Assemble the
Ingredients

Skye squirmed, trying to find a comfortable position on the wobbly plastic seat. She wasn't sure where the school had found these flimsy folding chairs, but they were not designed for a woman of her generous curves. She felt as if the chair was about to collapse at any minute, landing her on her butt. Skye was okay with her full figure, but situations like this reminded her that society had different expectations.

May and Skye had been the first to arrive. After their names were marked off on the list, they were given red and white checked aprons, a tote bag full of goodies — all products of Grandma Sal's Fine Foods and its subsidiaries — and had their picture taken with Grandma Sal. Then they verified their recipes and were sent to sit backstage to wait for the rest of the finalists to show up. Once all twenty-four contestants arrived they would be brought onstage and introduced to the media, and Grandma Sal would make her welcoming speech.

Skye wished she had brought a book. Her mother was chatting with Uncle Charlie, who had come in a few minutes after Skye and May. The woman sitting on the other side of Skye had been on her cell phone since she arrived — probably because she kept having to repeat herself over and over again, saying, "Can you hear me? Is this better? How about now?"

Skye contemplated telling the signal-impaired woman that Scumble River had more dead zones than a Stephen King novel, but decided against it. Telling her wouldn't do any good. Cell phone coverage was one of those life lessons — like a sign saying WET PAINT — that everyone just seemed to have to test out for themselves.

Skye yawned. She was *so* bored. Maybe she should go talk to her brother. Vince had come in ten minutes ago, causing a stir with his golden blond hair and male-model physique. Vince, May, and Skye all shared the Leofanti emerald green eyes, but Vince used his to better advantage. He had the ability to hypnotize any female between the ages of three and ninety-three.

Shaking her head, Skye decided this wasn't the time to chat with her brother.

The smitten women around him would not appreciate his sister diverting any of his attention away from them.

Skye counted the tiles in the ceiling. If something didn't happen soon, she was going to scream. It had been over thirty minutes since the last person arrived, and a quick tally of the people milling around the twelve-by-twelve room made it clear that they were all waiting for one last contestant. They had been instructed to arrive at ten a.m., and it was now closer to eleven.

Skye wrinkled her nose. The room smelled of makeup, sweat, and mold. Up until a few days ago the space had been used as a dressing room for the annual school play, and it housed the drama department's costumes during the rest of the year.

Uncle Dante must have persuaded Homer to have the room straightened up. The principal would never have thought of doing it on his own. Even the uncomfortable chairs, now arranged in four rows of six, would have been too much of a hassle for him. Homer had mentally retired from his job several years ago; he just hadn't bothered to turn in the paperwork.

Clearly everyone was beginning to get impatient. Some wiggled in their seats, others paced, and a few muttered about "talking to someone and finding out what's holding things up."

Skye hoped that one of the more vocal finalists would *do* something. Normally she would be leading the charge, but this was May's moment, and Skye had vowed not to ruin it for her mom, who preferred manipulation to confrontation.

To amuse herself, Skye turned her attention to the other contestants, trying to guess their day jobs. An attractive blonde a few years younger than Skye sat alone, her right leg encased in a Velcro brace and propped up on an empty chair. Small wire-rimmed glasses were perched on her nose, and she was reading the side of a prescription bottle. MONIKA was embroidered on the bib of her official apron.

This reminded Skye that her own name had been misspelled. Scowling, she looked down at the bright red thread reading, SYKE. The staff had promised to provide a corrected apron before the actual contest. If they didn't come through by tomorrow, Skye vowed she would put some sort of pin over the offending error.

Okay, where was she? Right, the blonde. *Mmm.* Either a teacher or a nurse.

Having made her guess, Skye turned her attention to a woman dressed straight out of the 1950s. She wore a wool dress with a full skirt and short matching jacket, high-heeled pumps, and even a little hat perched on her brunette pageboy, its peacock feather dipping over her right eye like an exclamation mark. Her apron sported the name DIANE. She sat erect in her chair, holding her handbag in her lap.

This was a tough one, but Skye guessed that Diane was either an executive secretary or the owner of an antique shop.

Next in Skye's line of vision was a woman built like a linebacker. She had to weigh at least three hundred fifty pounds, and it looked like solid muscle. Nothing jiggled as she paced the length of the small room. Her skin had a blue-black sheen, and her many long braids were pulled back and fastened at the back of her neck. She wore jeans and a T-shirt that said, KISS THE COOK. Her apron read, JANELLE.

Skye was stumped. Janelle could be any-thing from a professional wrestler to the owner of a construction company.

Before Skye could come up with a firm guess, the last finalist swept into the room, talking a mile a minute to the young man trailing behind her. "Darling, please don't forget to call my editor about the cover of SECRETS OF A HOTEL HEIRESS. Can you believe they thought green was right for my fabulous book? Clearly it should be pink." Without waiting for a reply, she went on, "Oh, and I forgot to pick up my new Vera Wang satin sandals. I'll need them for tomorrow, so call Juanita and have her run into Chicago and get them."

The woman paused to take a breath, and the guy said, "Gotcha, babe. Those shoes are bitchin'."

Skye squinted at the woman's chest and discovered her name was Cherry. Cherry, hmmm . . . well, she did have red hair, but it was chin-length, with ends flipped up and sticking out all over her head. The style reminded Skye more of a cactus than a fruit. The woman's floral wrap dress was unmistakably couture, and the cost of her Fendi tote could have paid Skye's salary for a month. It was hard to tell her age — there were slight creases around her eyes — but such extremely fair skin wrinkled easily. She might be anywhere from her late thirties to early fifties.

What in the world was she doing in a cooking contest, not to mention living in Stanley County? When Skye noticed Cherry staring at her, Skye looked away from the loud couple. It didn't really matter who her competitors were; Skye was pretty sure they could all beat her, even with one spatula tied behind their backs.

Skye was thinking about how awful her last attempt at the chicken casserole had been when the redhead's irritating voice penetrated her thoughts for a second time, and she glanced up. Cherry had sat down and was holding a small leather notebook in her left hand and a tiny gold pen in her right. The man, nodding, stood by her side with his hands in the pockets of a pair of long, baggy shorts. He looked like the quintessential California beach boy — blue eyes, rock-hard body, and deep tan.

Cherry continued, "And, Kyle, do tell Larissa to make sure the baby doesn't nap this afternoon. She claims she doesn't, but I think she lets him sleep as much as he wants when we're gone. I've told her again and again I need him to be tired by the time I get home."

Skye sucked in an audible breath and frowned. She had just read an article in the *School Psychologist Journal* about parents who kept their infants up during the day so they could sleep at night. There was a concern that interrupting the natural sleep patterns of the babies could harm their brain development.

Cherry's gaze fastened on Skye and she

glared, then turned back to Kyle and raised her voice. "We seem to have a Nosy Parker eavesdropping on our discussion. Please go over and tell her to mind her own damn business."

"Babe, that's totally bogus." Kyle ran his fingers through his blond curls. "Like, I'm sure no one cares what we're saying."

Cherry ignored him and stalked over to Skye. "You, there, Syke, my husband and I are having a private conversation. Back off."

"Where in this twelve-by-twelve room do you think I could stand and not hear you?" Skye was now completely annoyed. "There are twenty-four of us, which means we are each entitled to about six square feet. Since your *husband* isn't supposed to be here, you'll have to share your six feet with him."

Suddenly Skye felt a tug on her sleeve and looked down into her mother's angry scowl.

"What in the world is going on?" May whispered. "I turn my back on you for two minutes and you're already arguing with someone."

Skye, resuming eye contact with Cherry, said, "Go sit down, Mom. Everything is fine. Cherry and I were just discussing spatial relationships, and the fact that her ego is taking up more than its fair share of the available space."

May tugged Skye back a couple of steps and hissed in her ear, "I raised you right. You know better than to say things like that to someone's face — you only say them behind their back."

"Don't you think that's a little hypocritical?"

"No, I think it's good manners."

Before Skye could react, the door swung open and one of Grandma Sal's staff walked in. "Okay, now that everyone's here, please follow me onto the stage. Grandma Sal will introduce you; then you can answer some questions for the media."

The contestants hurriedly gathered their belongings and formed a loose line. Skye noticed that Cherry had managed to get into the number one spot.

Skye was surprised to see nearly every chair on the gym floor occupied and several TV camera crews jostling for position just beyond the footlights. Uncle Dante had been right: This was a major event and a good chance for Scumble River to get some positive PR.

A woman in her late seventies stood center stage. Her gray hair was arranged in a soft halo of curls, and her blue eyes twinkled behind wire-rimmed glasses. She wore a pink flowered dress and a matching hat

40

covered in artificial carnations.

Smiling at the contestants, she said, "Ladies and gentlemen, it is my pleasure to welcome you to the thirty-fifth annual Grandma Sal's Soup-to-Nuts Cooking Challenge." She waited for the applause to die down, then continued, "My name is Sally Fine, and I'm CEO of Fine Foods. Helping me with this contest are my son, Jared; his wife, Tammy; my grandson, JJ; and his brother, Brandon."

Skye looked over at the middle-aged couple and their handsome sons. Both young men seemed fairly close in age, somewhere in their twenties. JJ resembled Grandma Sal, a little pudgy, with blue eyes and curly blond hair, while Brandon looked more like his mother, athletic with dark hair and eyes. The couple and their sons waved politely, but none of the four looked pleased to be there. Skye remembered hearing that they lived in Chicago and, unlike Grandma Sal, were rarely seen at the Scumble River factory.

Grandma Sal waited for the clapping to die down, then said, "Our judges are Ramona Epstein, food editor for the *Chicago Post;* Alice Gibson, best-selling cookbook author; and Paul Voss, the restaurant critic for Chicago's leading radio station."

Skye studied the first judge. Even adding the weight of the gold and diamonds she was wearing, Ramona couldn't possibly top the scale at a hundred pounds. Skye wondered if the food editor ever actually ate anything.

Next to the tiny raven-haired judge, Alice looked almost hulking, although she probably was no more than a size twelve or fourteen. Skye nodded to herself in approval. If you were going to write cookbooks, you should at least look as if you tasted your own recipes.

The male judge stood a little apart from the women, his unnaturally blue eyes shooting sparks of disdain. Something about him reminded Skye of an evil Santa. She wasn't sure if it was the red pants, hat, and shoes, the white goatee, or the bowl-full-of-jelly belly.

After the judges came onstage, Grandma Sal turned to the wings and extended her right hand. "Now let's meet the contestants. First, Mrs. Cherry Alexander, a writer from Laurel Lake who is competing in Special-Occasion Baking."

Skye smiled. Good. She could avoid Cherry, since they weren't in the same category. It wasn't as if Skye would take first in her group and go up against the other three winners for the grand prize.

Several other contestants were introduced before Grandma Sal got to the attractive blonde with the injured leg. "Monika Bradley owns her own accounting firm and comes to us from Brooklyn. She is competing in the Healthy Foods division."

Dang, a CPA, not a nurse or teacher. So far Skye was zero for one.

A few more finalists had their fifteen seconds of fame; then the 1950s woman stepped forward, and Grandma Sal said, "Diane White is a cookie blogger from Clay Center, Special-Occasion Baking."

Okay, no one would have guessed cookie blogger for a profession. Skye's brows met over her nose in an irritated frown. What was a cookie blogger, and was it even a real occupation? Fine, she had one more chance.

The linebacker was the last contestant to be introduced, and before Grandma Sal could speak, a dozen or so men in the audience stood up, stamped their feet, and whistled. Skye couldn't see very well past the footlights, but the guys in the cheering section looked mighty big. Maybe the finalist really was on a football team.

Finally the crowd settled down, and Grandma Sal said, "Last but certainly not least is Janelle Carpenter from Granger.

Janelle is a prison cook and will be competing in the One-Dish Meals category."

Yikes! That was Skye's group. Could all those men cheering be ex-cons? If so, it was a good thing Skye didn't have a snowball's chance in hell of winning.

What seemed like hours later, Grandma Sal finally finished her welcoming speech, which had included the history of the company and a loving description of every division and every product sold.

As soon as the older woman relinquished the mike, Mayor Leofanti grabbed it. Skye cringed. Dante was less than five-six, and he carried all of his considerable weight in his chest and stomach. With his thick gray hair slicked back, red nose, and black suit, he looked like a penguin, only not as distinguished.

While Dante started, as expected, by thanking everyone and their dog for helping make this event possible, Skye's stomach growled. She'd had her normal breakfast of an English muffin and tea at eight o'clock, but it was already past noon, and they still had the media questions to face before they would be escorted to the luncheon being held at the Feed Bag, Scumble River's only sit-down restaurant. Wouldn't it be ironic if

44

she starved to death at a cooking contest?

Dante paused, then began his closing remarks. "Grandma Sal's Fine Foods has been a part of Scumble River for close to forty years. Mrs. Fine and her late husband built the factory here in the nineteen sixties, and pretty near saved this town from dying out. They have employed many of you, your parents, and grandparents, and have always been a good neighbor. Scumble Riverites have been able to depend on Grandma Sal's for jobs, charitable contributions, and a future. Because of this, we who have reaped their bounty want to thank them by hosting the best ever Soup-to-Nuts Cooking Challenge."

The crowd clapped and whistled, and Skye smiled at her uncle. He was not a particularly good uncle, and she knew from experience that he was a lousy boss, but he had turned out to be a great mayor. She was truly happy for him and her family that after so many years he had found his niche.

Dante waved, bowed, and then stepped back as Grandma Sal opened the floor to the media. The majority of the questions were addressed to all of the contestants, and anyone could answer. Skye noticed that Cherry usually managed to have the last say on most subjects. Grudgingly Skye acknowledged that the writer had a way with the audience. Her quips generally left them laughing and, more important, scribbling in their notebooks.

They had been standing on the stage for nearly two hours, and Skye was rocking from foot to foot, hungry, bored, and needing to pee, when the owner/reporter of the *Scumble River Star,* Kathryn Steele, asked the group, "What inspired your recipes?"

It took a moment for Skye to realize that her mother had stepped forward and was answering. It took another moment for her to grasp what May was saying.

"My entry was inspired by my daughter's upcoming wedding."

Despite Skye's pleas, the *Star* had run several stories about her crime-solving activities, so she was well-known among the paper's staff, and for some reason she couldn't fathom, they were fascinated with her personal life.

Kathryn's body language resembled that of a golden retriever that had just discovered a flock of ducks hiding among the cattails. "Who's the groom? Has a date been set?"

Skye didn't have time to think or plan what to say, but she knew she had to answer before her mother did. She leapt forward and, trying to keep the edge out of her voice, said, "Kathryn, you know Mom meant my eventual, sometime-in-the-far-far-future wedding." Skye held up her left hand, naked of any ring. "When I get married you'll see a rock the size of a Christmas-tree ornament on my finger." The audience laughed, and she wrapped it up with, "Who knows how many cooking contests Mom'll win before then?"

Skye shot a sideways look of warning to May, who had her mouth open but slowly closed it without speaking.

The rest of the questions were harmless, and Skye zoned out, concentrating on her increasing need for the ladies' room. Finally the contestants were dismissed. Several raced for the bathroom. Skye had the advantage of knowing the lay of the land and headed for the faculty restroom, located deep within the bowels of the building, which she was sure would be empty.

Whipping inside, she locked the door and was unzipping her pants when she heard loud voices coming from the other side of the wall. Hmm, that would be the teachers' lounge. Skye leaned closer to the wall, curious as to who had ignored the sign on the closed door that said, DO NOT ENTER. TEACHERS ONLY. THIS MEANS YOU.

"Listen up, sweet cheeks. You didn't give

me any data on her or her family other than what I already had. You guaranteed me that your information would be up close and personal. I have too much riding on this for your shoddy work to ruin things for me. You have until tomorrow morning to get me the dirt on her and her relatives." The woman's tone was angry.

"I sent you what Grandma Sal sent me. Can I help it if the old broad didn't give me what I asked for? She always does in-depth profiles of the contestants to make sure they're squeaky-clean." This second voice was deeper, but Skye couldn't tell if it belonged to a man or a woman. "I'll reach out to my sources tonight and have the low-down tomorrow at breakfast."

"You'd better. I doubt you want anyone to know what you're up to."

"Hey, I already got you into the finals. We both have secrets we don't want exposed."

"And I paid you good money for that."

Skye heard the door slam and hurried to finish up. She raced out of the restroom, but it was too late; no one was around. As she went back to wash her hands, she wondered who had bought their way into the finals, and which contestant they were so interested in and why.

CHAPTER 3
READ THROUGH
RECIPE

Skye and May were caught in the parade of cars driving the three miles between the high school and the Feed Bag. May's white Oldsmobile sparkled as the sun beat down on its hood. It looked as if it had just rolled off the assembly line, but in reality it was over ten years old. That it accrued less than six thousand miles a year and was rarely driven past the county line probably had something to do with the vehicle's pristine condition.

The Olds was sandwiched between Vince's Jeep and Charlie's Cadillac Seville. Looking into the side mirror, Skye could see her godfather scowling and shaking his fist. Scumble River did not usually have gridlock, and Charlie clearly wasn't enjoying the rare experience.

In contrast, Vince was bopping to whatever music was playing on the radio; or, knowing her brother, Skye wouldn't be surprised to learn that the beat was only in his head. Vince had been the drummer in local bands since he was fourteen.

As far as Skye could tell, May's attitude was somewhere in the middle — still excited to be a part of the contest, but worried she might miss something while she was stuck in traffic.

"Mom, I have a question for you." Skye figured that at the rate they were going it would take them at least fifteen minutes to get to the restaurant, which meant this was a good time to ask her mother about something that had been bothering Skye for the past few months. She was especially worried after her mom's performance at the press conference.

"So, ask it already."

"Why are you suddenly so intent on marrying me off?"

May hadn't been this determined to get Skye married in a long time. Had Skye's biological clock started ticking so loudly that even her mother could hear it?

May twisted the knob on the radio until she found the weather. "I don't know what you mean by 'suddenly.' I've always wanted to see you married."

"Well, you've wanted me to settle down with some nice guy and produce two-point-five grandchildren since I turned twenty-one, but the last few months you've ratcheted your efforts up about a hundred percent."

"Things have changed."

Skye turned off the radio and focused on her mom's face. "What has changed?"

"You and Wally." May's expression soured. Although she wanted Skye married, she wasn't keen on her marrying Wally, who was several years older, divorced, and not Catholic.

"What about Wally and me?" Skye asked.

"I'm worried that by the time you get Wally out of your system, Simon will have found someone else. I saw that nurse from your school, the one who dated Vince for a while, talking with Simon at church. And that new woman, the one who moved to town last summer with that wild daughter, was flirting with him at the gas station the other day."

"Mom, I don't want him back." Skye had dated Simon Reid, the funeral home director and county coroner, on and off for the past three or so years. Her mother's news that other women were flirting with him caused a twinge of jealousy, but Skye pushed it away. "I'm happy with Wally. Not that I necessarily want to marry him." She didn't want May to start planning that wedding either.

"You're going to be thirty-five this December!" May exploded. "It's time you settled down. Do you want to go to your kids' graduation in a wheelchair?"

"Mother!" Skye blew out an angry puff of air and crossed her arms. "A lot of women nowadays have kids well into their forties."

May muttered something about old eggs not producing a good omelet, then stared out the windshield. After several minutes of icy silence, she spoke as if nothing had happened. "Did any of the other finalists look sort of familiar to you?"

Deciding to let the Simon/Wally marriage issue go, at least until the contest was over, Skye teased, "Besides you, Vince, and Charlie?"

"Yes, smarty-pants, besides us."

Skye pictured the other twenty contestants, then shook her head. "No, I can't say anyone stuck out. I take it one did to you?"

"Sort of, but I couldn't place her. She's the one with short black hair that looks like a wig, and glasses with rhinestone frames. Her name is Imogene Ingersoll. I was only able to speak to her briefly — she was on the way to the bathroom — and she said we hadn't met. I didn't get a chance to talk to her again."

"Well, we'll all be together for the next couple of days, so maybe it will come to you, or she'll remember something."

"Maybe." May frowned. "But it's like a sore tooth. I keep poking at it."

"I hate when that happens."

May sighed, then asked, "What did you think of the other contestants?"

"It's hard to tell. I never got to speak to most of them."

"Yeah, we should have had a plan." May stomped on the brakes as the only stoplight in town changed from green to yellow. "We could have divided them up into four groups and gotten the scoop on each of them."

"Why would we want to do that, Mom?" Skye thought about the mysterious conversation she had overheard coming from the teachers' lounge. That person had wanted information on a contestant too; maybe May could explain why that data was so vital.

"It gives you a psychological advantage." May flipped down the visor and checked her hair.

"How does that help in a cooking contest?" Skye turned slightly so she could study her mother.

53

May eased off the brake and made a left. "Because if you can psych someone out, they might get so rattled they forget to add an ingredient, or they overcook their dish, or do something else that ruins their recipe."

"But that's not fair." May's primping prompted Skye to smooth her own wayward curls and apply a fresh coat of apricot gloss to her lips.

"All's fair in cooking and baking."

Her mother's attitude of "anything goes" made Skye wonder whether she should mention to someone in charge that one of the finalists had bought her way into the contest. After a few minutes' consideration, she realized that she had no idea who either of the two people she overheard was, and she could end up reporting the incident to the very person who was involved. She had been trying to learn that every problem was not hers to solve. This seemed a good place to start.

May eased over the bump leading into the restaurant's lot, then abruptly put on the brakes. "Shoot. The lot's full."

"Where are we going to park?" Skye asked. Her gaze swept the double rows on both sides of the building. All four were solidly packed.

May frowned. "We might have to park at

Vince's salon and walk back."

Great. Skye looked down at her new Ann Taylor zebra-striped pumps. She had splurged during a recent shopping trip in Chicago. Loretta had talked her into getting them, even though Skye knew there were limited places she could wear them without crippling herself. Now their pointy toes mocked her. Talk about shoes that *weren't* made for walking. She'd do better taking them off and carrying them than trying to hike a mile in the three-inch heels.

Skye was about to suggest her mother double-park — after all, everyone at the restaurant would be leaving at the same time — when she spotted a police car backed into a space right next to the restaurant's door. As she watched, Wally unfolded himself from the driver's side and approached the Olds. He had muscles in all the right places, and she enjoyed seeing him move.

She rolled down the window. "Hi, handsome. What are you doing here?"

He leaned in for a quick kiss, then answered, "I figured you might have some trouble finding a place to park, so I saved you a space." He leaned further into the car. "Hi, May. I'll pull out so you can pull in."

May nodded, but otherwise didn't respond.

Wally's smile cooled at May's cold shoulder, but it warmed back up when he turned to Skye and said, "Come ride with me. I need to talk to you for a minute before you go in."

"You don't have time." May's hand clamped down on Skye's wrist as she opened the car door. "We're on a tight schedule. You'll make everyone late."

"It'll be fine, Mom." Skye freed herself and stepped out of the car. She definitely had to make it clear to her mother that she needed to be nicer to Wally. After the contest they'd have a little daughter-to-mother talk, and May had better straighten up. "Go inside and save me a seat."

For a moment Skye was afraid that May would run them over when they crossed in front of the Olds, but she only revved the engine.

Wally helped Skye into the passenger side of the squad car, then slid into the driver's seat, started the engine, and pulled out. He was silent as he maneuvered the cruiser into the lot's lane of traffic and around the corner. He parked next to the Dumpsters in a space that said, RESERVED FOR DELIVERIES.

Skye bit her bottom lip. What was up? She studied Wally. He was a handsome man who filled out his crisply starched police uniform in exactly the right way. His warm brown eyes melted her heart, and his shiny black hair edged in silver made her itch to run her fingers through the waves. He also had a gorgeous year-round tan. But his most attractive feature was his kind and generous nature.

Now his expression was serious and unhappy. He half turned, took her hand, and opened his mouth, then seemed to change his mind and instead said, "Did I tell you how beautiful you look?"

Skye shook her head. "How could you? This is the first time you've seen me today."

"Mmm." He brought her hand up to his lips and nibbled on her fingers. "You taste good, too."

"That's because I haven't started cooking yet," Skye teased.

Wally continued to nibble. "When's your next time off from school?"

"Well . . ." Skye wasn't prepared for the question, and she stammered, "If you mean more than one day, that would be the end of school, which is June eleventh. Why?"

"We should plan a trip together." Wally's lips were now on the inside of her elbow.

"That'd be fun." Was this what he had needed to talk to her about? Skye glanced at the dashboard clock. She had to get inside pretty soon, or May would send the cavalry to find her — and her orders wouldn't be to hold their fire until they saw the whites of Wally's eyes. Skye prodded. "So, you had something important to discuss?"

"Right. Sorry. I know you don't have long. It's just that I wanted to tell you . . . that is, before someone else did . . . that, uh . . ."

He hesitated, then opened his mouth, but before a single word escaped his lips the radio squawked to life. "Chief, there's been an accident over by the I-55 exit. Car versus semi. Traffic is completely stopped, and the ambulance and fire truck can't get through."

"I'll be there in five." Wally had let go of Skye's hand to work the radio. Now he leaned toward her and opened the door for her. "Sorry, sugar — I'll explain when I pick you up for the dinner tonight. And remember, don't believe anything you hear until I get a chance to talk to you."

It almost felt as if he had pushed her out of the squad car. Skye's shoulders drooped. What in the world did he have to tell her? Whatever it was, she was pretty sure it wasn't something she wanted to hear.

■ ■ ■ ■

Scumble River might be a small town, but it wasn't quite small enough for the entire population to fit inside the Feed Bag, particularly since the maximum-seating-capacity sign read seventy-six. Still, it looked as if the residents had given it the old college try. When Skye entered the only way she could get to her table was by edging sideways and holding her purse above her head.

Once seated, Skye noticed that Tomi Johnson, the owner of the Feed Bag, was not her usual cool and in-control self. May reported to Skye that when Tomi had been introduced to Grandma Sal, the restaurateur had practically kissed the food manufacturer's ring. Now Tomi was rushing around bringing Grandma Sal bites of this, samples of that, and hanging on the CEO's every tidbit of praise.

In fact, Skye noted that a lot of Scumble River's citizens were acting out of character. They seemed more impressed by Grandma Sal and the contestants than they had been in the past by TV stars and supermodels. Why was that? Could it be that at some level the townspeople knew that nourishment was more important than glamour? Of course, it probably didn't hurt that Grandma Sal's picture was plastered on nearly every product her company sold, and many people saw her face at least three times a day.

The contestants were seated at four tables of six. Skye observed that Vince and Charlie had elected to sit separately, each the only rooster among five hens. Both men had self-satisfied looks on their faces that Skye's palm itched to slap off. She restrained herself, reasoning that once the cooking started and they burned their entries, those smug expressions would be erased with the first wisp of smoke.

Grandma Sal's staff had its own table, as did the judges and the media, which claimed the three back booths. The other diners were all locals, most of whom appeared to be more interested in catching a glimpse of Grandma Sal and the contestants than they did in eating. Skye was happy to see that Tomi had clipped an index card to the menus that read, MINIMUM ORDER PER PERSON $5.00. NO SHARING. NO DOGGIE BAGS. The restaurant owner deserved to make a profit from all this hullabaloo.

Skye had just bitten into her BLT when Butch King, their table's token male, tipped his head toward May and remarked, "So, both you and your daughter are from Scumble River?"

May nodded. "I grew up in Brooklyn, but ever since I got married I've lived here." Skye saw her mother peek at the man's left ring finger, which was bare, and flinched when she added, "I think a woman should live where her husband's work is, as long as it's not too far from her mother."

The man looked amused. He winked at Skye and said to May, "You sound like my mom. She was so happy when I tied the knot and moved into the apartment next to her."

"How wonderful."

Skye did not like the expression that had settled on her mother's face. She could tell that May was already picturing a house next to hers in the adjoining cornfield.

Hastily swallowing, Skye jumped into the conversation before her mother started drawing up the blueprints. "Where are *you* from, Butch?"

"Laurel." Butch cut a piece of his chicken-fried steak and forked it into his mouth.

"I was surprised that the contest was open only to Stanley County." Skye took a sip of her Diet Coke. "I had heard that Fine Foods has been enlarging its market."

Another contestant joined the conversation. "The scuttlebutt around cooking-contest circles is that this will be the last year there's a local contest. Fine Foods used to be strictly a Midwestern company, but the last couple of years it's been expanding to Southern and Western markets. There's a rumor that Grandma Sal is in negotiations with some big food conglomerate. If that company buys Fine Foods, the products will go nationwide and so will the contest."

"I wonder if that will affect the factory here." Skye worried that a lot of locals could be out of jobs if the company was sold.

No one seemed to have an answer, and a few minutes later May asked, "What made you decide to enter, Butch?"

"I didn't." His smile was boyish. "I'm a firefighter, and the guys at my stationhouse love my spaghechili, so they sent in the recipe."

"Spaghechili?"

"It's a combination of my Italian grand-mother's spaghetti recipe and my Mexican grandmother's chili recipe." Butch grinned. "I came up with it when I didn't have enough ingredients for either to feed the whole crew."

"Very clever," Skye complimented him.

"Clever, my eye," May muttered. "That's not a recipe; that's leftovers."

"Uh," Skye said quickly, forestalling May's next comment, "so you're a Laurel fire-fighter? Do you know our police chief, Wally Boyd?"

"Sure. He's a great guy."

"My mom works for him as a dispatcher."

"I'm a police, fire, and emergency dis-patcher." May's eyes narrowed. "My pay-check is signed by the mayor, not Wally."

"Oh, I see." Butch looked at Skye, then May. "I've probably heard you on the radio."

May nodded, then said, "I'll bet you know Simon Reid too, the county coroner."

"Right." Butch handed the waitress his plate and ordered lemon meringue pie for dessert. "Not well. He sort of keeps to himself, you know?"

"He's friendlier once you get to know him." May shook her head at the waitress's offer of dessert. "He's Skye's boyfriend, so we know him in a different way, of course."

"No, he isn't," Skye blurted out. "He and I stopped seeing each other six months ago. Actually I'm dating Wally now, but Mom refuses to believe Simon and I have broken up for good."

May harrumphed, nudging Skye. "Butch doesn't care about your love life."

Skye felt her face redden. "But you said . . ." Why did May always do this to her? Why did she start something, then make Skye feel like the one in the wrong? Skye stuttered to a stop. Anything she said to defend herself would make it worse. "Of course, sorry." When everyone else resumed the conversation, she hissed in her mom's ear, "You brought up the subject of Wally and Simon, so back off."

May harrumphed again, then turned her attention to another tablemate. "What about you, Monika? Did Grandma Sal say you were from Brooklyn?"

"Yes," the attractive blonde answered before pushing aside her nearly untouched plate. "I'm lucky it's only eight miles from here."

"I have a lot of relatives in Brooklyn," May said. "Do you know the head librarian, Jayne? She's one of my cousins."

"Yes." Monika reached into her purse and took out a Ziploc bag. "She's one of my clients."

May peered at the woman as she opened the plastic sack and started snacking from it. "Didn't you like your lunch?"

Monika hesitated, then explained, "I have severe food allergies and can't eat anything with dairy or gluten. I ordered a chicken breast broiled without butter, but they breaded it, and then I was afraid the fries had been in the same oil used to deep-fry other foods with breading."

"Such a small trace would be a problem for you?" May probed, a look of disbelief on her face.

"Yes, even a tiny bit could cause me to become extremely ill and possibly die."

"You poor thing." May patted the woman's hand.

Skye wrinkled her brow. If she had a food allergy that severe, would she be brave enough to come to a cooking contest, where someone's innocent crumbs could kill her?

As May had predicted, they were running late, but it wasn't Skye's fault. The responsibility lay with Grandma Sal, who was turning out to be a girl who just couldn't say no. All the townspeople in the restaurant and all the Feed Bag employees wanted an autograph and their picture taken with her. Skye had never seen anyone sign boxes of cake mix, tubes of biscuits, and packets of dry pasta before.

Finally, about three o'clock, a full hour after they were scheduled to have been finished with lunch, Grandma Sal's staff started moving the contestants out of the restaurant and into their cars. Everyone was instructed to follow Grandma Sal's limo to the factory, where they would be given a brief tour and then have a chance to do a trial run of their recipes.

Skye and May were in the last group to be ushered from their table.

As they stood to follow the contest staffer, May whispered to Skye, "Here are the keys. I'll meet you at the car. I have to go to the bathroom."

"Okay." Skye noted that a couple of women were lined up to use the only ladies' room, and wished she had brought a book to read.

Skye followed her tablemates out the door. Once they were in the parking lot everyone scattered toward their vehicles. Skye sorted through the huge ring of keys May had thrust into her hand. She had just found the car key and inserted it into the passenger-side door when she heard the first scream.

CHAPTER 4
BUTTER AND FLOUR
YOUR PAN

Skye froze. Did that sound like her mother?

The second scream propelled her into action. Over her shoulder she yelled to the few remaining people in the parking lot, "Call nine-one-one. I'll go see what's wrong."

Skye burst through the restaurant's door and skidded to a stop, searching for the problem. A third scream drew her to the back of the restaurant, where two women were engaged in a shoving match.

When Skye got closer she saw that one of the brawlers was Cherry Alexander. The redhead pushed her opponent and yelled, "You give it back to me right now!"

Cherry's shove moved the other combatant into view, and Skye cringed as she saw her mother raise both fists and shout, "I told you, I don't have your silly *secret* ingredient!"

Cherry pulled back her arm, aiming a slap

67

at May's face, but Skye grabbed the petite woman's wrist and said in her best playground-monitor voice, "No hitting. We're all adults here, and I'm sure we'll find whatever you lost."

"Get out of my way." May tried to thrust Skye aside, but her five-foot-two, one hundred twenty-five pounds was no match for her daughter, who had five inches on her, and quite a bit more weight. "I can fight my own battles."

"I'm sure you could beat each other to a pulp with no trouble whatsoever, but that would mean you would be kicked out of the contest." Skye raised an eyebrow. "Is that what you really want?"

As if someone had lowered the flame on a gas stove, both women went from boiling over to simmering in the space of a heartbeat.

"She started it." May thrust out her chin. "She accused me of stealing."

"If you didn't take it, who did?" Cherry theatrically rubbed the wrist Skye had released. "And I'd better be able to whisk tomorrow with this arm or I'm suing you."

Skye wanted to slap the asinine woman, but instead asked, biting off her words, "What did you lose?"

"You'd like to know, wouldn't you?"

Cherry's gaze darted among the women gathered around her.

Until then Skye hadn't noticed that the people who had still been in the parking lot had all come inside. Their presence reminded her that she had told them to call for help before going to investigate the scream. Now she asked, "Did anyone call nine-one-one?"

A woman nodded and held up a bright red cell phone. "They said they'd be right here."

"Shoot." Skye was angry with herself for jumping the gun. "Call them back and tell them we don't need them after all."

"Don't you dare!" Cherry forced her way past Skye and pointed at May. "I want this woman arrested."

Before Skye could react, the restaurant door slammed open and Officer Roy Quirk strode into the room. He immediately spotted Skye and asked, "We got a call about a woman screaming. What's up?"

Quirk was Wally's second in command and, since Skye had been hired as a psychological consultant to the Scumble River Police Department, one of her colleagues.

Skye pointed toward Cherry. "This woman claims her secret ingredient has been stolen, and she's accusing Mom of taking it."

Quirk spoke into the radio clipped to his shoulder, then approached Cherry and asked, "Ma'am, what exactly is missing?"

"I'm not saying." Cherry huffed, "Don't any of you understand the concept of *secret?*"

"Well, ma'am, how can I look for it if I don't know what it is?"

"It's in a white paper sack." Cherry crossed her arms. "And no one had better open the bag if they find it."

Quirk turned to May. "Is it okay if I look in your purse?"

"Sure." She thrust the large black satchel into the officer's arms. "I don't have anything to hide. I don't need a secret ingredient to win. I have talent."

Quirk opened the purse and upended it on a nearby table. He named the objects as he returned them to the bag. "Wallet, checkbook, comb, lipstick, pillbox, tissues, glasses, pen, pad of paper, and roll of mints."

Before handing the purse back to May he asked Cherry, "Are any of these your secret ingredient?"

"No," Cherry said curtly, her eyes burning with contempt and determination. "But that doesn't prove she doesn't have it. I want her strip-searched."

"Now, ma'am, we can't do that." Quirk pushed his hat back and scratched his head. "May, would you be willing to let this lady pat you down?"

May started to shake her head until Skye pointed out, "You both realize that if we don't resolve this matter here, you'll have to go to the police station, and you'll miss the tour and the chance to do a dry run of your recipes. Heck, maybe you'll even be disqualified."

"Both of us?" Cherry squealed, wheeling toward Skye. "She's the crook; I'm the victim. Why would I be disqualified?"

Skye exchanged glances with Quirk, who nodded his consent for her to go on. "If you make a formal report and we find nothing, we could arrest you for malicious mischief." Skye had no idea if this was really true.

"Fine, just forget it," Cherry said. "Once again the criminal goes free."

"Oh, no. You're not getting away with letting all these people think I'm a thief." May's jaw was rigid. "Cherry can pat me down, but if she doesn't find any paper bag, she has to apologize."

Everyone looked at Cherry, who finally shrugged and said, "Very well."

As she stepped toward May, May held her

arms perpendicular to her body and warned, "No funny business, now. I don't play for that team."

As soon as they arrived at the factory, Cherry cornered Grandma Sal's son and started complaining about her missing secret ingredient, which had not been found on May or anywhere else in the restaurant.

Skye stepped within listening range as Jared Fine tried to soothe Cherry by saying, "Don't worry, ma'am; we'll get you a replacement before tomorrow. Everything will be all right, I promise. Just tell me what it is you lost."

Cherry stomped her foot. "No. I'm not revealing the ingredient until I've won the contest. And I don't want you to go looking on my entry form and telling anyone, either."

"Then I'm not sure what I can do for you, ma'am." Jared backed away. "If you change your mind, let me know."

Cherry seethed. "It's not something you can pick up at any old grocery store. It needs to be special-ordered, you moron."

"Sorry, ma'am," Jared said. "Read your contest rules. We aren't responsible for missing ingredients that cannot be purchased locally."

Cherry pulled out her cell phone and stomped off, glaring at May as she passed her.

Skye realized that Jared had caught her eavesdropping. She made a face and joked, "Sounds like Cherry has a couple of issues."

"A *couple* of issues?" Jared shook his head. "She has the full subscription."

Even though they had wasted a good half hour searching for Cherry's secret ingredient, they had still arrived at the factory in time to join the last tour group. Skye and her mother donned the hairnets and hard hats they were handed and followed the group into the production area.

Their tour was being led by Brandon Fine. The handsome young man seemed less sullen than he had when he was first introduced at the press conference, and Skye wondered what had improved his mood. Maybe he had just been bored, or hungry, or had to go to the bathroom that morning. Skye certainly had experienced all three.

As they walked, Brandon said, "This is an older factory. Much of what you see is original equipment from when it was first built." He gestured to the left and said, "This is where the raw materials — such as sugar, powdered eggs, corn syrup, cocoa, and seasonings — are stored."

Skye poked her head into the enormous room and saw huge bins and sacks the size of refrigerators stacked on wooden pallets.

Next they were led to an area where Brandon pointed down. "The metal plate you see in the floor is actually a scale. While your recipes may call for two cups of flour, ours call for two hundred pounds."

As if on cue, a man wheeled an empty stainless-steel container onto the scale. He reached up to a pipe running above the tub and turned a valve handle, then walked over to a panel with digital numbers. Underneath the display was a series of switches. He flipped one, then another, and oil began to flow into the container.

May poked Skye in the ribs with her elbow. "Good thing your father isn't here to see this. Next thing you know he'd be running pipes for his beer into the living room."

The worker caught Skye's glance and snickered as he continued to add ingredients to the tub. When he was finished, he looked around and muttered, "Where did Shorty get to? I can't move this thing by myself."

"Never mind, Moose," Brandon said. "I'll give you a hand." He joined the factory worker, and they rolled the container over

74

to what looked like a giant milk shake machine.

As the group followed, Brandon said, "There is now over five hundred pounds of raw material in this vat."

As the ladies oohed and aahed, he reached up and grasped a switch.

Moose yelled, "No!"

But Brandon flipped the toggle to the ON position, and the huge mixer growled into life, catching the dangling cuff of Brandon's shirt in its beaters.

Before anyone else could react, Moose slammed down a big red button and all the machinery in the immediate vicinity went still.

The sudden silence was startling. No one said a word for a long moment; then voices rose in concern. Brandon waved away offers of help, inspected the damage to his shirt, and said, "Everything's fine. Moose, have them turn the power back on."

As soon as the machinery roared back into service, Brandon said, "It will take over thirty minutes to mix this batch, so we'll move on to the extruding area."

May held Skye back and whispered, "What do you think would have happened if they hadn't turned off the power?"

"He would have lost his arm, maybe his

life." Skye tugged on her mother's hand. "Come on. We'd better keep up. I don't want to take a misstep and become part of the frosting."

As they hurried past Moose, they heard the factory worker muttering to himself, "Those spoiled-brat gran'kids know just enough to be dangerous. We told 'em not to let 'em lead the tours."

Skye and May joined the group in watching what looked like unending rows of cake pans passing on conveyor belts. As the pans went under short lengths of hoses, batter was extruded into each one; then the pan moved into a long oven.

Skye commented, "Sure wish we had this setup for the next school bake sale."

"Yeah! And the family reunion, too," May added.

They ended the tour in the packaging area, where rows of women in white uniforms and hairnets placed the finished product into boxes, sealed the flaps, and stacked the boxes into cartons. There was another section of the factory in the far rear of the building that Brandon explained was called the Boneyard because it contained the out-of-date equipment and broken machinery that Grandma Sal couldn't bear to throw out.

As the tour group was led away, Skye noted that none of the workers was under fifty years old, and she bet that many of them had been doing that same job since they had graduated or dropped out of high school. What would they do if the company were sold to some big conglomerate that moved the factory away or modernized it or otherwise eliminated their jobs?

From the packaging area they were escorted back to the front of the factory, past a row of offices, then through a narrow corridor that led to an outside exit on the left side of the passage and a door leading into the warehouse straight ahead, where all the cooking would be done.

Four sets of six stoves had been arranged in two rows. Next to each stove were four feet of counters, a minifridge, a cupboard, and two drawers. Brandon explained that they'd run two miles of cable to provide the electricity needed for the setup. He also warned them that the room would be at sixty-five degrees to start with, but would warm up quickly once the cooking started and the spotlights were turned on.

The judges and the media were placed behind the kitchen stations. On the right the judges were shielded from sight by several folding screens, but on the left the media had an unobstructed view of the contestants.

In front of the cooking spaces, chairs for the audience had been positioned in rows with a central aisle. Skye was impressed by the professional arrangements and amazed at how efficiently the contest space had been designed. Before returning to Scumble River she had lived in apartments with less well appointed kitchens.

Contestants were grouped by their food category, which meant that Skye, Charlie, and Vince were all on their own. There was no way May could subtly help any of them with their recipes.

Because Skye and May were in the last tour, the other finalists had already begun to cook. Skye cringed when she heard her mother's voice.

"Brandon."

"Yes, ma'am?"

"Do you really think this is fair?" May gestured to the contestants busy at their stoves. "They've all had a head start."

"But, ma'am, this is just a trial run to make sure you have everything you need for tomorrow." Brandon glanced at the media area, a frown creasing his forehead. "It isn't timed or judged."

Skye followed his gaze and was relieved to see that the reporters' attention was focused elsewhere. She felt sorry for Brandon. First Cherry and her secret ingredient, now May and her sense of injustice. Skye bet this wasn't how this privileged young man usually spent his days.

"We're still at a disadvantage." May crossed her arms. "We all should have started at the same time."

"I'll mention that to Grandma Sal." Brandon backed away. "I'm sure she'll come talk to you about it."

May harrumphed, but allowed herself to be led to her cooking area.

Skye found her own stove, located between that of Butch the firefighter, and Janelle the prison cook. She nodded to them both as she stepped into her space, then let out a startled yelp.

The woman standing in front of the stove whirled around. Long fake red curls cascaded down her back to the low-riding waist of her skintight jeans. Lime Skechers matched the baseball cap worn backward on her head. She casually reached into her orange-and-green-striped tank top and adjusted a black satin bra strap, then shot Skye a wide grin.

Skye stood frozen. What in the world was

Bunny Reid doing at Grandma Sal's Soup-to-Nuts Cooking Challenge? Bunny was many things — Skye's ex-boyfriend's mother, a retired Las Vegas showgirl, and the manager of the town bowling alley — but she wasn't a cook. The only recipes she knew were the ones that called for crushed ice and a maraschino cherry.

Brown eyes twinkling, Bunny threw her arms around Skye and said, "I thought you'd never get here. I was just about to start cooking without you."

Freeing herself from the older woman's hug, Skye managed to ask in a neutral tone, "Bunny, this is quite a surprise. What are you doing here?"

"I'm your runner." She pointed to her sneakers. "See? I'm all set to get you anything you need."

"Oh." Skye stepped up to the counter, wondering if there was any way to trade runners. She didn't want to hurt Bunny's feelings, but since she herself was a novice cook, she really needed a helper who had actually stepped foot in a kitchen before.

Bunny trailed Skye like a piece of toilet paper stuck to her shoe.

Without turning around, Skye said, "Uh, you know, Bunny, since you and I are friends, I think maybe your being my runner is sort of cheating. The other contestants won't have their friends helping them."

"Honey, you really are *too* nice." Bunny tugged her closer until they were face-to-face, her body language turning suddenly hard. "You've got to be more ruthless in this world."

"No!" Skye nearly screamed. All she needed was cutthroat Bunny working for her. That would be like having a wererabbit for a pet. "I like to play by the rules."

"In that case there's no problem." Bunny relaxed her pose and hoisted her jeans up a fraction. "They asked all the runners if they knew the contestants, and almost all of them did to some degree or another, so they said it didn't matter."

"Great." Skye gave Bunny her best fake smile, all the while thinking, *Rats!* Excuses raced through Skye's mind, but she couldn't come up with any other good reason to object to Bunny as her helper. She was stuck with the redhead, and the last chance Skye had of producing an edible casserole had just hopped out the window.

Sighing, Skye took the recipe card and a pencil out of her purse, then stowed the bag in the nearly empty cupboard. Handing the card and pencil to Bunny, she said, "Read the ingredients off to me. I'll find them;

then you put a check mark next to them on the card."

"Okay." Bunny dug a pair of small reading glasses out of her pocket, settled them on her nose, and asked, "Ready?"

"Ready."

"Chopped chicken." Bunny looked at Skye over the top of her lime green frames.

Skye opened the minifridge and took out the Ziploc bag of cubed cooked breast meat. "Check."

"Elbow macaroni."

Skye reached into the low cupboard, but couldn't quite grab the box, which had been pushed to the back. Sighing, she got on her knees and stuck her head inside.

She had just curled her fingers around the package when she heard someone yell, "Son of a B! Who switched my sugar for salt?" The voice belonged to her mother, and May sounded as if she were ready to have a stroke — or all set to give one to someone else.

Skye sprang up and hit her head on the shelf. Flailing backward, she threw her arms in the air, trying to regain her balance, but failed and ended up sprawled on the wooden floor as macaroni rained down on her head like rice on a bride.

Before she was able to get to her feet,

May's shouts bounced off the walls of the warehouse. "I know you did this, Cherry Alexander, and you're not getting away with it."

CHAPTER 5
SIFT DRY
INGREDIENTS
TOGETHER

As Skye plucked noodles from her cleavage, she toyed with the idea of pretending she hadn't recognized her mother's voice or, even better, that she hadn't heard the screams at all. Which would have been a good plan if, just as Skye became pasta free, another yell didn't rip through the warehouse.

This cry was a wordless screech that somehow sounded more ominous than the ones before, and Skye gave up any idea of remaining uninvolved. Crunching over the dry macaroni, she ran toward May's assigned area.

Bunny followed, peppering her with questions. "Who's Cherry Alexander? Why would she switch salt and sugar? What's May going to do?"

Skye wished she knew. She was afraid May's retaliation might involve plucking poultry and heating up asphalt. Two things

May did not tolerate were anyone insulting her children, and anyone messing with her cooking. And as Skye knew from personal experience, rather than forgive and forget, May's specialty was to reprimand and remember.

When Skye reached the Special-Occasion Baking area, she recoiled. Cameras of all descriptions were pointed at the crowd gathered around her mother's stove. May stood in the center of the group waving a wooden spoon in the air. Two of Grandma Sal's employees, Charlie, and Vince were all dancing around her like orderlies at a mental hospital trying to put a straitjacket on a patient.

Another group restrained Cherry. Unfortunately they had not taped her mouth, and she was screaming, "First she steals my secret ingredient, and now she accuses me of sabotage. I demand she be kicked out of the contest."

Skye saw her mother's face go from red to magenta, and hurried forward. Stopping just out of wooden-spoon range, Skye raised her voice. "Mom, put down your weapon."

May sneered. "The only place I'm putting this is up Miss High-and-Mighty's a—"

Skye cut her off. "Just calm down and think. We'll find out who did this."

"I know who did it, and she's standing over there smirking." May pointed the spoon at Cherry, who did indeed have a smug expression on her face.

Before Skye could respond, a sweet female voice managed to project itself over the melee. "Oh, my heavens. What in the world is going on around here?"

The crowd around May and Cherry split open like a cracked egg, and Grandma Sal walked between the two angry women. Skye prayed fervently that no yolks would be broken.

Both May and Cherry tried to explain at once, but Grandma Sal raised a work-roughened hand and pleaded, "One at a time. My hearing's not so good anymore."

Hmm. That was odd. The older woman's ears had seemed to work just fine earlier. Skye thought she saw a roguish twinkle in Grandma Sal's eyes.

Both May and Cherry tried to speak again, and this time there was a quaver in Grandma Sal's voice as she begged, "Please, ladies, don't ruin my contest. If you do, it might be the last one we ever have."

Skye barely stopped herself from snorting. Grandma Sal was certainly laying it on thick, but it looked as if one of the angry women was buying it — at least up to a point.

May put the spoon on the counter and moved toward Grandma Sal. "We wouldn't dream of ruining your wonderful contest."

Grandma Sal clasped May's hands. "Thank you, my dear. That's so sweet of you."

"But . . ." May tightened her grip on the older woman's fingers. "We do have to punish the person who tried to ruin my recipe."

"Of course we do." Grandma Sal maintained her smile as she freed herself from May's grasp. "*If* it was intentional, but I'm sure it was just a mistake." She spoke to the crowd. "One of the reasons we have this trial run the day before the contest is to iron out any kinks, to find the mistakes and make everything perfect for the actual competition."

May narrowed her eyes and opened her mouth, but Grandma Sal gracefully cut her off. "When you are stocking twenty-four kitchens, there are bound to be mistakes, but let me assure you all that there was no malice involved. It was just an error that could happen to anyone."

The crowd broke into applause, and Skye read defeat in May's face. Sighing with relief that the incident had been averted, Skye turned to go.

She got about halfway back to her kitchen when she heard a male voice roar, "Dammit to hell! Who switched my sweet peppers for jalapeños?"

Skye closed her eyes and willed reality to change. If something was about to happen, please let it be Vince or Butch, not Charlie, whose ingredients had been messed with. Vince would grin and make the best of it, and Butch seemed like a laid-back guy, but Charlie would rampage through the warehouse like an angry hippo, chomping anyone who got in his way.

While Skye hesitated, another voice shouted, "My casserole is ruined. Who screwed with my timer?"

Within the next few minutes several other contestants added their complaints to the general din, including Monika Bradley, who had discovered that wheat flour had been substituted for her white rice flour. As she explained to Grandma Sal, in her case the switch would not only ruin her recipe, but also had the potential to kill her.

Whoever was sabotaging the finalists' recipes had moved from mere mischief to possible manslaughter. The question was — why?

It had taken hours for Grandma Sal's employees to straighten out the chaos. Those whose stations had been messed with had to be soothed, and new ingredients had to be obtained for everyone.

About half of the contestants were still trying to finish their recipes at six o'clock, when Grandma Sal made an announcement. "Due to the dinner being held here at seven this evening, we are asking you all to go home now so we can get the tables set up in time. Because of the technical problems we ran into this afternoon, you will all be allowed in early tomorrow morning to practice your recipe again. Your areas will be available to you from six until nine a.m. At that point the kitchens will be cleaned and restocked, and the contest will start at ten, as previously planned."

There was a smattering of applause, a few grumbles of complaint, and a couple of murmured conversations.

As Skye was putting away the ingredients she had taken out, her mother hurried up to her.

"Aren't you ready yet?" she asked. "I need to get home right away. I just talked your brother into doing my hair for tonight."

Briefly Skye wondered what Vince would do with May's short, wavy hair. Both its length and degree of natural curl precluded any new style Skye could envision, but she knew better than to ask. Hair was a touchy subject with her mother, and for once she pitied her brother, who was May's golden boy 99 percent of the time, but not when her coiffure was concerned.

Careful not to become involved, Skye said, "Go ahead without me. I need to clean up here."

"Can't your runner do that?" May's brows drew together. "Who is she, by the way? I got the middle school Home Ec teacher; isn't that great?"

"Great." Skye was not about to share with her mother that Bunny Reid was her runner. May had taken an unreasonable dislike to Bunny from the moment the redhead had arrived in Scumble River. "Mine's looking for a broom." Skye fervently hoped that Bunny would stay away until May left. May's favorite nickname for Bunny was the Trollop, and that was one of the nicer things she called her. "I'm sure she'll be back to help soon. You go ahead."

"How will you get home if I leave you?"

"Someone will give me a ride." Skye spotted her godfather chatting with someone she couldn't see. She pointed to him. "Uncle Charlie can drive me."

May's gaze followed Skye's finger and she nodded. "Okay. I'll tell him not to leave without you." May kissed Skye on the cheek. "Don't take too long here. You have to get dressed for the dinner, too."

"I won't. See you tonight, Mom."

"Do you want Dad and me to pick you up?"

"No, Wally's taking me."

May walked away shaking her head.

Bunny returned just as Skye finished cleaning up. They'd gathered their belongings and were approaching the warehouse door when two teenagers rushed through it. The boy was well over six feet tall, skinny, and wore horn-rimmed glasses. The girl was nearly his complete opposite — six inches shorter, well rounded, with long, wavy brown hair.

Skye's stomach tightened in concern. What were Justin Boward and Frannie Ryan doing here, and why were they running? Did it have something to do with their personal lives — Justin and Frannie had recently started to go steady — or was it about the student newspaper? Justin and Frannie were the coeditors of the *Scoop* and very competitive in their reporting.

The teens skidded to a stop in front of Skye and Bunny, and Justin said breathlessly, "Xenia is missing, and we think she kidnapped Ashley Yates."

Several questions crowded Skye's lips, but she finally managed to push one out in front of the others. "Why?"

"Because of the lawsuit," Frannie answered. "Xenia was way pissed when she heard Ashley's parents were threatening to sue the paper over the article she wrote."

Xenia's article had examined the politics of popularity, using Ashley as a prime example of the price girls were willing to pay to be one of the "in" crowd. Xenia had listed all the things Ashley had done to both gain and keep her popular status, including having sex with the entire boys' basketball team, one right after the other, in their locker room the night they won the championship.

"How would kidnapping Ashley make it better?" Skye asked before she could stop herself.

Both teens shrugged, and Skye could have slapped herself for asking such a stupid question. No one knew why Xenia did anything. Skye wasn't even sure Xenia did.

Backtracking, Skye asked what she hoped

was a better question. "What makes you think Xenia kidnapped Ashley?"

Justin and Frannie looked at each other. Finally he gave an almost imperceptible nod, and Frannie said, "The last post on her blog."

Before Skye could respond, Bunny jumped in. "A blog is like a diary that you write on the computer and let everyone see. All the kids do it."

"I know what a blog is," Skye retorted. "What I can't understand is why anyone would write on one that she had kidnapped someone."

Justin studied his sneakers and mumbled, "She didn't exactly write that, but we put two and two together and figured it out."

"Are you sure you did the math right?"

Frannie joined Justin in his intense interest in his shoe. "We're pretty sure, especially after Xenia's mom called looking for her."

"Why is that?" Skye had never pictured Xenia as a teen who reported her every move to her mom.

Justin explained, "Since we were off school, Xenia and her mom were going into Chicago to see a matinée of this play Xenia really, really wanted to see, then go to this super cool new restaurant for dinner. But she never showed up. They were supposed to leave their house at eleven this morning, and when Mrs. Craughwell knocked on Xenia's bedroom door to see if she was ready, she didn't answer. Mrs. Craughwell went in and she wasn't there, and she hasn't shown up all day."

"Oh." *Shit!* It sounded as if Scumble River's newest wild child might indeed have added kidnapping to her already long list of criminal acts. For a nanosecond Skye wondered if maybe Xenia herself was the kidnapping victim, but she quickly realized how unlikely that would be. No way would Xenia trust anyone enough to put herself in a position to become a victim.

Still, Skye held out one last hope that neither girl had been kidnapped. "Okay, the big question is whether Ashley is missing or not. Has either of you called her house to check?"

Frannie nodded. "I pretended to be one of her cheerleading friends." The teen's cheeks reddened. "I'm pretty good at imitating voices. Her mom was mad. Said she'd been looking for Ashley all day."

"Okay, so both Xenia and Ashley are missing," Skye acknowledged. "What did you say to Mrs. Yates?"

"Uh." Frannie swallowed hard. "Well, the thing is, I didn't know what to say, so I might have suggested that the cheerleaders had an all-day practice and a slumber party tonight. Which is why I was calling, since I couldn't remember where the party was. And that Ashley might have forgotten to mention it, since it was sort of a last-minute deal."

The muscle under Skye's right eye twitched, but she kept her cool. She reminded herself that Frannie had just been trying to keep things calm until she could talk to an adult she trusted. She wasn't really trying to cover up a crime. "I don't suppose Xenia's blog said where she was keeping her victim or anything useful like that?"

"Not that we could tell." Justin dug in his jeans pocket, pulled out a crumpled piece of paper, and thrust it into Skye's hand. "Here. I printed out the post for you."

"Thanks." Skye smoothed out the sheet and, with Bunny peering over her shoulder, read; *Crybabies should b careful. If u can't stand the heat, u need 2 b kooled off. Kept on ice. Get my drift?*

Skye felt even worse after reading the brief message. "Sounds like she was planning on stashing Ashley in a freezer somewhere."

"We thought of that," Frannie said, "but where is there a freezer big enough to hold

95

a person, where no one would notice that a frozen cheerleader had been added to their inventory?"

"I don't know." Skye started toward the door again. "But I do know we need to talk to the police."

After extracting a promise from Bunny not to tell anyone about the Xenia/Ashley situation, Skye sent her runner home. Skye didn't like the glint in Bunny's eye as she hurried out the door, but there wasn't much she could do about it.

Next, she found her godfather talking to a petite brunette half his age. At six feet tall, he towered over the woman. They were deep in conversation when Skye interrupted to tell him that Frannie and Justin were driving her home. He acknowledged her with a muttered, "Great," but his gaze never left the woman's face, and before Skye could add anything, he whispered something in the lady's ear that made her giggle and pat his arm.

Having taken care of Bunny and Charlie, Skye led Justin and Frannie out to the parking lot and borrowed Justin's cell phone — one of the few that mysteriously seemed to work anywhere in Scumble River. "Thea? This is Skye."

"Hi, honey. How's the cooking contest going? Your mom is so proud that you and Vince are in it with her." Thea Jones was one of the dispatchers who worked with May.

Thea was a grandmotherly type who knew everyone in town, and Skye acknowledged that there was no way to cut through the social chitchat if she wanted to keep Ashley's disappearance quiet, so she summarized the day's events, ending with, "We just finished, and I'm heading home to change for the dinner, but I wanted to ask Wally something first. Is he around?"

"Sorry, sweetie. He's not here right now. He's probably at home getting ready for your big dinner party."

"Thanks. I'll try him there. Bye." Skye hit the END button before Thea could ask any more questions, grateful she hadn't had to go through the whole "how are you, how's your family, isn't the weather nice" ritual.

While she dialed Wally's home number, Skye said to Frannie, "Start driving toward town."

From the seat of Frannie's father's pickup truck, Skye watched the trees sweeping by as her call went through. When she got Wally's answering machine she tried his cell phone, but he didn't answer that either. She left another urgent message, checked her watch, then said to Frannie, "Head toward my house. He's supposed to pick me up there at quarter to seven, and it's already six thirty."

Justin and Frannie were strangely quiet as they drove. Skye considered questioning them to try to gather additional information about Xenia, but decided to see what Wally thought before she did anything more.

It was only a few minutes to the old Griggs place, which Skye had inherited that past summer. The house was a little isolated, and a lot run-down, but Skye had felt an immediate connection with Alma Griggs, and had been touched when the elderly woman's will revealed she had entrusted Skye with her home.

During the six months Skye had owned the house, she'd been trying to fix it up. After hiring one horrible contractor, she had been lucky to find a great woman who had whipped the outside into wonderful shape. Skye admired the new siding, windows, roof, and sidewalks as Frannie pulled into the driveway.

The instant the truck stopped, Skye jumped out and headed up the steps, pausing on the wraparound porch to dig through her purse for the keys. Justin and Frannie caught up to her as she swung open the front door.

Inside, Skye had had the contractor fix the plumbing and wiring, but she had run out of money before she got to the cosmetic repairs, so she had been trying to do those herself. So far she had managed to paint the entrance hall, parlor, dining room, and kitchen, but the hardwood floors still need refinishing, and the drapes had to be replaced. She hadn't even begun to touch the upstairs, except for removing a loathsome moose head from the wall of the master bedroom.

Now, as she stood in the freshly painted foyer, she tried to decide what to do about the present situation. Should she change into the clothes she had planned to wear for the dinner? Should she even attend the dinner? She had no desire to sit through a formal banquet, but if she didn't May would demand to know why, and that would mean news of Ashley's disappearance would be all over town. Maybe Wally would want her to go to the party just to keep things quiet. If that was so, she'd better get dressed. He was due in less than five minutes and was rarely more than a minute or two late.

Turning to the teens crowded behind her, Skye pointed to the kitchen and said, "Why don't you guys help yourselves to some sodas and snacks while I change? When the doorbell rings, make sure it's Chief Boyd; then let him in. I'll be back in a few minutes."

"What are you changing clothes for?" Justin demanded, looking her up and down.

"Shut up," Frannie hissed, elbowing him in the side. "I'll explain later."

Skye ignored both teens and took the stairs two at a time, shutting the bedroom door behind her. Kicking off her shoes, she wiggled out of her slacks and yanked her blouse over her head. Luckily she had already selected a dress to wear, and she grabbed it from its hanger.

As she pulled it over head and started to shimmy into it, she heard the phone ring. The dress was a straight black sheath, and required some time to get on. Hurrying was not an option, and before she was able to poke her head out of the draped neckline, there were two more rings.

Skye rushed to the phone by her bedside, another improvement she had finally made to the house. Previously the only phone was in the parlor.

Grabbing the receiver, she heard Wally say, "Skye —" Then an extremely loud buzzing sound interrupted, and she couldn't make

100

out a word.

She shouted into the mouthpiece, "Hang up and call back."

After returning the receiver to its cradle she waited, wondering if this was one of her ghost's latest tricks. She and Wally had just about given up trying to spend any time at Skye's house. It seemed that whenever they started to get intimate, something would short out the power, cause the plumbing to spew like a fountain, or blow up. Secretly — she had never shared this thought with anyone — Skye thought the ghost of the previous owner was behind the mischief.

Mrs. Griggs had taken quite an interest in Skye, and Skye was pretty sure that Mrs. Griggs didn't want Wally around. Skye wasn't sure if that applied to all men she might date or just Wally, since she'd been broken up with Simon before taking owner-ship of the possessed house.

The phone rang again, but this time when she tried to answer it nothing happened — no voice, no buzzing, just empty air, so she hung up. When it didn't ring again, she tried Wally's home and cell phones, but couldn't reach him on either.

Grinding her teeth, Skye finally gave up and went back to dressing. It took her only a few minutes to finish. She slipped on black patent-leather sling-backs, brushed some bronzer on her face and mascara on her lashes, combed her hair into a smooth page-boy, and stuffed her jewelry into her evening bag to put on later.

Skye looked at her watch as she descended the stairs. It was a few minutes past seven and she hadn't heard a doorbell. Unless the teens had let Wally in before he had even rung the bell, he was late, which wasn't at all like him.

What could be keeping him? Perhaps if she had been able to hear him when he phoned she would know.

CHAPTER 6
CREAM SUGAR AND
BUTTER

Skye listened in exasperation to Wally's message on her answering machine. "Skye, sugar, what's wrong with your phone? I sure hope you get this. I'm really sorry, but I've had an emergency come up and I can't take you to the dinner." There was a pause and she could hear a muffled voice in the background; then Wally said, "I'll call you tomorrow morning before you leave for the contest." There was silence, but she could tell he hadn't hung up; then he added, "Oh, I almost forgot to tell you, my cell phone's not working. Bye."

"Damn!" Now what was she supposed to do? Skye wished Trixie hadn't gone away for spring break. Come to think of it Trixie had a knack for being away when things at school imploded.

Skye's head felt as if it were about to fly off her shoulders. Did Wally's emergency involve Ashley's disappearance? Clearly he hadn't gotten either of her earlier messages. Should she go to the police station? Should she go to the dinner? Or maybe she'd go to bed and let everyone deal with their own problems. "Shit! Shit! Shit!"

Justin had sidled into the parlor without Skye noticing. "Uh, Ms. D, are you okay?"

"I'm fine." She took a deep breath and forced herself to smile calmly. "Just a little frustrated."

Frannie edged in and stood next to Justin, taking his hand. "Are you mad because Chief Boyd broke your date?"

"No." Skye sank into the sofa, feeling strangely like crying. "I'm upset because I'm not sure what to do."

"You'll think of something," Frannie soothed. "Take a deep breath."

Skye looked at the girl and realized that Frannie had come a long way since she first met her over two years ago. Back then Frannie had been insecure and obsessed with her own problems. Now, as Skye looked into the teen's confident and caring brown eyes, she saw the woman Frannie would become.

"You're right." Skye inhaled and instantly felt a bit calmer. "Thank you."

"So, what are we going to do?" Justin paced in front of the settee. "If Xenia kills Ashley, the superintendent will get rid of the paper for sure."

Skye fought a flicker of irritation at Justin's self-absorption, reminding herself that he was almost a year younger than his girl-friend, and had had a much harder life.

While Frannie had a loving and supportive father, Justin had pretty much raised him-self. Mr. Boward was in nearly constant pain and lived from day to day, which had caused Justin's mother to sink further into a depres-sion that rarely allowed her to leave the house.

"There's not a lot I can do until I can reach the chief," Skye said, and stood up. "Maybe the emergency he was talking about was Ashley's disappearance." She turned to Frannie. "When you talked to Mrs. Yates, did you get the impression she was going to call the police?"

"No. Probably not after I made up the story about the cheerleaders having a slum-ber party."

"Shoot. I had forgotten about that." Skye scooped up the cordless phone and strode into the kitchen. "So she won't be expect-ing Ashley until sometime tomorrow?"

Frannie nodded.

"Okay. First I'll call the police station and see if Ashley or Xenia has been reported missing. I doubt Xenia's mom will involve the cops, considering her daughter's history, but I want to make sure."

Skye punched in the nonemergency number for the PD and said, "Thea? It's Skye again. Have you heard from Wally?"

"Isn't he with you?" Thea's voice rose in alarm. "You're both supposed to be at the dinner. Your mom will be real upset if you aren't there."

"I'm on my way. Wally left me a message saying he had an emergency, but I really need to talk to him."

"Sorry, he doesn't have a radio with him and isn't in a squad car. How about his cell?"

"He said it's not working. I guess I'll try his house again." Skye bit her lip, then asked, "By the way, you haven't had any reports about a missing teenager or two, have you?"

"No. Who's missing?" Thea demanded.

"Uh, I'm not sure. Oh, someone's on my other line. Gotta go." Skye hung up, feeling guilty. No one else was phoning. She didn't even have call waiting.

She turned to Justin and Frannie, who had been listening. "Well, that settles that. Mrs. Yates has not called about Ashley, which means I'll have to tell her Frannie was lying."

Both teens protested, but Skye remained firm. As much as she didn't want to risk the student paper, she knew Mrs. Yates had to know the truth. With Wally AWOL, Skye had no choice. She couldn't ask one of the other officers to look for a girl they didn't have an official report on and whose parents had no idea she wasn't where she was supposed to be.

A few minutes later, after reaching Mrs. Yates and explaining Frannie's deception, Skye held the handset away from her ear. Ashley's mom was not taking the news well. Not that Skye had expected her to. Skye made soothing sounds as the woman ranted and raved, and threatened another lawsuit. Just before she hung up, Mrs. Yates said she was phoning the police.

Although Skye was relieved that at least now someone would be looking for Ashley, she still had to bite back a pithy comment or two about parents keeping control of their own children, and not expecting the school to do the parents' jobs for them.

The call to Mrs. Craughwell went even more poorly. She did not believe Xenia was involved and claimed her daughter was in her room as they spoke. Of course, even if Xenia was there, it didn't mean she hadn't kidnapped Ashley earlier and stashed her somewhere. The best Skye could do was make another phone call to the police and leave a message about Xenia's blog entry.

All of this took surprisingly little time. After Skye sent Justin and Frannie home, she looked at her watch and saw it was only seven forty-five. If she left right away, she could still make the dinner. There was nothing else she could do for Ashley or Xenia, and according to the schedule, cocktails were at seven and the food would be served at eight. Skye would be just in time for the soup, which might be soon enough to keep her out of hot water with May.

"Babe, I promise, I'll totally tell her as soon as this contest is over. She'd grease us both if she barneyed because we messed with her mind." A low, smoky male voice drifted over the racks as Skye stepped into the center of the coatroom, an area in the back of the warehouse that had been partitioned off with two folding walls, and furnished with a dozen or so metal frames with poles suspended horizontally between them.

Skye stood in the middle of the rows. She hadn't realized anyone else was in the room until she heard the voice. Should she cough to indicate her presence, or should she just quietly leave? The tricky part would be moving silently among all the dangling hangers.

Before she could decide, a distraught female voice said, "You always have some excuse. I can't go on like this. Either you tell her about us by this Sunday, or I'll tell her."

"No!" the man shouted, then took on a cajoling tone. "Sorry, babe, I didn't want to tell you this, but I can't bail on her. We have an ironclad prenup. She'd get everything, including custody of the baby."

"But what about us?"

Skye cringed, hating to eavesdrop on these future guests of *The Jerry Springer Show*. She took a step backward and froze when she bumped into a rack, causing a tinny clunk.

"Did you hear that?" he demanded.

"Hear what?" the woman asked between sobs.

There was a long moment of silence while Skye fought to remain quiet.

"Guess it was nothing," the man answered, then said, "I'd better get back to the table. We'll dial in on all this tomorrow while the queen's busy cooking. Her Highness will be wondering what's taking me so long. I swear, she even times me when I take a leak."

A soft giggle hiccuped through the tears.

"You're so funny, Kyle."

Skye raised an eyebrow. So, half of the amorous couple was Cherry Alexander's husband, Kyle. She wondered who his lover was.

"And you'd better get back before Juanita complains to Cherry about having to do your job and hers too."

"I didn't leave the baby with Juanita."

Ah, the nanny. How clichéd. Skye shook her head. Did every rich father sleep with his child's nanny?

"What?" Suddenly the male voice was no longer cajoling. "Who's watching him?"

"He's in the car."

"By himself?"

"Yes." The girl's voice quavered. "He's in his car seat asleep and the doors are locked."

"You skank!" All traces of Kyle's prior charm had drained away, and his tone was now utterly harsh. "Never, ever leave my son alone again."

"But . . . but, Kyle. What about us?"

"Just get out of here, Larissa. We'll talk later."

It took Skye a moment to realize that the couple would have to come her way to get out of the coat area, and another second to figure out what to do. Hoping that their own movement would be blamed for the noise,

110

Skye wedged herself between two racks, pulling the coats in front of her as camouflage. Thank goodness she was wearing black.

Larissa came first. She was crying too hysterically to notice if an armed Roman gladiator popped up in front of her. Kyle was close on the girl's heels, looking straight ahead, nearly pushing the distraught nanny out of his way. Luckily for Skye he was too angry to care who might be around.

Once the couple left, Skye found a hanger, hung up her coat, and smoothed her hair and dress. As she made her way into the large area that had been set with circular tables, she shook her head. She would never have guessed that surfer-dude Kyle would turn into Romeo Kyle, then morph into protective-father Kyle. That scene had sure been an eye-opener.

The tables were packed, and servers were scurrying around delivering bowls of steaming soup, bringing baskets of fragrant bread, and filling glasses with wine. Skye's stomach growled. She hadn't had anything to eat since a BLT six hours ago.

She scanned the chairs, looking for her mother and dad, but couldn't spot them. Finally, one of the servers asked, "Can I help you find your table, ma'am?"

"Are there assigned seats?" Skye was a little surprised, wondering how Grandma Sal's staff had decided who sat with whom.

"Yes, ma'am. Are you a contestant, media, judge, or Grandma Sal's staff?"

"Contestant."

"The contestants are seated two to a table with their guests and their runners and their runners' guests." The young man pointed to a group of twelve tables in the front of the room. "Starting from the right side, the places are arranged alphabetically."

"Thank you." Skye nodded at the server and walked toward the area he indicated.

She found her place at the third table. Her mother and father sat with the middle school Home Ec teacher, whom Skye was acquainted with, and a man Skye assumed was the teacher's husband. On the other side of her parents were two empty seats, and next to the vacant chairs were Bunny and her son, Simon.

Skye paused only a second before turning to leave, but it was a second too long. May saw her before she moved.

As Skye searched her mind for options, she saw her mom stand up, wave her arms, and yell, "Over here!"

What in the world had Vince done to their mother's hair? All the natural curl had been gelled out, and it was plastered to her scalp like a rubber Halloween wig. May looked as if a vat of cooking oil had been poured over her head and left to congeal.

"Why are you so late?" May demanded as Skye slipped into her chair. "You certainly don't look as if you spent the extra time primping."

"Thank you, Mom. You look nice, too." Skye fought to keep the sarcasm out of her voice and to prevent her gaze from drifting to her mother's new 'do. "I'm not late. I just had a rescheduled arrival time."

"You sound like those teenagers you spend too much time with." May's tone was disapproving.

"Hi, everyone." Skye ignored her mother. "Sorry I wasn't here on time."

The others said hello and murmured that her tardiness wasn't a problem.

"I was worried something had happened." May reached up and tucked a stray curl behind her daughter's ear. "What kept you?"

Skye had taken the empty chair nearest her mother, as her other choice was the vacant seat next to Simon. Now she wondered if she had really chosen the lesser of two evils. "A situation with the school newspaper came up, and it took me a little longer to deal with it than I estimated."

"What situation?" May narrowed her eyes.

"Oh, nothing I couldn't refer to someone else."

The others had remained silent through the exchange, but as May paused in her interrogation and Skye sipped a spoonful of soup, Bunny piped up, "Where's your date, Skye?"

Skye closed her eyes and counted to ten. "He had an emergency and had to cancel." Sitting at a table with both Bunny and May was almost like having two mothers to irritate her. It was odd how different the women were, but they could certainly both drive her crazy. Of course, considering how this day was going, all it would take was a short putt.

May dabbed her lips with her napkin. "He seems to have a lot of emergencies popping up lately."

"He is the chief of police." Skye counted to twenty. At this rate she'd be up to a hundred before the entrée was served. "He's bound to be occasionally called away."

As usual, Skye's father, Jed, was silent while the women talked, and the other two tablemates appeared determined to appear as if they hadn't heard a word of the discussion.

Skye saw Simon open his mouth, but then

close it without speaking.

They all finished their soup, and the server replaced their bowls with salads. May lowered her voice and asked in a hopeful tone, "Are you and Wally breaking up?"

"Not that I know of. Have you heard something?" Skye matched her mother's low volume. "Or is this just wishful thinking on your part?"

"You rush in here an hour late, disheveled and dateless. It's not much of a stretch."

"Everything's fine between us," Skye assured her mother, but wondered herself what was going on. Determined to change the subject, she raised her voice and asked the middle school Home EC teacher, "Barb, what made you decide to volunteer to be a runner?"

"When I didn't final in the contest, I thought maybe seeing the whole process up close and personal would give me a hint about what to enter next year." The stylish brunette leaned forward. "How about you, Bunny? Are you looking for ideas for next year's contest, too?"

"No. I'm not very good in the kitchen." The redhead jerked up her strapless aqua minidress, fluffed her curls, and fluttered her lashes at the teacher's husband. She giggled. "I'm better at keeping the bedroom sizzling. After all, I'm still a hot babe. But now it comes in flashes."

Simon's handsome face reddened, and Skye gave him a sympathetic look that clearly said, *Mothers!*

His hazel eyes softened and he smiled, nodding his head in agreement.

After the entrées were served, and everyone turned to their food, Simon leaned close to Skye and said quietly, "Frannie mentioned that some disgruntled cheerleader's parents are suing the school newspaper. Does that have anything to do with why you were late?"

Skye hadn't intended to let anyone know what had happened, especially before she could talk to Wally, but she found herself nodding.

"Anything I can do to help?" His soothing tenor made Skye relax for the first time since Justin and Frannie had told her about Ashley's disappearance.

"I don't think so, but thanks for offering."

Once they finished their entrées and the tables were cleared, the room was darkened and a masculine voice boomed over the loudspeakers, "We have a special treat for you tonight. Instead of a traditional dessert, our factory has constructed the largest chocolate fountain in the country." A spotlight aimed at the center front of the room flared to life, illuminating a tublike vessel about the circumference of a child's wading pool and nearly as tall as a refrigerator. From its four spouts chocolate flowed in a continual stream.

After a second of silent appreciation, applause and excited chatter broke out among the audience. Flashbulbs went off as newspaper photographers took pictures. Even TV cameramen jockeyed for good shots.

Once the noise and activity decreased, the voice said, "Tables one through four are invited to come up and get your dessert now."

May was the first one out of her seat. From the table near the fountain she piled her plate with slices of banana, small squares of angel food cake, and a small mountain of strawberries.

Simon was behind Skye, and as he made his selections he murmured to her, "I can think of something I'd rather drizzle chocolate over than this stuff."

Her face flooded with warmth, but she pretended not to have heard him. They had broken up at the end of last summer because she thought he had cheated on her. At the time he had refused to explain himself, and Skye had not learned until Thanksgiving that the woman she had discovered him with was his half sister, not a girlfriend. By then Skye had become involved with Wally, and Simon's explanation involving family secrets was too late.

Since finding out Simon's big secret, she had seen him here and there, but hadn't spent any time with him. Skye considered their relationship over, and she wasn't ready to be just friends. Was Simon saying he felt otherwise? Was he just flattering her or was he intimating that he wanted her back?

Before she could figure out his intentions or decide what to do about them — she really was very happy with Wally — a voice came over the PA system.

Clearly the person speaking didn't mean for the whole place to hear him when he said, "What do you mean, you might not sell Fine Foods? You can't pull out of a deal like this. They'll sue us, you crazy old woman."

Grandma Sal's voice was easily recognizable. "I haven't signed anything, and behavior like this won't get me to. You'd better watch your manners and remember who owns the majority of Fine Foods."

"I've slaved my whole life for this company. You'd better not try to screw me out of my share now."

"It's not your name and face on the products; it's mine, and I have to do what I think is right for both the business and its employees."

"And I have to do what I think is necessary for me. I'm warning you that if you get in my way on this deal, I'll be forced to get rid of you."

CHAPTER 7
ADD EGG YOLKS

No human being should be forced to get out of bed at five in the morning. Skye stuck an arm out from under the covers and thumped her squealing alarm. She usually woke to the sound of music, or at least a deejay's serene baritone, but she had purposely changed the setting to buzzer, knowing that anything less wouldn't rouse her at this ungodly hour.

May was picking her up at ten to six. She'd insisted they needed the full three hours allotted for practice, and while Skye didn't disagree, she knew her mom hadn't taken into consideration the fact that no amount of preparation would make Skye's cooking edible.

Skye had tried to talk May into meeting her at the factory, intending to arrive later in the morning, but May knew her too well and had vetoed that suggestion. At the time it had seemed too much trouble to argue, but now that she actually had to get up at the crack of dawn, Skye wished she had insisted on driving herself.

It was too late to change things now, and Skye set a new personal record for showering, dressing, and gulping down a cup of Earl Grey tea. She was waiting on the porch when her mother pulled into the driveway. She slid into the passenger side of May's Oldsmobile and slumped back on the seat, closing her eyes.

"Good morning," May chirped. Skye winced.

"Morning," Skye mumbled, refusing to call anything that started this early "good."

"Isn't this a beautiful day?"

"If you like the wind whipping down the plains." Skye squirmed in her seat. "My poor tulips have been stripped of all their petals."

"You sound grumpy." May expertly backed out of the long drive. "What's wrong? Are you sleepy, hungry?"

"No. And I'm not Happy, Dopey, or any of the other Seven Dwarfs either."

"Then what's up?" May ignored Skye's feeble attempt at humor.

"Nothing. I'm fine. You know I'm not a morning person. Just give me a chance to wake up."

May huffed, but was silent for only a few seconds before saying, "Who do you think that was arguing with Grandma Sal over the PA last night?"

Skye forced open one eye. "Who else could it be but her son, Jared?"

"Yep, that's what everyone else I talked to on the phone this morning is thinking too."

It didn't surprise Skye that May had already polled people about the incident. Her mother's group of friends got up before the birds, and had a better communication network than AT&T.

May was silent for another couple of seconds, then changed the subject, a dark look clouding her usual sunny expression. "All I can say is that if Cherry Alexander messes with my ingredients today, I'll make cherries flambé out of her."

"Mom, you don't know that Cherry was behind the salt/sugar mixup."

May ignored Skye's interjection. "Yesterday my cake turned out flat as a training bra. That won't happen again. Today I'll check everything as soon as I get there, and no one will get near my kitchen."

Skye closed both eyes again. "Sounds like a plan, Mom."

Before Skye could doze off again, May commented, "You and Simon seemed to be pretty cozy last night."

Skye shrugged, keeping her eyes shut. Simon was not a subject she was ready to discuss before she was fully awake and armed with all her senses.

May continued, "Barb and her husband commented on how well you two danced together."

Darn! After the dinner the front area had been cleared for dancing. A local band had been hired to provide the music. In a moment of weakness and — Skye might as well admit it — pique at Wally's absence, she had agreed to one waltz with Simon.

Skye shrugged again, then realized she'd better nip May's fantasies in the bud before they grew into Barbie's Dream Wedding. "Simon and I have had a lot of practice dancing together. It doesn't mean a thing. After all, he danced with several of the women present."

"They were all married or old enough to be his mother." May put on her turn signal and slowed down, then eased the big car into the nearly empty factory parking lot.

As soon as May stopped the Olds, Skye leaped out and hurried toward the warehouse entrance. She had to get away from her mother and clear her mind. It was time to become one with the casserole.

May lagged behind, hefting a box and two canvas bags she'd taken from the trunk. Skye watched as her mother struggled under her load. What in the world did she have in the box, not to mention the bags? Grandma Sal's people were providing all the ingredients, pans, and utensils, although they had said it was okay to bring your own.

Skye was torn between giving May a hand and completing her escape. Just as she was about to go back and help, someone dressed in a dirty factory jumpsuit, wearing both a hairnet and a net over the lower half of his face, rushed past May. Skye couldn't hear what her mother said, but the worker stopped, turned around, and took the box from her mom's arms.

Skye's mouth hung open as she saw the person close the lid of the trunk and allow May to lead the way. Her mother was truly amazing. She could guilt nearly anyone into doing nearly anything.

Smiling, Skye turned back to her original goal, and sprinted the last few steps to the warehouse entrance. As she reached for the handle the door smashed into her. She teetered backward, trying to regain her balance, but before she recovered her uncle Dante rushed out of the building shouting something unintelligible. In the process he slammed into her and she fell onto her derriere.

May was his next victim. Dante hit her like a champion in a belly-bucking contest. The two bags she was carrying flew upward, spreading kitchenware in an impressively large arc. A sudden gust of air caught the lighter articles and carried them away.

The person carrying May's box dropped it and took off running like the space shuttle blasting into orbit.

As Skye struggled to her feet and hurried over to her downed relatives, she wondered if May's helper could outrun the wind. "Are you okay, Mom?"

"I'm fine." May had already gotten to her knees and was retrieving the cooking items from the grass.

"Uncle Dante." Skye squatted down level with the mayor, who was still sitting, stunned, on the sidewalk. "What happened?"

At first his response was gibberish, but finally Skye made out a few words. She heard him say, *woman, dead,* and *chocolate.*

The last explained the wet brown stain on Dante's ample shirtfront, but that still left the most important question: Who was dead? Was it Grandma Sal? After all, they had all heard her being threatened by her son last night.

Her heart pounding in alarm, Skye looked around. Her mother hadn't heard Dante's mumblings — she was still picking utensils out of the grass — and no one else was in sight. The guy in the jumpsuit had not returned, and Skye figured he was probably late for work or didn't want to get involved with the crazy people. She checked again, but no one else had materialized, which left her in charge.

She brought her attention back to her uncle and asked, "Who's dead? Are you sure they aren't just hurt? Did you call for help?"

Dante was rubbing at the chocolate on his shirt, muttering something that sounded suspiciously like, "Out, out damn spot," and didn't seem to hear Skye's questions or feel her shaking him.

Deciding that he would be of no help for quite some time, Skye reached around him and unclipped the cell phone from his belt. Dante frowned momentarily, but didn't stop in his stain-removal efforts.

Rising to her feet, she dialed 911. Due to May's absence, the PD was shorthanded and Thea was on duty again, but this time Skye cut off her social chat and said, "Thea, Skye here. We have a problem at the Grandma Sal's factory. Send the police and an ambulance. I'm not sure exactly what the situation is. My witness isn't coherent at the moment."

The dispatcher instantly snapped into professional mode. "Someone will be there in a few minutes. Don't hang up, in case you need help."

"Fine." Skye left the line open, but wanted her hands free. She had no pockets and was afraid that if she put the phone into her tote bag she'd never find it again. Shrugging, she slipped it into her cleavage. The little antenna sticking out from her chest looked a tad strange, but there was nothing normal about this situation.

Skye's mother had finally retrieved all her belongings and noticed that Dante was sitting on the sidewalk in a nearly catatonic state. Now that her whisk was safe and her measuring spoons out of harm's way, May focused on trying to snap her brother out of his stupor, but he still wasn't putting together coherent sentences.

Since Skye was the new Scumble River Police Department psychological consultant, she would no doubt be assigned to debrief her uncle once Wally arrived, but for now she felt that securing the scene of the crime was more important.

She positioned herself in front of the door,

determined to keep anyone from entering before the police arrived. Dante's exit had jammed the door into an open position, and the wind was blowing debris from the yard inside. She chewed her lip, wondering if she should close the door.

The longer Skye waited, the more she second-guessed herself. Maybe she should have checked to see what Dante was mumbling about before calling 911. What if he'd had a psychotic break, and there was nothing wrong inside the building?

Before the police had employed her she would have gone in and scoped out the situation, but now she felt obligated to be more restrained and professional.

While she was considering her next move, an earsplitting scream from just beyond the warehouse doors prodded her into action, and without thinking Skye rushed inside. As she ran she dug through her purse until she found the pepper spray she always carried. Holding the canister at the ready, she followed the sound of the screams.

Last night the party had taken place in the rear of the warehouse. Although the tables had been cleared, they were still arranged as they had been for the dinner, facing the back wall near the dessert station and dance floor.

As Skye wound her way through the table maze, she saw that the dance floor was clear, but to her left, standing frozen by the chocolate fountain, was Diane White, the cookie blogger. She stood in the famous *Home Alone* pose, hands to cheeks with mouth and eyes rounded into giant Os.

Looking past the shrieking woman, Skye saw a pair of five-hundred-dollar Vera Wang sandals sticking up from the chocolate fountain. They weren't moving. Skye approached Diane warily, not sure what role the blogger had played in this particular tragedy. Was she the innocent witness, or was she the diabolical killer, sneaking back to clean up her tracks?

Skye was pretty sure the woman in the fountain had been murdered. Suicide by chocolate or natural death via cocoa was a bit of a stretch, even for Skye's active imagination.

"Diane, calm down. Everything's fine. The police will be here any minute." When the blogger continued to shriek, Skye's palms itched to slap her, but luckily for the finalist the Scumble River police force arrived, and Skye stepped back and allowed them to handle the hysterical woman.

Wally, gun drawn, raced into the warehouse, followed by Anthony, one of the part-time officers who also had his firearm at the ready. Both men aimed their weapons at Diane, who swallowed a scream in midscreech and promptly began to choke.

Without taking his eyes from the suspect, Wally asked Skye, "Are you okay?"

"I'm fine."

"What about her?" He indicated the coughing woman.

"I heard her start to scream a minute or two ago, which was several minutes after Dante came running out of here covered in chocolate and muttering about a dead woman."

Wally nodded. "Anthony, pat her down, then get her out of here and have the paramedics take a look at her, but don't let her leave."

The officer complied. He didn't find any weapons on the blogger and took her outside.

As soon as they were gone, Wally rushed to Skye and took her in his arms. "Are you sure you're okay?" He smoothed the hair off her forehead. "Thea was hysterical. She said you didn't answer her, and all she could hear on the phone was screaming."

Guiltily Skye reached into her bra and withdrew Dante's cell. "I . . . ah . . . forgot I had it on. Once the yelling started I followed my instincts."

As a pair of EMTs ran in, Skye reluctantly withdrew from the safe haven of Wally's arms. He kissed her on the temple, gave her one last squeeze, and then joined the paramedics at the chocolate fountain.

Suddenly Skye felt dizzy and sank into a nearby chair. Her view was a bit obstructed, but it was clear from the snatches of conversation she heard and the body language of the EMTs that the woman in the fountain was dead.

There was a short argument between Wally and one of the paramedics, who was obviously inexperienced. The newbie wanted to remove the body from the chocolate, but Wally insisted they wait for the coroner.

Skye cringed. It was obvious to her that Wally's legendary patience was growing thin. She could see the irritability on his face and the way his shoulders twitched. Unfortunately the EMT didn't seem to notice, and Skye was afraid that Wally would take a swing at the guy, whose persistent questions were as annoying as a two-year-old demanding a toy at Wal-Mart.

Fortunately, before Wally decided to deck the guy, Simon rushed in, and, as county coroner, took over.

Skye watched Wally step aside and speak into the radio clipped to his shoulder. She guessed he was calling the county crime scene techs. For a while Scumble River couldn't get assistance from the county because the sheriff blamed Skye and Wally for opening an investigation into his conduct on a previous case. But a few weeks ago the old sheriff had finally been removed, and his temporary replacement was a reasonable man who didn't hold a grudge.

A quick glance at her watch told Skye that it was nearly six thirty. She knew it would take at least three-quarters of an hour, maybe more, for the techs to arrive. They were based in Laurel, the county seat, which was forty-five miles of secondary roads away.

Pulling herself together, Skye rose from her seat and walked over to Wally. "Is there anything you want me to do while we wait for the techs to get here?"

"I've called in all off-duty and part-time officers, and they're keeping the perimeter intact and rounding up anybody they find nearby. Luckily only you and your mother were here promptly at six for the practice. The other contestants have been showing up a few at a time, and my officers have been able to stop them at the gate."

"Except for Diane," Skye reminded him.

"I wonder when she arrived."

"Good question. May said that you two got here just a few minutes before the mayor came running out." Wally paused until Skye nodded her confirmation. "Dante and the screamer are still not making any sense."

"Do you want me to try to talk to them?"

"Might as well give it a try." Wally nodded toward the chocolate fountain. "I'd like to know if they saw anything or only stumbled across the body. Ms. White was too clean to have committed the murder — unless she did it naked and then re-dressed."

"Now there's a picture I could have done without." Skye winced.

"Sorry." Wally patted her arm. "We've called for Grandma Sal to come out and identify the body."

"Do you want me to look?" Skye hated to do it, but knew that the sooner they knew who the victim was, the better their chances of solving the case.

"It would be a help, but you don't have to. We can wait." Wally put an arm around her shoulders.

"No, I can do it." Skye gazed into the warm depths of Wally's eyes and gained strength from them.

"Okay." Wally led her to the chocolate fountain.

Simon had laid the victim out on the floor. The rest of the crime scene belonged to the county techs, but the body was the coroner's domain. He was taking a temperature reading to help determine the time of death, and Skye tried not to notice the sharp probe going into the body's liver. Instead she concentrated on the face. She leaned forward and looked closely. As she had suspected from the expensive sandals, the chocolate-covered corpse was Cherry Alexander.

CHAPTER 8
ADD VANILLA

"Uncle Dante?" Skye found the mayor sitting on a bench, clutching a gray wool blanket around his shoulders and staring into space.

It wasn't like her uncle to remain on the sidelines — he was too fond of the limelight to wait for someone to seek him out. His normal MO would be to charge into the crime scene, try to order Wally around, and generally make a nuisance of himself. Clearly he wasn't okay.

May sat next to her brother, patting his hand and murmuring soothing words. When Skye approached, May looked up with a worried crease between her eyebrows. "I saw Simon go in. Who's dead? What happened?"

"Cherry Alexander," Skye answered, then wondered if she should have kept that information to herself. "Don't tell anyone else. Treat the info as if you heard it while at work — confidential." Skye answered her mother's last question: "We don't know what happened. How's Dante? Has he said anything?"

"I can't get him to talk. I even tried to get a rise out of him by mentioning that this would probably be the end of the good publicity for Scumble River, but he still didn't respond."

"Have the EMTs looked him over?" Skye didn't see an ambulance in the parking lot.

May shook her head. "They had their hands full with that cookie blogger. She was screaming and twitching and causing all sorts of commotion. I heard they thought she was having a stroke or a seizure or some such thing, so they're transporting her to the hospital."

It crossed Skye's mind that Diane might be putting on an act in order to get away from the cops. "Did Anthony go with her?" It would be a lot easier to escape from the hospital than from the police station.

"I think so." May's voice was taut, her fingers twisted in a knot. "They asked if Dante was okay, and I said he wasn't hurt, so they gave me a blanket for him and then left. Did I do something wrong?"

"I don't know." Skye squatted in front of her uncle and studied him closely. His breath was coming in small, fast gasps, his

136

skin was blotchy, and the area around his mouth had a bluish cast. Skye chewed her lip, then handed Dante's cell phone to May. "Mom, you'd better ask for another ambulance. I think he's going into shock."

May fumbled a little, but eventually managed to turn the phone on and dial. "Thea? It's May. We need another ambulance at Grandma Sal's."

Once Skye was sure May was making the call, she tuned out her mother's voice and focused on her uncle. "Dante, everything is okay now. The police are here and you're safe." She pressed him back so that he was lying on the bench and elevated his feet by putting them on May's box of utensils. "Just forget what you saw and relax." She kept her voice a hypnotic tone as she loosened his shoelaces, belt, and tie. "Think of your favorite place."

Dante didn't react. He appeared to be conscious, but completely unresponsive.

"The ambulance from Brooklyn is on its way," May reported.

"Good." Skye unbuttoned Dante's shirt, then without looking away asked May, "Do you have a gallon-size Ziploc? One that hasn't been used?"

"Yes." May dug through the canvas bags next to the bench, found the unopened box, and extracted a bag. "Here's a brand-new one."

"Hold it open," Skye instructed as she eased her uncle's shirt off him and carefully put it into the bag. "Close it up and don't let it out of your sight."

May nodded, closed it, then stared at the plastic sack as if it might sprout wings and fly away.

Skye turned back to her uncle, and as she pulled the blanket higher around Dante's shoulders she noticed that his undershirt was soiled, too, and this spot didn't look like chocolate. She lifted the white cotton tee and examined his upper torso; there was a jagged wound smeared with dried blood just above his belly button. The chocolate on the front of his outer shirt had masked the bloodstain. Dante had been stabbed!

Skye was torn between staying with her uncle and finding Wally to report this new development, but before she could decide she heard an ambulance siren. In minutes a man and woman rushed over to them and began issuing orders and firing questions.

As Dante was being wheeled away, he suddenly became alert and grabbed Skye's hand, saying, "Don't let them cancel the contest. Promise me you'll make Grandma Sal keep it going."

She was saved from answering when the EMTs lifted the gurney into the ambulance.

"Here, take this." Skye's mother shoved the Ziploc bag containing Dante's shirt into her daughter's hands. "I'm going with him." May grabbed her purse and hurriedly climbed in beside her brother, clutching his cell phone and muttering, "I need to call Olive and Hugh, and you need to get hold of your father." She aimed the last bit at Skye.

"No!" Skye swallowed back a frustrated shriek. "Call Olive, but don't tell her what happened. Just say that Dante's injured and going to the hospital. Do *not* say anything else and do *not* call anyone else."

May nodded distractedly, and Skye wondered if her mother had even heard her. Since May was armed with a cell phone and knew how to use it, Skye decided she needed to fill in Wally ASAP, or the news of Dante's wound would be all over Scumble River before the chief of police even knew about it. Wally had been a little cranky lately, and Skye didn't think being scooped by the town gossips would improve his mood.

Skye passed Simon and his assistant, Xavier Ryan, wheeling a gurney bearing a black body bag down the sidewalk toward the parking lot. She nodded to both men, but kept walking.

While she had been with her uncle the county crime scene officers had arrived, and the warehouse was buzzing with voices and activity. She found a tech she knew and handed him Dante's shirt, explaining how it came to be in her possession. He put the Ziploc into his own evidence bag, noting the information she had given him on the outside.

Circling the crime scene, Skye made her way over to the table in the rear corner of the dining area, where Wally was seated, talking to Grandma Sal and Jared. JJ and Brandon were at a table in the opposite corner of the room. Both young men had cell phones pressed to their ears, but neither seemed to be having much luck with reception as they took turns yelling, "What? Say that again. No, I said dead, not bread."

Skye caught Wally's eye, then made a questioning face. Should she join them or wait somewhere else? He nodded and indicated a chair next to him.

Skye sat down, and Wally introduced her. "This is Ms. Denison, the psychological consultant for our police department."

Grandma Sal smiled. "You're also one of our finalists. Right?"

"Yes, ma'am."

"Then maybe you can help me convince my boy here that the contest must go on."

Skye was caught by surprise. That was the last thing she had expected to hear the older woman say. "Well, I hadn't given it much thought." In fact, she had figured that Grandma Sal would be horrified by the murder, and would want to put as much distance between it and her company as possible.

Grandma Sal's son spoke up before Skye could say more. "Going on with the contest would be disrespectful to Ms. Alexander, and put an undue burden on the rest of the contestants. We certainly can't expect them to do their best under these conditions."

Wally looked at Skye. "What do you think? The techs say they'll be done by this afternoon, and I would like to keep everyone together until we figure out what happened here. If we cancel the contest, all the participants will scatter. I can't order that many people to stay put. Their lawyers would be all over me."

"I think the challenge should go on, for several reasons." Skye paused to gather her thoughts. "First, as you say, it's better for the investigation if everyone stays around. Second, it isn't really fair to the finalists who have worked so hard to get here to have it canceled. And third, going on with the contest will provide some closure to the people involved. Perhaps you could even give out an extra prize, the Cherry Alexander Award for something or other."

"Perfect." Grandma Sal clapped her hands. "We'll push everything back a day. I'm sure no one will mind sticking around an extra twenty-four hours." She turned to her son. "Jared, you and the boys make sure everyone gets the word that we're going ahead, and the cooking starts at ten a.m. tomorrow. You can use the phones at the factory, and I'll meet you there when I'm done here."

Her son shook his head, but stood up and walked over to JJ and Brandon. Neither of the "boys" looked pleased with Jared's news, but both followed him out the door.

Wally asked Grandma Sal a few more questions, then rose and held out his hand. "Thank you for your cooperation."

Grandma Sal shook Wally's hand, nodded to Skye, then headed toward the exit.

As soon as Grandma Sal was out of sight, Skye said, "We need to talk."

He picked up his pen. "Shoot."

"When I went out to check on Dante, I found a stab wound on his stomach. He's

142

on his way to the hospital."

"Son of a bi . . . !" Wally stammered to a stop. His jaw worked for a while, but he finally said, "What happened?"

"He's in shock and not able to communicate, except to order me to make sure the contest goes on."

"He and Grandma Sal are two of a kind."

Skye shook her head. "Let's just hope they aren't a 'dying' breed."

"So, he didn't mention that he'd been stabbed, and you have no idea how he got the wound?"

"That pretty much describes the situation."

"Any guesses?"

"It depends." Skye shrugged. "We arrived here at six o'clock on the dot, and Dante came running out of the warehouse maybe thirty seconds later. Was Simon able to give you a time of death for Cherry?"

Wally consulted his notes. "Reid said the body temp was ninety-seven-point-four. Bodies cool at about one and a half degrees per hour, and she was one-point-two degrees below normal. Which means she could have been killed just a few minutes before you were knocked over by Dante."

"I take it that the chocolate fountain wasn't heated at the time?"

"No."

"But then" — Skye narrowed her eyes — "why wasn't the chocolate hard?" She had noticed it was in liquid form when she was trying to calm down Diane.

"Grandma Sal said the fountain chocolate is like the syrup you pour over ice cream. It never solidifies."

"Okay, then it's my guess that Dante wrestled with the killer and was cut by him or her. Was Cherry stabbed or drowned or both?"

"The only injury Reid found was at her hairline above her right eye. There were lacerations and a depression in the skull, indicating she had been hit on the head with something like a hammer or mallet." Wally tapped the table with his pen. "Unfortunately, Reid can't say yet if it was the blow or the chocolate that killed her."

"Why not?"

"Drowning is a diagnosis of exclusion. If the medical examiner doesn't find any other cause and there's fluid in her lungs, he'll call it a drowning."

"Maybe once they wash the body they'll be able to tell us more. Hard to see bruising while she's covered with chocolate."

"Yep. Let's hope Reid missed something." Wally pushed back his chair. "I guess I'd better get to Laurel Hospital and see if the mayor is talking yet."

Skye followed him as he headed out and waited as he had a word with the techs and his officers, but as he reached his squad car she put a hand on his arm and said, "We really need to talk. Did you get my message about Ashley Yates's disappearance?"

"Yes. Quirk moved on it last night. He didn't find her, but her mother admitted that this isn't the first time Ashley has gone missing for a couple of days."

"Really?" *Gee.* What a shock that Mrs. Yates hadn't mentioned that to Skye, instead blaming the school. "But how about Xenia and her blog?"

"Xenia was home, just like her mother claimed, but — surprise, surprise — when Quirk questioned her she claimed the blog wasn't hers, and it has since disappeared into cyberspace." Wally's expression showed his disbelief. "Quirk's got the county computer expert looking into that."

"Good. Xenia bragged to the other kids about the blog, so I'm sure she's lying about it not being hers. Not to mention she's quite a hacker, which is how she got her story about Ashley into the newspaper without Trixie or me catching it. So she wouldn't have any trouble getting rid of the blog if she wanted to." Skye let go of Wally's arm. "Was that why you couldn't make the dinner last night? Was that the emergency you mentioned?"

He shook his head, the expression on his face strained. "No. That was something else."

She opened her mouth to ask what, but Wally was already sliding into the driver's seat and closing the door.

He rolled the window down and, as he started the engine, said, "I don't have time to get into it right now. Are you free tonight?"

She nodded, a feeling of alarm making her chest hurt. What was going on? Was he breaking up with her?

"Okay. Unless something else happens I'll be at your place around seven, and I'll bring supper." He stuck his arm out the window and took her hand, raising it to his mouth for a kiss.

The touch of his lips sent a flame into the pit of her stomach, and the warm expression in his brown eyes curled around her heart.

She sensed his reluctance to let go, but when he did he said, "Everything will be fine. I promise."

As Skye watched the cruiser drive away, it

occurred to her that Wally had said he'd come to her house. That was odd. Although they'd never voiced their concern, it seemed that every time she and Wally even touched each other anywhere in her house, something exploded or caught on fire or flooded. Since Thanksgiving they'd been spending most of their time together at his house.

Why did he suddenly want to meet at her house? She frowned. Was Wally planning to tell her something that would end their relationship for good, and so had no intention of touching her? She blinked back a tear and forced herself to think positive thoughts.

When Skye finally turned away, she realized that she needed a ride. Her mom had left with Dante, taking the keys to her car with her. And all newcomers were being turned away at the factory's gates, which were being monitored by the police.

Shoot. She'd have to go over to the plant, ask to use a phone, and get someone to pick her up. But who? She had no idea where Uncle Charlie or Vince was, since they were also contestants and would have been turned away at the gate a couple of hours ago. Her dad refused to answer the phone.

Skye thought for a moment. Heck, anyone she called for a ride would expect her to tell them everything that was going on, which she couldn't do. Maybe her best bet was to go to the gate and see if anyone she knew turned up. It would be easier to be evasive with an acquaintance than a friend.

Slinging her tote bag over her shoulder, she started toward the main road, about a quarter mile away. She kept to the pavement, not wanting to get her new running shoes dirty. About halfway there she noticed a swathe of white caught in the bushes that lined the driveway. It was probably just garbage, but something about it seemed familiar.

She stepped closer, trying to avoid the mud. Just as she reached out to touch it, it fluttered in the wind, and Skye realized she was staring at a discarded factory jumpsuit that was smeared with chocolate, and maybe blood. *Oh, shit.* This must belong to the man she and May saw running in the parking lot that morning. Darn. In all the confusion she'd forgotten to tell Wally about the guy — and he *could* be the killer!

What to do now? Better to let the techs get it, but did she dare leave it? What if it blew away? Okay, she'd wait until someone came in or out, and ask them to get a tech. This kind of situation made her wish for a cell phone.

Twenty minutes later her plan to wait didn't seem like such a good idea. Finally an elegant black Lincoln limousine coming from the direction of the factory purred into view. Skye waved it to a stop, and leaned in as the passenger window eased down. Inside were Grandma Sal, Jared, JJ, and Brandon.

Skye explained her dilemma and asked them to go back and get a crime scene tech. After a bit of an argument as to whether it would be faster to call the Scumble River PD and wait for the message to be conveyed to Wally, or just to drive back the quarter mile, driving back won.

That decision led to a discussion about who should do what. In the end Brandon and JJ got out of the car to stay with Skye while Jared and his mother were driven back for the tech.

While they waited Skye tried to make conversation. "Do you both work for the family business?"

JJ, the pudgy, blue-eyed blond, ducked his head shyly. "I'm Grandma's assistant."

"Where'd you go to school?"

"I graduated from Loyola a year ago with a degree in business."

"Good school." Skye turned to the dark-haired one. "How about you, Brandon?"

"I'm the head of the company's legal department."

"Does that mean you do *all* the legal work for the company?"

"No." Brandon smirked. "I supervise the people who do it."

"My, you seem so young for such a responsible position."

"Yes. Pays to have family connections. Right, JJ?"

The young man nodded.

Skye nodded too, having benefited from nepotism herself when Uncle Charlie got her the school psych job in Scumble River. Still, she'd bet JJ was making five times what she did, and Brandon probably made ten times her salary.

Skye was uncomfortably aware that they were standing in silence. Neither young man seemed able — or willing — to chat.

She searched for something more to say, wishing the tech would arrive. "Sounds like you're both tried-and-true Chicagoans. Do you get out to the Scumble River factory very often?"

"We work mostly out of the Chicago building." JJ stared at his shoes. "Grandma comes out here a lot, and she insists we maintain duplicate offices for all the departments here, but they're rarely used."

"Why does she do it, then?" Skye asked,

intrigued at the way big business was run compared to the school, where she was lucky to have a single cramped office, let alone a spare one.

"Grandma says she feels closer to Grandpa here than anywhere else," JJ answered.

Brandon rolled his eyes. "She gets to be the queen bee out here. That's why she likes it."

Skye sighed with relief as the unmarked county car pulled up, followed closely by the Fines' limo. Skye showed the tech what she had found. She was about to explain that someone wearing a factory jumpsuit had been running past the warehouse that morning, but something stopped her and she decided to tell Wally first.

The Fines offered her a ride home, and she gratefully accepted. As she sat cradled in the soft leather seat of the luxury car, she wondered what it would be like to know that you were going to inherit millions and millions of dollars. Of course, everyone said that money couldn't buy happiness. Still, she might enjoy the chance to see for herself.

CHAPTER 9
SLOWLY ADD DRY MIXTURE TO CREAMED

Skye wasn't surprised to find several messages on her answering machine when she got home. Most of the callers wanted to know what had happened, and a couple asked how Dante was, but the one she returned immediately was from Frannie, who had called to ask if Ashley had been found.

Skye cradled the receiver between her shoulder and ear so she could change into jeans and a sweatshirt as she phoned the teen. There was no answer at Frannie's house, and Skye was in the process of looking up Justin's cell number when her doorbell rang.

She hurried down the stairs, looked out the peephole, and opened the door. "I was just calling you."

Frannie and Justin stood on her welcome mat. Frannie looked upset, and Justin's expression said that he was itching to punch something really, really hard really, really soon.

"What's up?" Skye ushered them inside and steered them toward the kitchen.

Frannie flung herself in the chair Skye offered, but Justin ignored the proffered seat and paced.

Skye raised an eyebrow, then ducked her head into the refrigerator to hide her expression. As she gathered meat, cheese, and condiments she asked, "Are you hungry? I'm starving. That's the problem with getting up at five a.m. — you're ready for lunch by ten."

Frannie giggled politely, but then drooped back into her original dejected posture.

Justin sneered and kept pacing.

Skye knew from past experience that Justin wanted her to beg him to talk. She also knew that if she did, he would close up tighter than a shrink-wrapped CD case.

Instead she asked, "So, who wants a snack?"

Frannie's well-mannered, "No, thank you," was a sharp contrast to Justin's negative growl.

Skye shrugged and assembled a sandwich. She was just cutting it on the diagonal, because even TV chef Alton Brown said sandwiches tasted better that way, when

Bingo sauntered into the kitchen.

The cat had an uncanny ability to appear when food was being prepared or eaten. He could be anywhere in the house, from the attic to the basement, and still manage to arrive before Skye could take the first bite.

This time Bingo ignored Skye and her sandwich, walked over to where Justin was pacing, and started doing figure eights between his ankles.

Skye watched carefully while pretending to be engrossed with shaking potato chips into a bowl. Justin had come a long way from the angry and depressed eighth grader she had originally seen for counseling, but she still wasn't sure he wouldn't lash out, given the right circumstances.

At first the teen snarled at the feline, but Bingo ignored him and revved up his purrs to jet-engine volume. Finally Justin stopped moving, and the cat immediately sat down on his feet, looking up at him with a questioning meow.

Skye took a quick peek at Frannie, who had straightened and was staring with her mouth slightly open.

The scraping of a chair on linoleum brought Skye's attention back to the boy and the cat. Justin was sitting with Bingo on his lap. The teen's expression was still angry, but his shoulders had relaxed and his hand rested lightly on the cat's soft black fur.

Skye nonchalantly made her way to the table, putting the bowl of chips in the center and sitting down with her plate. Just before taking a bite she asked again, "What's up?"

Frannie glanced at Justin, who shrugged and kept petting the cat.

Slumping once again, Frannie sighed and said, "It's Xenia."

Skye's throat tightened, but she forced herself to say lightly, "What about her?"

"She's being a real bitch," Justin blurted out.

"In what way?" Skye wanted to ask how being a bitch was new behavior for the girl, but controlled the urge. She couldn't say that about one student to another, no matter how great the temptation or accurate the observation.

Frannie took a chip and crumbled it in front of her. "She's claiming that she didn't write that blog, and is acting like we betrayed her by even thinking she had kidnapped Ashley. She's turned a bunch of the kids on the newspaper staff against us."

Ah. Skye nodded her understanding. Both Frannie and Justin had had friendship issues in the past. Neither had been accepted by the "in" crowd, and they had gotten to the point of forming their own circle of friends only within the last couple of years. Add to this that their group consisted of the other newspaper kids, and Xenia's duplicity took on a whole new meaning.

Before Xenia's arrival in the fall, Frannie and Justin had been the undisputed leaders of that crowd, but Xenia had challenged them at every turn for that position.

Justin broke off a piece of potato chip and offered it to Bingo, who sniffed, took a delicate lick, then regally accepted the offering.

Skye took the opportunity to swallow before saying, "When the truth comes out the kids will see who their real friends are. Xenia has a lot of charisma, but it isn't something that can sustain a relationship for long."

Frannie nodded. "That's true. Remember, she tried to get everyone on her side when she first came here, but it didn't last long. This is just another lame attempt to be elected editor next year."

"Easy for you to say." Justin shook his head. "You'll be away at college next year. I'll be the one stuck with her."

Skye's internal warning bell went off. This was the first time either Frannie or Justin had acknowledged that Frannie would be leaving next fall, and the pair would be separated.

She stole a peek at Frannie, who swallowed a couple of times before saying, "Maybe you and Xenia will team up and not miss me at all."

Justin scowled but didn't verbalize his reply.

Finishing the last bite of her sandwich, Skye pushed the plate away. "You do realize that Mrs. Frayne and I have to approve whoever is elected student editor?"

"You wouldn't say someone couldn't if he or she was elected, would you?" Justin asked.

"In a flash, if we thought they'd cause trouble." Skye poured three glasses of Diet Coke and put one in front of each teen, keeping the third for herself. "But that's next year, and a lot can happen between now and then. So, any idea where we can look for Ashley? Or did you both forget she's still missing?"

"I didn't forget, but there's nothing I can do about her, and it's not as if we were her pals or anything." Frannie shook her head. "When she came into the newspaper office to complain about Xenia's article, she looked right through me. Then, when she thought she could use me, she tried to pretend we were best friends. So I asked her my name, and she didn't have a clue. Heck. We've been in classes together since third grade."

"Yeah." Justin nodded his agreement. "Ashley thinks she's such hot shit, but she only stinks."

In a sympathetic but firm tone, Skye said, "Be that as it may, we can't let Ashley get hurt just because we don't like her. It's our duty as decent people to help find her if we can."

Justin shrugged. "Whatever."

Frannie snorted.

Skye took that as agreement. "Let's start with the blog message you showed me. Maybe I'm not reading it correctly. Let's see if your interpretation is any different from mine." She grabbed a couple of legal pads and a few pens from the junk drawer and reseated herself at the table. "The message read: 'Crybabies should be careful. If you can't stand the heat, you need to be cooled off. Kept on ice. Get my drift?' Right?"

Both teens nodded.

"Okay. Is there any other meaning to the word *crybabies,* beside whiner or complainer?"

"The kids use it to mean tattletale, but that's sort of the same thing," Justin offered.

"Has anyone told on someone lately?"

"No." Frannie frowned. "No one I can think of." She looked at Justin, who shook his head.

"Any ideas on what the blogger meant by the next section?" Skye underlined it with her pen.

"Just, if you can't stand the problems you've caused, you should fix things." On her scratch pad, Frannie doodled monsters with huge open mouths and pointy fangs.

"How about the 'cooled off and kept on ice' part?"

Justin looked away, then muttered, "Some of the wannabe gang kids use that term to mean kill and get rid of the body, but I think Xenia might mean it more like keeping Ashley away from her friends until she cools off and stops her parents and their lawyer from harassing the paper."

Skye's breath had gone out with a whoosh when Justin mentioned murder, but she was able to inhale by the time he finished his thought. "And the last bit? Anything with the word *drift?*"

Both kids shook their heads.

"Have you had any ideas since yesterday

about where Xenia might be keeping Ashley?"

More head shakes; then Frannie added, "We've looked in all the places we knew that either of them hang out."

"We even checked the school — you know, like the cafeteria's freezer and the pantry, and the closets and lockers — in case she was hiding her in plain sight." Justin leaned forward, and Bingo jumped off his lap with an annoyed yowl.

"Ashley pretty much hung out with the cheerleaders, and they pretty much hung out at each other's houses during the winter and at the rec club beach during the summer." Frannie put her hand down to pet the cat, but he stalked away.

"Where would one teenager hide another?" Skye muttered almost to herself. "It would have to be either completely isolated, like a hunting cabin, or a place with so many people going back and forth that no one would notice a couple more."

"Xenia is new in town. She doesn't have any uncles or cousins around here with shacks in the woods," Frannie pointed out.

"Right, so it's got to be the other choice." Skye and the teens were silent, thinking. Finally she said, "I'll call Officer Quirk and see if he's had any luck."

It took her a while to track Quirk down, but she finally got through to him. "Roy, this is Skye. I'm calling about Ashley Yates. Is she still missing?"

"Ten-four. Parents have not reported her return."

"I've been going over the blog message with a couple of my students, and we wondered if Xenia had access to any hunting cabins or fishing shacks." Skye wanted to double-check before crossing that possibility off her list.

"That's a negative. And we've searched the school and both the vic's and the suspect's garages."

"Any other ideas?"

"No, we put out an AMBER Alert right away, but there haven't been any legitimate tips."

"Thanks, Roy." Skye didn't want to keep him any longer, knowing how busy he'd be with the morning's murder.

She relayed her conversation to Frannie and Justin, who remained quiet.

Finally she stood up and said, "Sorry, guys, but I have to get ready for an appointment, so you'll need to be going."

The teens shuffled to their feet and headed toward the front door. Skye heard Justin

161

whisper the word *date* to Frannie, who giggled.

Once the kids were gone, Skye phoned the hospital to see how her uncle was faring.

Her mother was put on the phone "Uncle Dante is fine. He lost some blood and is a little shocky, but the wound was superficial."

"That's a relief." Skye hadn't realized until just then how worried she'd been about her uncle. "Did he say how it happened?"

"No. Wally's been trying to get him to make sense, but no luck. The doctors say Dante should be back to normal in a couple of hours."

"Okay. Thanks, Mom." Skye looked at her watch as she hung up. It wasn't even noon yet. She had seven hours before Wally was supposed to show up. She could probably finish painting the sunroom. And maybe as she painted, an idea about Ashley's whereabouts might pop into her head.

By the time she spread the drop cloths, taped the windows, and picked up a brush, she was feeling calmer. Skye loved the delicate moss green color she had chosen for the walls. She couldn't wait until the painting was finished and she could have the new hardwood flooring laid and the floral window treatments hung.

She painted in contented silence, not even putting on a radio, letting her mind wander from mystery to mystery. Who had killed Cherry Alexander and why? Where had Xenia hidden Ashley, and how had she managed to subdue the cheerleader? What did Wally have to tell her, and why at her house instead of his, their usual meeting place?

Hmm. If the body had been Grandma Sal, after that argument that went out over the PA system last night, Skye would have thought her son did her in. But there was no way Cherry could have been mistaken for Grandma Sal.

What did she know about Cherry? She was self-centered, annoying, and married to a surfer dude who was boinking Mary Poppins. All of that certainly gave the husband and the nanny motive.

Skye got down from the ladder, balanced the brush across the open paint can, and grabbed a pen and paper from the end table. She made a note of her thoughts about Kyle and Larissa.

While she was at it, she added the guy in the soiled jumpsuit who had helped May that morning. Who was he, and what was on his clothes?

This time when Skye got back to painting, Xenia and Ashley popped into her mind. Had Xenia drugged Ashley? But surely someone would notice one teenage girl hauling an unconscious friend around. Especially since Xenia's preferred mode of attire was gothic-punk sex kitten.

Was there any way Xenia could have persuaded or tricked Ashley into going with her? But what did Xenia have that Ashley would want? Certainly not her spiked dog collar or stiletto granny boots.

Okay, forget how; concentrate on where. Skye paused to move the ladder, then picked up where she had left off. Where? It took several minutes, but suddenly an idea came to her mind. Could "kept on ice" equate to ice cream?

The local soft-serve drive-in, the Dairy Kastle, closed at the end of September and didn't unbolt its wooden shutters until the beginning of May. Surely they would have a freezer, even if it wasn't running.

As Skye finished the last wall and put away her equipment, the idea of Xenia keeping Ashley at the Dairy Kastle grew stronger and stronger. Xenia wouldn't hesitate to break into a locked building. The drive-in was on the edge of town, and the gas station that was next to it was out of business, so Ashley could scream her head off and no one would hear. Yes, Xenia could be hiding

Ashley at the Dairy Kastle.

Skye hurried to the parlor and grabbed the phone, dialing as she ran upstairs. *Shit!* Quirk was still at the warehouse questioning suspects, Wally was in Laurel informing Cherry's husband of her death, and the dispatcher couldn't help her contact either one. Thea said that there was no officer at the police station at that moment, and asked whether it was an emergency, or if Skye would like to leave a message.

Skye wanted to declare it an emergency, but somehow couldn't bring herself to do so. After asking Thea to tell Quirk to call her, she tried to let the idea go, but couldn't.

She looked at the clock. It had taken her a little over five hours to finish the sunroom and talk to Thea at the PD, so she still had two hours until Wally was due. She'd check out the Dairy Kastle herself.

Should she get ready for their date first or go look first? Look first. If Ashley was there it wasn't fair to keep the girl locked up any longer than necessary. Besides, Skye might get dirty if she had to smash down a door or something. Good thing she hadn't gotten paint all over herself.

Considering that she might have to break through a lock, she gathered a hammer, screwdriver, and flashlight from her basement workbench, then grabbed her keys and coat and took off.

At the edge of town most of the businesses were closed, and not just for the winter. Many buildings had been razed, but there were enough deserted relics left intact to make the area creepy.

Skye parked nearest the back entrance of the drive-in and got out of the car. She shivered despite the warmth of her wool pea jacket. The door was locked, not that she had expected anything else. Still, it would have seemed silly not to try.

She used the handle of the screwdriver to knock, calling, "Ashley, are you in there?"

Silence.

Skye knocked harder and yelled again.

Maybe the teen was gagged. "Ashley, if you can hear me, make some noise."

Nothing.

Skye listened intently; still no sound. Okay, what if she couldn't move? What if she was unconscious? But breaking down a door based on nothing but a hunch was not a good thing. She'd better wait and talk to Wally or Quirk.

Turning, she took a step toward her car. Suddenly she heard a rattle and dashed back to the building. She put her ear to the cold metal. Nothing. Nothing. Then she heard it again: a distinctive rattling sound. If that was Ashley, it would be unconscionable to leave her locked up for one more minute.

The lock was a dead bolt — nothing a credit card would open. There had to be another way in. She circled the building and discovered that the front serving windows were covered with wooden shutters nailed on in four places.

Moments later, using the claw end of her hammer and working patiently, Skye lifted off one of the wooden rectangles. The darkness inside was too deep to penetrate even with her flashlight, so she hoisted herself up on the metal counter and swung her legs over the other side.

She slid down to the floor and called reassuringly, "Ashley, it's Ms. Denison. Don't be afraid. I'm here to rescue you."

The only response to her announcement was another rattle. She thumbed on her flashlight and aimed it toward the sound. There in the back of the twelve-by-twelve space, between cans of strawberry sauce and buckets of peanuts, two glowing yellow eyes stared at Skye.

She screamed, scrambled back over the counter, and ran for her life.

CHAPTER 10
MIX UNTIL SMOOTH

Skye checked her watch as she tore up the stairs. Less than a half hour before Wally was due to arrive. Shedding her clothes in the middle of her bedroom floor, she dashed into the bathroom and turned on the shower.

Even with the new plumbing it took forever for the water to get hot, and as she waited the humiliating memory of her latest escapade nagged at her. What would Wally say when she told him she had broken into the Dairy Kastle to save Ashley, who wasn't there, then had been frightened away by a rat?

She knew exactly what Simon would say. His lecture would begin with the consequences of breaking and entering, segue to the fact that she had not found Ashley, and end with a scientific explanation as to why she couldn't possibly have seen a rat. He would have coolly pointed out that the rodent she'd had eye-to-eye contact with was merely a harmless field mouse. All of which made her glad she wasn't dating him anymore.

But the million-dollar question: Would Wally react any better? A couple of months ago she would have said yes, but lately he'd been behaving oddly.

Skye hurried through her shower, debating whether she really even had to tell him about her little adventure. She had returned to the drive-in and nailed back the shutter, so she doubted anyone would know the building had been broken into. Maybe she could "forget" to mention how she had spent the latter part of her afternoon.

As she blew her hair dry, a little voice nagged at her, insisting that if this was the man she might want to spend the rest of her life with, keeping secrets from him was not a good idea. Even though the voice sounded a lot like her mother's, she listened anyway.

This meant she had to figure out the best way of imparting the news, and time was running out. As she applied bronzer and mascara, she rehearsed how she would tell Wally about her afternoon activities.

She finished polishing her speech as she wiggled into a pair of black jeans, then chose a baby pink off-the-shoulder knit top that displayed her cleavage to its full advantage. She hoped her décolletage would sweeten her words, or at least take the sting out of them.

The doorbell rang as she was slipping on pink Skechers, but she took time to put on lipstick and take one last glance in the mirror before going to answer it. Wally's recent history of breaking dates suggested he was taking her for granted lately. It wouldn't hurt him to cool his heels on her front porch for a few minutes.

After passing her own inspection, Skye made her way downstairs, took a quick look out the peephole, and opened the door. Her welcoming smile faded as she noted that Wally was in uniform. That he hadn't changed meant either he was still on duty or had been so busy he couldn't get home before coming over. Either scenario did not bode well for a relaxing evening.

At least he held a pizza box. She was starving, and the only ingredients she had on hand were those that went into her contest entry. And she was pretty sure they were both sick and tired of Chicken Supreme.

Wally silently handed Skye the pizza, strode through the door, and shed his jacket. He hung it and his gun belt on the foyer's coatrack, then took the pizza back and tossed it on the table.

Finally he turned toward her and said, "It seems like years since we've spent more than five minutes together." Without waiting for her response, he swept her into his arms and added in a lower, huskier tone, "Damn, I've missed you so much."

As his lips claimed hers, Skye caught a glimpse of his expression. Passion and something she couldn't quite read warred in his dark eyes. Deciding not to worry about it for the moment, she put her arms around his neck and buried her hands in his thick black hair. She loved the crisp feeling of the strands as they feathered through her fingers.

His kiss sent the pit of her stomach into a wild Tilt-A-Whirl ride, and she pressed closer, her body tingling from the contact.

Wally groaned and parted her lips, his tongue exploring the recesses of her mouth.

He tasted sweeter than her favorite chocolate, and she wanted to devour him. She forgot about the murder, the kidnapping, and all her other worries and enjoyed the moment.

Wally's fingertips were icy as his hands crept under her shirt, but his palms were fiery hot when they cupped her breasts.

She caressed the planes of his back, and they moved as one toward the stairs.

Skye blindly stepped backward, expecting to encounter nothing but hardwood floor. Instead her shoe came down on a throw rug, which somehow wrapped itself around her ankle, causing her foot to slide out from under her.

She was about to do the splits in slow motion, but Wally grabbed her upper arms, trying valiantly to keep both of them upright. There was an instant when it seemed he had succeeded; then the rug slithered farther away, and Skye toppled over.

At the last minute Wally thrust himself sideways to avoid landing on top of her, and for a split second their fall seemed frozen in time, like some bizarre ballet routine. Then, as her back and head hit the edge of the stairs, the hurt swept away all of her fanciful thoughts.

Skye had no idea how long she lay there absorbed in pain, but when she was able to focus she looked to where Wally lay sprawled motionless on the hardwood floor. In saving her it appeared he had hit his head on the newel post. Her heart stopped, and she couldn't swallow the lump that had risen in her throat.

Whimpering, she raised herself on one

172

elbow. "Wally, sweetheart, are you all right?"

It seemed like forever, but he finally sat up, fingering the back of his head. "I'm fine. How about you?"

"I'm not sure." The room was spinning, and she was slightly nauseous.

He immediately leapt to his feet. "Stay right there." Staggering a little, he rushed to her side. "I'll call an ambulance."

"No. Wait." She put her hand out. "Help me up."

"You shouldn't move if you're injured."

Skye ignored him and got to her knees. The pain in her back made her gasp, but she forced herself to her feet. "See? I'm fine. Just a little shaken up."

He wrapped an arm around her waist and they hobbled into the parlor. Lowering themselves onto the settee, they both let out sighs.

"What the hell happened?" Wally cradled Skye against his side.

"It's this house." Skye shook her head, and the pain shooting through her skull made her realize that movement of any kind was a bad idea. "For some reason it doesn't want us to be together."

"That's ridiculous." Wally touched the bump on the back of her head. "Maybe we should let a doctor take a look at you. You're not being rational."

Skye jerked away from him, the stab of pain that surged up her spine reminding her once again that quick movements equaled suffering. "Don't start that rational stuff on me, or I'll think you're channeling Simon. And we wouldn't want that, would we?"

"That was a low blow." Wally scowled.

Skye raised an eyebrow. "If the personality trait fits . . ."

"Okay, forget rational. It doesn't feel like the house hates me. There aren't any cold spots. The lights don't flicker. The doors don't lock me out."

"Maybe not, but I swear that rug was not at the foot of the stairs when I came down to let you in, and it's not the only time something bad has happened." Skye scrunched up her face, thinking. "There was the first time we kissed in this house and the kitchen faucet did an impression of Old Faithful." Skye held up her index finger. "Then there was the mirror that smashed to smithereens the first time you tried to take my bra off, and the space heater that blew up the next time things got hot and heavy between us." She wiggled three fingers at him.

"It's an old house," Wally stated, but sounded less sure as he added, "Things are bound to go wrong."

"Right. So, why have we spent all our time together at your house since the explosion?"

He shrugged. "Coincidence."

"And since we're on the subject, why didn't you want to meet there tonight?"

"Well . . ." Wally's face clouded with uneasiness. "That's one of the things I wanted to talk to you about."

Suddenly Skye didn't want to hear what he had to say. "I'm starving. I bet you are too." She hated surprises. "How about we heat up the pizza and talk while we eat?" She popped up off the settee, ignoring the ache in her back. "I'm pretty sure the house will let us eat in peace. It just seems to dislike it when we touch."

"Okay." He looked puzzled by her abrupt change of mood, but stood up. "I'll grab the pizza from the hallway and meet you in the kitchen."

"Great. You want a beer or are you still on duty?"

"They'll only call me if something comes up with the murderer or the missing girl, but I guess I'd better stick to Diet Coke just in case."

Skye nodded and scurried into the kitchen. She set the dial on the stove at three-fifty to preheat, then got two glasses

175

from the cupboard. She was already pouring the soda over ice when Wally came in carrying the now-cold pizza.

After she wrapped it in foil and put it in the oven to reheat, she sat down and immediately started telling Wally everything she could think of regarding the murder and Ashley — up to the point where Skye had broken into the Dairy Kastle.

He listened and took a few notes, but the only thing she had to say that got a rise from him was her news about the person who had helped May that morning, and finding the factory jumpsuit. "Do you think your mom got a good look at the guy when he was helping her with her box?"

"I doubt it." Skye pursed her lips. "The lower half of his face was covered with that net thing the workers use if they have beards or mustaches, and he had another hairnet on his head. The only thing exposed was his eyes."

"What color were they?"

"He was never close enough for me to see." Skye bit her lip. "Mom may have noticed."

"Did you tell anyone about seeing this guy?"

"No. I forgot to tell you this morning, and then I wanted to talk it over with you first."

"Good." Wally absentmindedly started to pat her hand, but snatched his away as if he had been burned.

Skye lifted her chin. "I thought you didn't believe the whole haunted-house thing."

"I don't." The tips of his ears turned red. "I just didn't want to distract you." He cleared his throat and added, "We'd better make sure May doesn't tell anyone either. If it was the killer, we don't want him to think she can identify him. It was a him, right?"

"I think so, but Mom probably got a better impression than I did." Skye wrinkled her brow. "I guess the reason I thought it was a male was the net thingy on his face. But I couldn't see if he really had a beard or mustache, so maybe that was just used as a sort of mask."

"I'll talk to May first thing tomorrow." Wally made a note. "Your dad picked her up at the hospital just as I was leaving, and she said they were going to stop for supper at the new Culver's in Laurel, then head straight home, so she shouldn't tell anyone between now and then."

"Are you kidding?" Skye snickered. "May is gossip central. She'll probably hit the phone as soon as she gets home. No way would a Culver's butter burger and a custard keep her from broadcasting on the

Scumble River ten-o'clock news. You'd better call her right now."

Wally's hand went to the clip on his belt where his cell phone should have been, and he cursed when he realized it was not there, then got up and grabbed the kitchen phone.

Skye tuned out his conversation as she set out plates, napkins, and silverware.

As soon as he hung up he said, "May hasn't told anyone and promises she won't. She didn't see the color of his eyes, and isn't sure if her helper was a he or a she."

Skye blew out a frustrated breath, then took the pizza from the oven and put it on the table.

After they practically inhaled the first pieces, she asked, "Did you ever get Uncle Dante to tell you who stabbed him? And why he was at the warehouse, anyway?"

"Dante said he was there as a favor to Grandma Sal to help make sure everything went smoothly and that no one played any more pranks."

Skye made a disbelieving noise.

"*Anyway,* he was supposedly inspecting the cooking areas, heard a noise in the back of the warehouse, went to check on it, and saw feet sticking out of the chocolate fountain. When he bent down to look more closely, someone threw a tablecloth over his

178

head, spun him around, and stabbed him in the stomach." Wally took a swallow of Diet Coke before continuing. "By the time he got clear of the tablecloth his assailant had run away, and when he saw the blood he started to feel woozy, so he ran out of the building looking for assistance."

"Shoot." Skye licked her fingers. "So, Dante was no help at all."

"Right. His attacker could be anyone. Dante's not a big man, so most women could handle him in that situation." Wally helped himself to another slice. "The county crime techs found the tablecloth when they drained the fountain, but say they doubt there's any trace evidence on it after being submerged in chocolate."

"Did they find any other evidence?"

"Nothing yet. The ME has the body, and we should get word tomorrow on cause of death, but he did confirm she'd suffered a blow to the head."

Skye wiped her mouth with a paper napkin. "So, what's the plan?"

"Once I knew that it would be a while before Dante was in any shape to talk, I went over to Cherry's house to break the news to her husband. But contrary to my instructions, someone leaked Cherry's identity to the press. Reporters had descended and told him about her death. At which point Alexander became hysterical, his doctor was called, and he was given a sedative. So he's on the top of my list to interview tomorrow morning."

"You'll probably want to chat with Larissa, the nanny, too," Skye suggested. "She and Mr. Alexander are having an affair. I overheard them arguing about it at the dinner last night. She wanted him to leave his wife for her."

"Right." Wally made a note. "I also need with talk to the other contestants again, and anyone else having to do with the contest who we didn't get to today."

"Do you want me to do anything?" Skye's face lit up. "Maybe I should drop out of the challenge to help you."

"No, I think you'll be more valuable hanging around and hearing what everyone has to say." Wally took her hand and kissed her wrist. "Besides, I don't want your mom any madder at me than she already is."

"Chicken." Skye picked up a slice of pepperoni and popped it into his mouth. "Will we have a lot of problems with the media? I remember when that model was killed at Thanksgiving. They were so obnoxious they even stole people's garbage."

"Grandma Sal's PR people are handling

it. They're putting out a statement saying that Cherry Alexander was discovered dead this morning, but so far there is no cause of death. We're holding back the whole chocolate-fountain part."

"But Cherry was a best-selling author. Won't the media be looking for a better story?"

Wally devoured the last piece of pizza, which Skye had slipped onto his plate, figuring he probably hadn't had any lunch. After he finished he said, "An author isn't really a celebrity. Unless they're Stephen King or Danielle Steel or someone like that, most people don't even recognize them. You read a lot. Did you recognize Cherry?"

"No. But from the title she mentioned while we were waiting for the opening ceremony, she writes tell-all books about celebrities, which I don't read."

Wally shrugged. "Well, if the media is more interested than I'm guessing, Dante said the mayor's office would take care of any spillover Grandma Sal's people can't handle."

"That's a relief. The press was a darn nuisance on our last case." Skye thought about the Thanksgiving murder for a moment, then asked, "Any news on Ashley's disappearance?"

He shook his head. "The county and state police are looking for her, and all the area police departments have her picture. But no one's seen a thing."

"Well, I had an idea this afternoon, but it didn't pan out." Skye looked at him from under her lashes. He seemed only mildly interested, so she quickly gave him the rehearsed and sanitized story, ending with, "But she wasn't there, so I nailed the shutter back."

"Too bad." Wally wiped his fingers, crumpled up his napkin, and threw it on top of his empty plate. "But what was causing the noise if it wasn't her?"

"Just a mouse." Skye kept her face down so he couldn't read the real answer in her eyes. She didn't want to go into the whole rat versus mouse issue. "Still, I feel like an idiot for tearing over to the drive-in when she wasn't even there."

"Why would you feel like an idiot for following a logical lead?" Wally cupped her cheek. "You would feel a whole lot worse if she was found there later and you'd disregarded your hunch."

Skye turned her face and kissed his palm. This was why she was with Wally and not Simon. Simon's insistence that she act as coldly logical as he was drove her nuts. Wally's acceptance of who she was, with no desire to change her, made her feel cherished.

Wally scooted back his chair and started to clear the table. Skye ran hot water in the sink — she hadn't been able to afford to install a dishwasher yet.

"So we're all caught up on the murder and Ashley, right?" Wally asked.

"I think I've told you everything I wanted to." Skye squirted detergent into the water. "Xenia's blog — which she now claims isn't hers — my idea that fell flat, and the runner wearing the jumpsuit. Yep, that's it."

Skye plunged the dishes and silverware into the bubbles, trying to come up with more information to stall him, but before she could think of anything Wally said, "There's something I need to tell you, and I'm not sure how you're going to take it."

Skye's stomach clenched. Had his ex-wife come back? Had he met someone else? Was he sick?

When she didn't speak, Wally continued. "I know you've wondered what's been up these couple of months. Why I've had to cancel out on you so many times."

She nodded, but couldn't force any sounds past the lump in her throat.

"Well, you know how I don't like to talk

about my family or my past?"

"Yes." Her voice quavered, but she managed to squeak out the single word.

"I told you it was because after my mom died, my dad and I didn't have anything in common, since he didn't like me going into law enforcement, right?"

"Right."

"Well, that's true, but not the whole truth." Wally's eyes were wary.

"Okay." Skye dried her hands on a dish towel and walked back to the table. She had a feeling she needed to sit down for this.

"The reason my dad was so upset with me for becoming a cop rather than getting my MBA was because I'm an only child, and there was no one else to take over the family business."

"I can understand that. My dad feels the same way about Vince not taking over the farm. He's been a little better about it the past few years, since he's seen how happy Vince is with the hair salon, but it still bothers Dad."

Wally moved closer to Skye, taking her hands. "Imagine how your dad would feel if the farm wasn't five hundred acres, but five thousand."

"Your dad owns five thousand acres?"

"He owns a lot more than that." Wally

squatted in front of Skye. "I'm from a little town in west Texas. My grandfather was a rancher, and then when my dad was in his late teens, oil was discovered on their land. My dad parlayed the oil money into an international company with concerns in almost every kind of manufacturing."

Skye's mouth opened, but nothing came out. What do you say when your boyfriend tells you his father is a multimillionaire?

CHAPTER 11
BEAT FOR TWO
MINUTES

Skye jerked her hands from Wally's grasp, pushed back her chair, and jumped to her feet. She felt light-headed, and the room seemed to spin out of focus. Her mind raced as she tried to figure out what to do, what to say. She needed to be alone for a couple of minutes to pull herself together. The bathroom. That was it. He wouldn't follow her in there, and she *was* slightly queasy.

As she fled the kitchen she said over her shoulder, "I need to use the restroom. I'll be right back."

She staggered up the stairs and into the master bath. Once inside she slammed the door, snapped the lock, and leaned against the thick wood as if guarding it against a marauding Mongol horde.

When she was sure Wally hadn't followed her, she moved from the door to the sink and got a damp washcloth for the back of her neck. She still felt a little shaky, but her heart rate had returned to normal and the pizza was no longer threatening re-appearance.

A few seconds later her brain kicked back into gear and began working again. The first coherent thought it produced was a question. *If Wally's a gazillionaire, but has never revealed that fact before, why is he bringing it up now? And, most important, does that change anything between us?*

Skye had a bad feeling that it might. After all, she was a farmer's daughter from Po-dunk, Illinois. Wally's father was the CEO of an international conglomerate, and probably had homes in Paris, London, and St. Kitts.

Not to mention how poorly the whole rich-boyfriend thing had gone the last time Skye found herself in this situation. Been there, done that, had the T-shirt repossessed right off her back. Her ex-fiancé Luc had proved to be a shallow, bigoted, self-centered bastard. How often did a guy have to dump her for being a country bumpkin before she caught on?

No, wait. That wasn't fair to Wally. She'd known him for eighteen years, and she'd never seen any trace of Luc's awful charac-teristics in him. He was thoughtful, fair, and always put others' needs ahead of his own.

Could money change that in a person?

And, hey, he didn't say his father had died and left him the money. He and his father weren't even on good terms. Maybe Mr. Boyd had cut his son out of his will, and that was what Wally had been leading up to.

She was being silly, jumping to conclusions. Just because Wally had finally told her about his family didn't mean that his father had persuaded him to resign as the Scumble River police chief, move back to Texas, and take over the family business. Did it?

Skye stared in the mirror. A thirtysomething woman with too-generous curves and hair that tended to revert back to Shirley Temple curls at the slightest hint of humidity looked back at her. Her only remarkable feature — large emerald green eyes — clouded with worry.

She bit her lip. No matter how hard she tried, she couldn't see herself on the arm of a tuxedo-clad millionaire attending charity balls and making small talk with all the other trophy wives. Did Dior even make an evening gown in her size?

Praying that Wally wasn't about to shuck his old life, including her, and become a star on *Lifestyles of the Rich and Famous,* Skye splashed cold water on her face, freshened her lipstick, and treated herself to an extra spray of Chanel. Then she squared her shoulders and went back downstairs.

She found Wally pacing in the sunroom. When she entered, he rushed over to her. "Are you okay?"

"I'm fine." She perched on the edge of the chair. "I'm sorry I took so long. You sort of threw me for a loop, and I needed time to think."

"And have you?" His dark eyes were intense.

"Yes." Skye sank back, feeling a little dizzy again. "And I am ready to hear the rest of what you have to tell me." She paused, and when he didn't say anything she prodded, "There is more to this than just a sudden urge to tell me about your family, right?"

Wally nodded and sat back down on the settee, then became interested in one of Bingo's squeeze toys. He studied the little rubber mouse as if he had never seen one before. Finally, without looking up from the plastic rodent, he said, "It all started the beginning of January. My father called to wish me a happy New Year, then mentioned he was in the area on business and asked if we could get together."

"That would have been the first time you canceled a date with me."

"Yeah." Wally turned the molded toy over

189

and ran his finger along the seam. "I figured this was a onetime visit on his part; he'd never been to Scumble River before, and I didn't see any reason to go into my whole complicated family situation with you."

"Yeah. You wouldn't want to do that unless you were in a serious relationship." Wally tried to protest, but Skye cut him off. "Except it wasn't a onetime visit. He's been back . . . let's see . . ." She thought backward, counting the missed dates on her fingers. "He's been here five more times, including last night, right?"

"Yes." Wally gripped the mouse, and its loud squeak in the silent room startled them both. "He dropped by twice in February and twice in March."

"And you still didn't think to mention him to me or introduce us?"

A muscle below Wally's right eye twitched, and he said, "I just don't trust him. I was afraid he'd do something to hurt you, or that knowing him would make you think less of me."

She ducked her head so he couldn't read her face as she considered what he'd said. Did she believe it? Or was there something else he wasn't telling her? She braced herself and asked another question. "What about last night?"

"That was different." Wally finally put down Bingo's plaything and looked at Skye. "Previously he's called from Chicago and then driven down, or I've met him in Joliet for dinner. Yesterday afternoon after I got off work I took the Thunderbird to the gas station near I-55 to fill it up so it would be ready for our date that night, and there he was, filling up his rental car. I figured he was going to surprise me, so I explained how I couldn't cancel our date this time, since you were counting on me as your escort, and he said that was fine; he'd see me today for lunch."

"So, what happened?" Skye tilted her head. "I mean, you did stand me up, so . . ."

"Well, he seemed to be acting odd, like he hadn't really expected to see me and didn't want to. And he almost looked as if he were in disguise."

"How so?"

"He had shaved his head and was wearing cheap mirrored sunglasses, and his rental car was a Ford Escort."

"I'm guessing he has a beautiful thick head of hair like you, usually wears designer sunglasses, and always rents a high-end automobile." Skye tapped the armrest of her chair. "Could he be sick? Maybe he didn't shave his head. Maybe his hair fell

191

out because of chemo treatments?"

"I considered that, too. In fact, I thought maybe the reason he'd been in Chicago so often was for treatment. That could explain his suddenly wanting to see me too."

"But?"

"But then I saw him pull into a cabin at Charlie's motor court and throw a tarp over his car."

"Hmm." Skye scrunched up her face, thinking. "That is odd. First, how did he get a reservation? Charlie's been booked up for this weekend since January. And second, why would he protect a rental car with a tarp?"

"Unless he was trying to hide from someone." Wally ran a hand through his hair. "So, I decided I'd better watch him."

"Did he do anything suspicious?"

"Nope. He didn't leave the motor court. I watched until eleven, when the lights went out, and he was there the next morning when I got the call about Cherry's death. I drove past on my way to the factory."

"What did he say when you had to cancel lunch with him today?"

"Not much. Said he'd catch me next time. But I was afraid he might show up at my house tonight before I could tell you about him, which is why I suggested we meet here."

"I see." Skye tucked her legs under her and got more comfortable. "You know, it's pretty weird that he would drive all the way down here from Chicago without checking to see if you were free. It had to take him at least ninety minutes to two hours, depending on traffic, and then he wasn't upset when you couldn't see him. Is he usually that easygoing?"

"No. He expects everyone and everything to revolve around his convenience."

"Since he said he'd catch you next time, I'm assuming that means he's left town."

"That's what you would think, isn't it?" Wally's brows met over his nose. "But I had a funny feeling about it, so I came past the motor court on the way here, and his car was still there."

"Why would he stick around and not tell you? Unless he meant he'll see you tomorrow."

"That can't be it. If nothing else he's always extremely precise in what he says."

"When you've gotten together these past few months, what has he talked about?" Skye plucked a pen and pad from the end table. "Was there a theme — the good old days, your childhood, current events?"

Wally bent forward and put his elbows on his knees. "A lot of it was just general stuff. We hadn't seen each other in years, and it seemed to me he was mainly trying not to start an argument."

"You never asked what he was doing in Chicago so often?" Skye's massive curiosity couldn't imagine leaving that question unanswered.

"No. I figured it was business, and I didn't want to get him started on how much I had disappointed him by not taking a job with the family company."

"Maybe he's thinking of remarrying. Did he sound you out about how you'd feel about a stepmother?"

Wally shook his head. "My father has a lot of traits I don't particularly care for, but he loved my mother with a passion that never faded. He would never remarry. No other woman could take her place."

"Never is a long time. He's been a widower for what, eighteen, nineteen years?" Skye tried to put it delicately. "A man has needs."

"Tell me about it." Wally raised a brow, and his chocolate brown eyes invited her to fall into their depths. "I'm not saying he didn't have an occasional lady friend, but the Boyd men are like wolves — there is

194

only one true mate for us. And once we find her, no matter how short a time we have together, there is no one else."

Skye caught her breath. Wally had been married for over ten years before his divorce two years ago. Was Darleen his true mate, and Skye just someone to meet his needs?

Before she could figure out how to phrase that question, Wally had pulled her up from her chair and settled her on his lap, tucking her curves neatly into his own contours as if they were two pieces of a jigsaw puzzle.

The muscles that rippled under his uniform shirt as he lifted her quickened her pulse, but she tore her gaze away and raised it to his face. Smooth olive skin stretched over high cheekbones, and his strong features held all the sensuality he usually kept hidden. He was a devastating package, and Skye yearned to tear off the wrapping.

Lightly he fingered a tendril on her cheek, then slid his hand down to caress her neck and bare shoulders. Hypnotized by his touch, she tingled under his fingertips, her growing arousal erasing all her questions and doubts.

Suddenly, as if he couldn't wait any longer, he crushed her to his chest. Her body tightened from the contact, and she wound her arms around his neck and lifted her face to his, basking in his hungry gaze. His kiss was urgent, devouring her and making her forget everything but him.

He freed one hand and was sliding her shirt off when she heard the first yowl. Skye stiffened, but either Wally hadn't heard it or he was ignoring it.

A few seconds later an even louder howl, this one sounding almost like a baby's scream, penetrated his passionate fog, and he tore his mouth from hers. "What in the hell was that?"

A third yowl ripped through the house, followed by a thud and another howl.

Skye scrambled from Wally's lap. "I think that's Bingo, but he's never sounded like that before." She raced in the direction of the noise, which seemed to be coming from above them.

Wally followed her as she ran up the stairs and into her bedroom. They both skidded to a stop and gaped at the agitated feline. The black cat's fur was standing on end, making him appear twice his normal size. He was arched by the balcony doors, hissing at what Skye at first thought was an elderly woman, but a moment later realized was just a bunch of rags being blown against the glass by the wind.

As they stared, Bingo gathered himself up

and launched himself at the door. His bounce off the pane and onto the floor produced the thud they had heard in the sunroom.

Skye leapt forward and tried to grab the cat, afraid he could hurt himself or break the window.

When Bingo evaded Skye's grasp, Wally snatched up an afghan draped over a chest at the bottom of the bed, snapped it open, and threw it over the cat, scooping the disturbed feline up like a sack of fireworks about to go off at any minute.

Skye took the squirming cat from Wally's hands and cuddled him to her chest, murmuring reassuring words.

Wally strode over to the doors and flung them open, surveying the balcony. He stepped outside and picked up the bundle that had been beating against the glass and examined it. It was a faded housedress wrapped around a tree branch.

Skye joined him. "Where do you think that came from?"

"It must have blown off someone's clothesline. It's been really windy the past couple of days."

"It sure has." Skye turned and leaned against the railing. "I noticed it was really bad at the factory this morning."

"That's the one thing I hate about Illinois springs." Wally put an arm around her and cuddled her to his side. "The high winds drive me crazy."

"Yeah. I can take the snow and the cold, but the wind gets on my last nerve." She shivered. "You know, for a minute there, when we first ran into the bedroom, I could have sworn it was Mrs. Griggs pounding on the balcony door."

"You have quite an imagination," Wally teased.

"True, but that's the kind of dress she wore, and I find it odd that one so similar not only got wrapped around such a large branch, but also found its way to my balcony."

"You live on the river in the middle in a flat area. All sorts of trash blows through here."

"Maybe." Skye shrugged.

They were quiet for a few minutes; then Wally said, "I bet this is old Mrs. Calvert's dress. She's your nearest neighbor, and she wears clothes like this."

"Sure. It couldn't possibly have been another of the house's attempts to keep us apart."

"Of course not."

"It's getting cold out here." Skye separated

herself from Wally. "I'm going back."

"Yeah." Wally opened the door for her and stepped inside as she crossed the threshold.

Bingo had recovered from his trauma and was curled in a ball on top of the bed, snoring lightly. Skye gave him a pat as she walked by, and Wally followed suit.

Once they were resettled in the sunroom, Skye felt restless. Wally tried to resume their kissing, but she shrugged him off and paced. Finally she said, "Let's get out of here for a while. The paint smell is driving me crazy."

"Okay. Where do you want to go?"

She was about to suggest they get a drink somewhere, but caught back the words when she remembered that Wally was still in his uniform. Where could they go? There weren't a lot of entertainment options in Scumble River.

"How about McDonald's?" Wally asked. "I'll buy you a hot-fudge sundae."

"Perfect."

McDonald's was crowded. It was a favorite hangout for the teens, several of whom greeted Skye. It was nice to see that quite a few of them also said hi to Wally, and that none of the kids seemed to feel awkward in their presence.

After getting their sundaes, Skye and Wally

settled into a back booth. They were still in the process of taking the lids off their ice-cream containers when Skye stiffened and put her finger to her lips.

Wally shot her a questioning look.

She jerked her chin to the booth on the other side of theirs, then cupped her ear.

He nodded and leaned forward.

A group of girls from the high school was seated there, and two were arguing. Skye immediately identified the dominant voice as that of Bitsy Kessler, a preppy cheerleader who wrote an advice column for the school newspaper. Skye didn't recognize the other girl.

Bitsy's tone was scornful. "I can't believe you losers think that Ashley has really been kidnapped. I'll bet you still leave milk and cookies for Santa, too."

The other girl murmured something too low for Skye to hear, but Bitsy's next words were loud and clear. "Yeah, right. Poor little Ashley. The victim of the Scumble River Snatcher. She's probably holed up in a motel room with some guy, laughing her ass off at all of us."

"Why would you think that?" the other girl challenged.

"Ashley's the biggest social climber since Cinderella. This whole negative article in

200

the newspaper and her parents' insisting on suing over her little indiscretion with the basketball team pissed her off.

"It just pointed out that her family is so blue-collar. You don't see Paris Hilton's mother suing when her sexploitations are printed in a newspaper. All the knockoff Vera Bradley purses and last-season Emma Hope sneakers in the world can't change who your parents are. Even her North Face jacket is last season's from a secondhand shop."

"But how does running away help?" The other girl sounded confused.

"What better way to get back at everyone? Her parents are worried sick. The girl who wrote the nasty stuff about her is suspected of the kidnapping. And the superintendent is threatening to shut down the newspaper. All things Ashley would love to see happen."

Skye shot Wally a meaningful glance.

His look said it *was* a plausible explanation.

"But where would they be hiding?" Ashley's defender sounded less sure than she had at first.

"Where else is there around here but Mr. Patukas's motel?" Bitsy paused, and Skye heard the sound of a straw sucking up air rather than liquid. "It's not like Ashley would go camping."

Once the teens moved on to another subject, Skye scooped a spoonful of ice cream covered in chocolate into her mouth, then asked in a low voice, "What do you think?"

Wally finished his sundae, wiped his mouth on his napkin, and answered, "Maybe we should stop by Charlie's and see if Miss Ashley is in residence."

"All but one of the cottages are rented for contest personnel, and don't we think your father has that one?"

"Who knows?" He lifted a shoulder. "Someone could have canceled."

"True." Skye plucked the cherry from the bottom of her dish. "Doesn't it seem like the contest and the kidnapping and the murder have all been going on forever?"

"Uh-huh. Hard to believe how short the time really has been. Ashley's only been gone a day and a half, and the murder took place this morning."

Skye popped the cherry into her mouth, slid out of the booth, and walked toward the wastebasket with their trash. "And with that in mind, I think we should get moving and kill two birds with one stone."

Wally followed her to the exit. "You mean . . . ?" He held open the door.

"Exactly. Let's go look for Miss Ashley and then pay your father a little visit."

CHAPTER 12
SET ASIDE BEATEN
MIXTURE

Skye and Wally pulled into the Up A Lazy River Motor Court a few minutes after ten. The red neon NO VACANCY sign glowed steadily, and of the dozen cabins that formed a horseshoe around the parking lot, the front windows in all but number twelve were pitch-black. Scumble Riverites went to bed when the WGN nine-o'clock news ended, and visitors soon fell into the same routine.

Skye stared at the darkened motel, feeling her investigative fervor waver. "Maybe we should come back tomorrow morning. We don't want to wake people up, do we?"

Wally jerked his chin toward the well-lit office-bungalow that blossomed like a pimple on the lip of the frowning row of cottages. "Looks like Charlie's still up. Let's see what he has to say."

"Right. Surely he knows who he rented his cabins to."

When there was no response to her first knock, Skye hesitated. Maybe Uncle Charlie had fallen asleep in front of the TV. She hated to wake him.

Wally clearly had no such concern and reached around her to knock a second time on the old wooden door. This time they heard the creak of the La-Z-Boy as the footrest was lowered, then heavy steps approaching where they stood. The blue gingham curtain was snatched aside, and Charlie's face appeared in the little window, his round head looking like a jack-o'-lantern floating in the glass.

Abruptly the cotton cloth dropped back into place and the door was swung open. "What's wrong? What are you two doing here at this time of night? Is it May?"

Skye had never quite figured out how her mother and Charlie had become so close. In the past she'd even wondered if they'd once had an affair, but she'd finally realized that Charlie's love for May was paternal, and May reciprocated with daughterly affection. Both fulfilled a need in the other. Charlie had never married or had children, and May's father had died while she was still a teenager.

"Mom's fine, Uncle Charlie," Skye hurried to reassure him. "Sorry to give you a scare. We just have a few questions about a couple of your guests."

Charlie stepped away from the doorway and gestured for them to come inside. "This have something to do with the murder?" He pointed to the sofa and settled himself in his lounger.

"No, with the missing girl." Wally sat down and leaned forward with his hands dangling between his legs.

Skye sat next to him. She watched her godfather as Wally told him what they had heard at McDonald's. Charlie had been one of the very few people in town who had not expressed his views about Skye breaking up with Simon and starting to date Wally. It had been unusual for him not to wade in with an opinion, and now she wondered what he thought and why he had kept silent.

Something flitted through her mind, but before she could figure out what, she tuned in to what Charlie was saying.

"There's no way that girl could be here, unless one of those contest people is hiding her, and I can't quite see Grandma Sal stashing her in her bathtub, can you?"

Skye started to shake her head, but then took a second to think of the people involved before saying, "Well, you know, those media people would hide a teenager in a flash if she could convince them there would be a big story. And Brandon and JJ might have other reasons for sharing their room with a cute cheerleader. But you're probably right about the judges, Grandma Sal, her son, and her daughter-in-law being in the clear."

Before Charlie could respond, Wally asked, "Wouldn't the lady who cleans the cabins for you mention an extra person? I mean, I know you charge more for additional guests."

Charlie nodded. "That's true normally, but Grandma Sal is paying for the whole block of cabins, so I gave her one rate. And I had to hire a couple extra ladies to help with the cleaning, so they might not think to mention something like that. I can give you their names and you can ask them."

"I'll have Quirk talk to them tomorrow morning. What time do they get here?"

"They start at eight."

Charlie picked up a cigar and ran it between his sausagelike fingers. He had given up smoking a couple years ago after a health scare, but Skye knew he still liked to hold a cigar, especially when he was agitated. What could be bothering him?

"Uncle Charlie, have you seen anything out of the ordinary? Maybe an incident that, now that you think about it, might have something to do with the missing girl or the murder?" Skye asked, trying to cover all the bases. Charlie wouldn't lie to her, but he might not volunteer information. She knew her godfather had his secrets.

"No, can't say as I have." Charlie put the cigar down and took a pull on his beer can. "You want a Budweiser?"

"No, thanks, Charlie." Wally leaned a little closer to the older man. "Sorry to bother you so late, but we have one more question."

"Oh?" Charlie picked up the cigar again.

"It's about the twelfth cabin." Skye leaned forward too. "I thought you told Uncle Dante that it had been rented for four months straight by somebody, and that's why you couldn't let the contest people have it."

"Yeah, that's right," Charlie said, narrowing his eyes. "What about it?"

"Well, then, why did you let some guy rent it yesterday?"

"I didn't. I mean, the guy who's in cabin twelve is the guy who's rented it since January." Charlie relaxed. "He got a new haircut and is driving a different kind of car, that's all."

Wally and Skye exchanged a long look; then Wally asked, "What's his name?"

"Brown, Charles Brown."

Another long look passed between Skye and Wally, but this time she spoke. "How did he pay for the room?"

"Cash on the barrelhead. Thirty dollars a night times one hundred and twenty nights: three thousand, six hundred dollars in hundred-dollar bills." Charlie smiled in fond remembrance. "Between Mr. Brown and the contest, the Up A Lazy River is going to have a good first quarter."

"So you didn't see the guy's ID?" Wally stated.

"No, why would I need to?"

"And you didn't think it was a little comical that Charlie Brown was renting your cabin?" Skye asked, exasperated with her godfather's nonchalance. "Did you check to see if he had Snoopy with him?"

"There's nothing funny about thirty-six hundred dollars. And you know I don't allow pets."

For the second straight day, Skye woke to a buzzing alarm at the appalling hour of five a.m. Once again she hurried through her morning ablutions and choked down a cup of scalding tea — burning her tongue in the process, which added to her bad temper.

Why in the world had she agreed with

209

Wally when he had encouraged Grandma Sal to continue the contest? Right now she could still be curled up under the covers, dreaming that she and Hugh Jackman were dancing cheek-to-cheek on a white sand beach in the Caribbean.

But no. Instead she was standing in the cold wind waiting to be picked up by her mother in order to go cook a dish that had yet to come out of the oven in an edible state. And to top it all off, last night had not ended well.

When she and Wally had left Charlie's they'd walked over to cabin twelve, which still had a lamp burning in its front window. But as soon as Wally rapped on the door, the light was snapped off and the drapes drawn. Finally, after half a dozen knocks, each more insistent than the one before, Skye had persuaded Wally to give up.

By then neither had been in the mood for romance, and he had dropped her off at her house with only a quick good-night kiss. Not exactly how she had expected her Saturday night to end.

Now Sunday morning felt like déjà vu to Skye as she slid into the passenger side of May's Oldsmobile, slumped back on the seat, and closed her eyes.

At least this time May's voice wasn't

chirpy when she said good morning.

Skye opened one eye and muttered a greeting.

May drove a mile or so in silence, then said, almost as if she were desperate for a topic, "I didn't see you in church last night. Did you forget you wouldn't have time to go this morning?"

Skye nodded, unwilling to go into a full explanation of what had distracted her. "Maybe I can cut cooking practice short and run over for eight-o'clock Mass."

"If you go to confession God will forgive you for missing Mass, but Grandma Sal won't forgive your macaroni being rubbery no matter how many prayers you say."

Skye knew that May was intent on one of her recipes winning the contest, but she had thought that the state of her immortal soul might sway her mother. Clearly May was willing to take a chance that Skye might burn in hell if it meant taking home the gold.

After a few minutes of blessed silence, Skye asked, "How's Uncle Dante?"

"Fine. They're letting him out of the hospital this morning, and he's holding a press conference at city hall to inform everyone that he nearly lost his life while trying to help Scumble River grow."

211

"Better tell him to spread the word that he didn't see his attacker."

"Why?" May's head jerked toward Skye. "Do you think whoever did it might try again?"

"Duh." Sometimes Skye forgot that her mother had taken up permanent residence in the land of denial, and that almost nothing could make her apply for a passport out of that realm. "It's also why you have to keep quiet about the person who helped you yesterday morning. If anyone asks, you don't remember a thing."

"So I've been told." May scowled. "I'm not as dumb as you think, missy."

Skye bit her lip before something sarcastic slipped out. If her mother didn't win the contest she'd be looking for someone to blame, and Skye wasn't about to paint a bright red target on her backside by upsetting May right before she started cooking.

They were both quiet until they pulled into the factory parking lot. Then, as she shut off the car's engine, May asked, "Do you think any of the contestants will drop out?"

"No." Skye stepped from the Olds. "In fact, I heard that Grandma Sal offered Cherry's slot to the runner-up, and that person snapped it up."

"Anyone we know?" May's voice came from inside the trunk of the car as she leaned in to get her belongings.

"I didn't ask." Skye plucked a box from her mother's arms as May emerged. "But probably not." She took a step toward the warehouse, then turned to look at May. "Unless you entered a fifth time."

May shushed Skye. "Keep your voice down. Are you deliberately trying to get us in trouble?"

Skye raised an eyebrow. "I thought we weren't doing anything against the rules."

"We aren't, but I don't want them to write any new ones," May retorted as she hurried through the door.

In the cooking area, Skye put the carton on her mother's counter. Not surprisingly, they were the first to arrive, but even as Skye headed toward her own space, she heard the door open and a voice she recognized stopped her in her tracks.

"Earl, you are stupider than an idiot. If I didn't need it for my secret recipe, I'd knock you into Tuesday with my cast-iron skillet."

Skye cringed. It couldn't be. Slowly she turned her head and looked behind her with slitted eyes. *Shit!* Just what they needed. As if the murder, the missing teenager, Wally's father, and the contest weren't enough, standing at Cherry Alexander's cooking area, dressed as if she were about to sing a duet with Johnny Cash, was Glenda Doozier.

Kneeling at Glenda's cowgirl-booted feet was Earl Doozier, Glenda's husband and the patriarch of the Red Raggers. Skye ducked behind a stove and edged away from the pair.

The Red Raggers were hard to explain to anyone who hadn't grown up in Scumble River. They were the ones your mother meant when she warned you not to go into certain parts of town. They were the ones who were most often complained about in the newspaper's "Shout Out" column — but only by people who never signed their names, because no one was foolish enough to purposely get the Red Raggers sore at them. In short, they were the ones whose family tree didn't branch — and that single trunk was full of dry rot.

Skye had a special relationship with the Dooziers. In the past she had protected them from bureaucratic school rules, and they had protected her from her own naïveté, but she didn't like to press her luck.

While Earl was firmly in her corner, there was no love lost between her and Glenda. Thank goodness they weren't competing in the same category. Speaking of category, if Glenda was taking Cherry's place, that meant she was in the Special-Occasion Baking group. What on earth could Glenda produce that would be fit for a special occasion? Possum Pie? Roadkill Jubilee? Or maybe a Squirrel Sundae?

Once Skye reached her cubicle she put the Dooziers out of her mind and began to assemble the ingredients for her recipe. While she worked, more finalists began to appear. They came in all shapes, sizes, and ages, but everyone wore the same determined look.

This was *the* day. Either they'd take home thousands of dollars and bragging rights for the next year, or they'd leave with nothing, and be forced to say over and over again, "Oh, I'm not disappointed I didn't win. It was just an honor to make the finals." Those words might quickly become harder to swallow than Skye's cooking.

As the warehouse started to fill with the sounds and smells of food being prepared, Skye slid her practice Chicken Supreme into the preheated oven. She set the timer, checked the clock on the wall, and looked at her watch. The dish had to come out in exactly fifty minutes, just as the cheese started to bubble, but before it started to brown. At that point she would sprinkle the top with buttered bread crumbs and then cook it five minutes longer.

Skye frowned as she adjusted her apron; they still hadn't gotten her one with the right spelling of her name. She was tempted to take a Magic Marker and make the correction herself, but instead she set off to visit her competition and see what everyone was saying about the murder.

She couldn't exactly take notes as she chatted, but she did tuck a small spiral pad in her pocket to jot down anything relevant as soon as she was out of a contestant's sight. She was hoping to overhear discussions, but would start one if there was no alternative.

The first row of six stoves that Skye approached was the Healthy recipe entrants. She noticed that one cooking space was empty. Where was Vince, and how come May hadn't picked him up and hauled his butt to the six a.m. practice? Skye ground her teeth; Vince had always been their mother's favorite.

Pushing away her jealousy, she concentrated on what the other five Healthy recipe finalists were saying. The first conversation she tuned in to was between two women cooking next to each other. One of them was the contestant that May had thought she knew when they first gathered on Friday, Imogene Ingersoll.

This time Skye saw what her mother meant; there was something familiar about Imogene, but thick glasses, heavy makeup, and what was obviously a wig made identification difficult. *Hmm . . .* Skye bit her lip. Maybe Imogene had lost her hair undergoing chemotherapy. A couple of months ago Skye'd given a ride to a student who worked part-time at the Laurel Oncology Clinic and that might be where she'd seen Imogene.

Skye's focus was brought back to the two when Imogene said, "After they turned us away at the gate yesterday, I thought for sure they'd cancel the contest, or at least postpone it." She tied on her apron while continuing to chat. "I didn't see the message on my cell that the contest was still on until I came home from Mass; then I flew over here."

Skye recognized the other lady as the one with the injured leg. What was her name? She squinted at the apron pocket. Right, Monika. Now she remembered — Monika Bradley, the CPA from Brooklyn.

As Skye watched, Monika nodded. "Yeah, I was surprised, too. But my husband can never let a phone go unanswered, so I got

217

the news yesterday afternoon." She slid a pan into her oven, then said, "I guess the show must go on."

"Well, not to speak ill of the dead, but she wasn't very nice."

"That's an understatement. She reminded me of my cousin's poodle. It was a pretty little thing, all bright eyes and curls, and it would come up and rest against your leg like it wanted to be petted. But the minute you reached down to stroke it, it would bite your fingers clean to the bone." Monika set the stove's timer. "Did you hear her yelling in the restaurant? Someone stealing her secret ingredient, my eye. I saw her put that little sack she was carrying on about in the garbage can. She shoved it in way to the bottom."

"Really? Did you say something to her?"

"Sure." Monika crossed her arms and leaned back against the counter. "At first she denied it, but then I threatened to go to Grandma Sal and she admitted she pulled the whole stunt to try to get May Denison kicked out of the contest."

"No!"

"Yes. Cherry said that May was her biggest competition, and she always tried to get her main rival disqualified."

Imogene pushed her glasses up. "Why

didn't you turn Cherry in?"

"Because they were going at each other tooth and nail. I was hoping both of them would get kicked out. If Cherry had ended up winning the grand prize and I had a chance at winning it, I would have turned her in then." She sniffed. "Instead they let the next runner-up take Cherry's place. Damn!"

Skye snickered softly and moved on to the Snack recipe row. Here Charlie was holding court, waving a spatula and talking loudly. He wore his usual gray twill pants, white shirt, and red suspenders. His three-hundred-pound bulk took up nearly every inch of space in his cubicle, and made him look like a sumo wrestler squeezed into a pair of size-A panty hose.

Charlie's booming baritone echoed off the warehouse walls. "If I hear any of you say that again, we'll be suing you for slander."

Skye slipped behind a pillar. She wanted to know what he was talking about, but not enough to be drawn into the fray.

"Oh, shut your yap, you old fool." A bird-like woman marched up to him clutching a whisk. "All I said was that the dead woman had a fight with May Denison. You can't sue me for stating the facts. I'm not saying May killed her."

A dignified woman whom Skye recognized as a math teacher from Scumble River High shook her head. "Besides, Mr. Patukas, I think Ms. Alexander had words with at least a dozen or so people. I saw her yelling at Grandma Sal's son just after we finished dinner."

The others in the area joined in, and Skye quickly scribbled names and motives in her notebook. It seemed as if Miss Cherry had argued with nearly everyone in the place.

Skye looked at her watch; she had ten minutes before her dish had to come out of the oven. Hurriedly she moved on to the Special-Occasion Baking row. Here all was quiet. May was intently making frosting roses on what looked to Skye like a tiny lazy Susan.

Next to her the cookie blogger, Diane White, concentrated on a chocolate creation that looked something like the fusion of a truffle, a tiramisu, and a brownie. Skye licked her lips. As she watched Diane started to sprinkle chocolate shavings on the dish's surface. Just then the blogger's assistant arrived, gliding into the kitchen area.

Diane's back was to the entrance, and when the assistant spoke, the blogger threw up her hands and squeaked in fright. The bowl of chocolate flakes slipped from her fingers, spilling its contents on the ground, and Diane sank to her knees, screaming.

Wow, she certainly was high-strung. Was she afraid she might be the next victim, or was she on edge because she was the killer? She had been poking around the murder scene yesterday. In fact, she'd had to be escorted out due to her hysteria. But maybe that had been a ruse to escape the scene of the crime without arousing suspicion. Could the cookie blogger be a coldhearted criminal?

CHAPTER 13
BEAT EGG WHITES
UNTIL STIFF

Shit! Skye glared at her watch. If only sheer willpower could make the hands move backward. It was nearly five minutes past the time her casserole was supposed to come out of the oven. Just what she needed — another ruined mess.

But surely anyone would agree that finding out who murdered Cherry was more important than creating the perfect entrée. Skye paused and bit her lip. Well, anyone but her mother. With May's angry yet disappointed face in mind, Skye turned on her heels and raced across the warehouse to the One-Dish Meals area. Making a tight turn at the end of the row, she skidded into her cubicle.

The first thing Skye saw was Bunny sitting on a folding chair painting her nails, wearing a red leather minidress and matching ankle boots laced with white silk ribbons. Not a good look for someone Bunny's age, but the redhead had never appeared more beautiful to Skye. Surely Bunny would have taken the dish from the oven when the timer went off.

Skye's smile faltered when she realized the counter was empty — no sign of the Chicken Supreme. Still, the timer wasn't pinging, so Bunny must have stopped it.

Skye let her gaze slip to the oven just in time to see twin columns of smoke curl upward like elephant tusks. She yelped, ran forward, and twisted the dial to the OFF position. Seizing a potholder, she flung open the door and grabbed the Corning Ware dish.

This time her scream was louder than a the tornado siren, as the casserole slipped from her hands to the floor; elbow macaroni, chunks of chicken, and cheese splattered the cubicle. Skye gazed at the oozing cabinets and closed her eyes. The orange and white mess was revolting!

As she tried to pull herself together, the smell of scorched Velveeta clogged her throat. Her eyelids flew open and she whipped around to look back at the stove. The smoke had turned from gray to black and was billowing toward the ceiling. Somehow, although the arrow on the dial was aligned to the word OFF, the oven's broiler had been ignited.

Damn! Damn! Damn! Some of the ingredients must have bubbled over while baking and were continuing to burn. Before she could react, the overhead sprinklers chirped, then spurted like exploded water balloons.

Bunny bounced off her chair and popped out of the cubicle like refrigerator biscuits from a tube. Skye covered her head with both arms and dashed after her. The shrieks of Skye's neighboring finalists accompanied her flight.

Within seconds contest staff came running from the four corners of the warehouse. The first to arrive slid into Skye's booth as if he were making a grand slam home run; others followed, looking like cars piling up on I-55 in a snowstorm.

Grandma Sal's son, Jared, picked himself up from the heap and turned on Skye. "What the fu . . ." He caught himself and took a deep breath. Speaking between clenched teeth, he gritted, "What happened?"

He drummed his fingers against the partition as Skye explained, pointing to the offending dial. When she finished he said under his breath, "Great, another prank." Then, looking out at the gathered reporters, who were firing questions faster than a Xerox machine spitting out copies, he pasted a fake smile on his face and announced, "We've had a little mishap. No big deal. It only affected three workspaces, because Fine Foods went to the added expense of wiring the sprinklers in small sections. And, since the contest hasn't started, I'll get a cleanup crew here right away, and these people can get back to cooking."

While Bunny and Skye waited for their area to be put to rights, Skye picked bits of green pepper and red pimento off her arms. Without looking at the older woman, afraid that if she did she might smack her, Skye asked in her best psychologist voice, "Bunny, why didn't you take the casserole out of the oven when the timer went off?"

"Yesterday you told me not to touch it."

"But you did turn off the timer?" Skye wondered how the woman had managed to remain both spatter-free and dry.

"Well, yeah. I had to do that." Bunny adjusted her black-and-white-checked thigh-high stockings. "It was as annoying as a poor man begging for a kiss."

"Didn't you think that the timer might be set to indicate something? Like maybe when the casserole was done?"

"Nah." Bunny resumed painting her nails. "Thinking causes wrinkles."

"So does death," Skye muttered as she continued to scrape burned food from herself.

"What?" Bunny peered up at Skye.

"I said, please get me some wet paper towels."

"Sure. As soon as my nails dry."

"You know, Bunny" — Skye jammed her hands in her pockets so she wouldn't strangle the redhead, but she couldn't resist a verbal jab — "that outfit you have on is a bit on the young side for you. Don't you think?" She attempted to twist the knife. "How old are you, anyway?"

Bunny, clearly impervious to Skye's criticism, deposited the nail polish bottle in her purse and started to wave her fingertips in the air as she replied, "Age is just a number, and mine is unlisted."

At ten o'clock Grandma Sal blew a whistle and the Soup-to-Nuts Cooking Challenge officially started. Each contestant would have six hours to produce three identical dishes. One would go to the judges for tasting, one would go to the photographers for pictures, and the third would be cut into bite-size pieces and put out for the audience to evaluate. It was up to each finalist to determine which of their dishes went where.

Skye knew her mother would be among the most pressed for time. Not only did May have the mixing and baking to contend with, she also had the decorating. On the other hand, she also had a recipe she had successfully produced many, many times, while the best casserole Skye had ever managed to create ended up looking like drowned roadkill on the warehouse's floor.

As Skye set to work putting together her first official Chicken Supreme, her mind drifted to what had been happening in the outside world while she had been chained to a hot stove.

When Quirk talked to Charlie's cleaning crew, had they told him anything about the missing teenager? Had Wally found his father or figured out why he was checked into the motel under the assumed name of a cartoon character? And most important of all, had the police found out who killed Cherry Alexander?

Skye finished the first casserole and popped it into the oven. She couldn't start on the second one until the first was nearly done. May had warned her that each dish had to go into the oven as soon as it was finished. It could not be refrigerated nor sit at room temperature.

This left Skye between thirty and forty minutes to investigate. But what would she do about Bunny?

She glanced beneath her lashes at the redhead, who had settled back into the folding chair and was leafing through an *In Style* magazine. "Hey, Bunny, do you want anything? I'm going to take a walk and get a Diet Coke."

"Yeah, bring me a cup of coffee. Two creams and three fake sugars."

"Okay." Skye slipped out of the kitchen area, then poked her head back, praying Bunny wouldn't decide to come with her. "Listen, if I get held up and the timer goes off, take the casserole out of the oven, okay?"

"Sure." Bunny didn't look up from the glossy page. "I've got you covered."

Skye vowed to be back before the first ding.

Most of the contestants would be too busy to be talking about Cherry's murder, so Skye headed back to the hospitality lounge, a walled-off section furnished with tables and chairs. Coffee, tea, and soft drinks were provided, along with small pastries and sandwiches.

Two women and a man were the only occupants besides Skye. They sat at a table against the back wall, deeply involved in a conversation. Skye immediately recognized the trio as the contest judges.

Skye smiled to herself. This was perfect. She couldn't approach them, but it made sense that they would be in the lounge, since they wouldn't have anything to judge for the first hour or more.

She concentrated on being invisible, silently choosing a can of pop and a bear claw. Careful not to make eye contact, she selected a seat off to one side. She wasn't facing them, but they were in her peripheral vision. Someone had left the Books section of the Sunday *Tribune* on the table, and Skye opened it in front of her face.

As she hoped, the judges paid no attention to her and continued their discussion.

The first thing Skye heard was the male judge, Paul Voss, say, "I doubt they'll ever figure out who killed that woman. The cops here are straight out of *Mayberry R.F.D.* Barney Fife questioned me yesterday and could barely spell my name correctly."

"You needn't sound so pleased," Alice Gibson, the cookbook author, chided him. "All that means is that someone gets away with murder." She poked Paul in the ribs with her elbow. "Unless, of course, you're the killer."

"Very funny." Paul took a swig from a water bottle. "It was probably the husband. It's always the husband. Or the lover, if she had one."

"Whoever it was, they did us a favor," Ramona Epstein, the food editor, said. "That woman was the most annoying contestant I've ever run into."

"True." Alice fingered her napkin. "If flattery and bribes didn't work, she tried blackmail."

Paul straightened. "What'd she have on you?"

"Nothing I couldn't handle." Alice raised an eyebrow. "How about you two? She told me she had something on all of us."

Ramona and Paul both said, "Nothing," at the same time; then Paul added, "Well, we may be happy she's gone, but Fine Foods sure must be upset."

"Why?" Alice asked.

Ramona answered before Paul could. "Because Fine Foods is in the midst of a big buyout deal. This is not the time for Grandma Sal's to look bad in the press."

"So, Fine Foods wants the murderer caught and the case closed and forgotten ASAP?" Alice asked.

Paul nodded. "Sure, it's just like when you

sell your house — you make sure the lawn is mowed, the carpet is vacuumed, and the windows are sparkling so you can get the best price."

The two women nodded.

He looked at his watch. "We probably should be getting back to the judging booth. If a dish comes in and we're not there, Grandma Sal will kill us."

After the judges left, Skye wrote down what she had heard. She'd been having some remarkable luck in eavesdropping on conversations about Cherry. On the other hand, what else would anyone be talking about the day after the murder?

Interesting that Cherry had been able to come up with information to threaten all of the judges. Of course, everyone had their secrets, but how had Cherry known about them? Did she have a private investigator on her payroll? *Hmm.* That wasn't as wild an idea as it might seem, considering the type of books she wrote. She'd need someone to dig up the dirt on her latest victim . . . er, subject.

Skye made a note to find out who Cherry was writing about in the book she was currently working on, then checked the clock. She had several minutes until her casserole was due out of the oven, but not wanting a

231

repeat of that morning's disaster, she hurried back to her workspace.

After handing Bunny her coffee, Skye clicked on the oven light. Her casserole looked perfect. A couple more minutes and she'd top it with the buttered bread crumbs and finish baking it. Meanwhile, she'd start on the next one.

As she worked, she casually said to Bunny, "Have you heard anything about the murdered woman?"

Bunny got up and leaned a hip on the counter. "Not much. She made big money from those tell-all books she wrote about famous people. Her husband is at least twelve years younger than her, screws any woman who is breathing, and his only job is as her manager."

"Wow." That certainly gave him motive. "Where did you hear all that?"

"People talking at the bowling alley." Bunny fluffed up her red curls. "And the husband's been hanging out at the bar, hitting on any female who crosses his path."

"Anyone take him up on his offer?" Skye finished with the second casserole and put the topping on the first one, returning it to the oven so the bread crumbs could brown.

"Not that I saw." Bunny adjusted her bra strap. "He may be good-looking, but there's something missing in him. Even me, with my bad luck with men, can tell that."

"Yeah, I noticed a certain coldness behind his eyes," Skye agreed, then chewed on her bottom lip. Kyle was looking better and better for his wife's murderer.

After a few minutes Skye took her first casserole out of the oven. It looked surprisingly good. The cheese was melted, the sauce bubbled, and no little elbows of macaroni were sticking up, waving their burnt arms. Now the question was whether to send it to the judges or the photographer. Each could award a dish up to forty-five points. The audience had a mere ten points, and it was mostly stacked with friends or relatives of the competitors, so Skye's getting their points was unlikely.

If only she could taste the casserole. But she couldn't, and she had to make a decision soon. Once it cooled off it wouldn't be good for either the judges or the pictures. Okay, she'd send this one to the photographers. It really did look perfect.

After delivering the dish to the photo area, Skye returned to her workspace and checked her watch. Once again she had nearly half an hour until the second casserole came out of the oven — plenty of time to find a telephone and make contact with the outside world.

She repeated her previous instructions to Bunny and headed out of the cooking area. There were no public phones near the judges or behind the workstations. She spotted a few reporters in the media quarters, but they were all using cell phones.

Skye tapped her foot. She really wanted to talk to Wally. Maybe he had some news about the murder or the kidnapping, or at least what the heck was going on with his father.

She wandered around for another fruitless ten minutes, at which point she was ready to scream. How could there be no public phones in the whole place? Did they really assume that everyone had a cell, or, more important, that a cell would work when they needed it?

Blowing a curl out of her eyes, Skye decided she'd have to go over to the factory. Surely they'd have regular phones there. Unfortunately, a peek at her watch informed her that she had only ten minutes left. Realistically, could she get from the warehouse and back in time not to risk her dish?

No. She'd just have to wait until after she made her third casserole. Maybe she could borrow Bunny's cell phone, but it seemed sort of sleazy, using her ex-boyfriend's mother's phone to call her present significant other. *Crap.* Maybe it *was* time to buy a cell of her own.

The second casserole emerged looking as good as the first. Was there a chance she might actually win? Skye took this one to the judges. Her mother's Chicken Supreme was superb. If by some chance Skye had managed to reproduce the recipe, it could very well be one of the best dishes in the category.

As she assembled the third and last casserole, Skye daydreamed about what she would do with her half of the five-thousand-dollar prize. Two thousand would go for more home repair and remodeling, but she was taking the other five hundred and going shopping for spring and summer clothes. And she could actually go to Von Maur and Nordstrom, rather than Target and Kohl's.

Four hours into the contest Skye put her third dish into the oven. As long as nothing went wrong she'd finish with nearly an hour to spare, but right now she had thirty minutes available, and this time she was finding a phone.

Neither her mom nor Uncle Charlie had a cell, so that left Vince. He was doing May's Healthy Pasta Primavera, and Skye wondered how her brother was making out. As far as she knew Vince ventured into a kitchen only to grab a beer and a bag of pretzels. May brought him lunch at his salon every day, and if he wasn't going out in the evening, he ate supper at his parents'.

Not surprisingly, when Skye arrived at Vince's workstation, a group of women was gathered around the entrance. Skye elbowed her way through the adoring masses, announcing, "I'm his sister. Family business. Step aside."

The throng parted reluctantly, and she finally made her way to the edge of the inner sanctum. She could see Vince bent over his stove, his assistant standing a few steps behind him holding a spoon as if it were a scalpel ready to be slapped into his waiting hand.

Vince's helper was a stunning brunette who Skye remembered worked as a fitness instructor at her mother's health club. Somehow Skye didn't think her presence was a coincidence. The instructor had probably heard May talking about the contest and thought this would be a good time to spend some quality time with her client's handsome son. Girls had been plotting similar schemes since Vince had turned fourteen.

Skye dredged her mind for the assistant's name. Skye remembered that besides being May's fitness instructor, the woman had been the roommate of a suspect in a murder Skye had investigated a little over a year ago. But what was her name? It had something to do with a TV game show. Ah, Price, as in *The Price Is Right*. And her first name was . . . yes, Nikki, since she helped nick those inches away.

Clearing her throat, Skye said, "Nikki, hi, I'm Skye, Vince's sister."

"Shhh." The brunette frowned and put her finger to her lips, then whispered, "He's almost done."

Skye waited impatiently while Vince tossed whole-wheat spaghetti with cottage cheese, then topped the mixture with sautéed vegetables.

He turned with a flourish and bowed to the crowd, holding up his dish for everyone to admire. "Ta-da!"

After the applause died down, Skye finally got her brother's attention. "Do you have your cell phone with you?"

"I did, but Ma took it a few minutes ago. She said she had information that might help solve the murder."

237

CHAPTER 14
FOLD EGG WHITES
INTO BATTER

For once Skye was eager to talk to her mother. She was hurrying over to May's cubicle when she noticed the time. Once again the minutes had ticked away, and her dish was in danger of burning if she didn't hustle back to her oven. Interrogating her mother would have to wait.

This was why she hated cooking. It felt as if she were shackled to the stove and, as soon as she got a certain distance away, someone removed a few links from the chain and yanked her back.

As she rushed toward her workstation, Skye plotted her escape. This was her last casserole; as soon as she browned the topping and gave the dish to the contest staff supervising the audience tastings, she'd be free. And once she was liberated she would find May, and then she'd call Wally.

She was nearing the beginning of the One-Dish Meals row when she heard a commotion. Several male voices battled to be heard, but a loud alto drowned them all out. "I'm gonna pop all you upside the head if you don't shut the —"

A tenor cut her off. "Why you bustin' our chops, Janelle? We was stickin' up for you."

Skye tiptoed forward and put her eye to the gap where the cubicle partitions didn't quite meet. Once she got used to peering through the crack she could see Janelle Carpenter, the prison cook from Granger, surrounded by guys from the opening ceremony's cheering section. They looked even bigger and more menacing close up.

There were four of them, ranging in size from elephant to manatee. Skye guessed that the manatee had been the one to interrupt Janelle, because the cook had hold of him by his shoulders and was shaking him like a dust mop.

"Get outta my face, chump, before I kick your ass. There's only an hour or so left, and I ain't even got my third dish in the oven yet."

The elephant stepped forward. "Can you cook and listen? This is important."

She shrugged, but let go of the smallest guy. "Make it quick. My first one didn't turn out so good, so I had to send it to the audience tasting. The next one looked good, but I wasn't sure if I forgot the salt or not, so it had to go the photographers. That means this one gotta be perfect, 'cause it gotta go to the judges."

"Gotcha." Mr. Elephant nodded. "But you'll want to know this."

"Okay." Janelle's red flip-flops flapped against the soles of her feet as she turned back to the counter. "Go ahead, but you best not be wastin' my time."

The rhino, the second-largest of the quartet, said, "We was jes' kickin' — you know, waiting for more food to be brought out to taste — when this cracker tried to hustle us."

"How?"

"He offered us papes to give our points to his bitch's entry."

Janelle swung around holding a butcher knife. "How many times do I gotta tell you about using that word when you're talking about women?"

"Chill, Janelle, and check out the rest." Mr. Elephant shoved Mr. Rhino aside.

Janelle narrowed her eyes but went back to cooking. "So, what happened?"

"Dude —" The manatee started to talk, but the wildebeest, the third in line, size-wise, interrupted.

"That punk not only tried to bribe us; he

240

usin' fake money to do it with."

"How you know that?" Janelle looked over her shoulder. "You take him up on his offer? You gonna give someone besides me your points?"

All four men backed away, protesting their innocence, but still putting at least a knife's length between them and Janelle.

Mr. Elephant, plainly the leader of the group, cleared his throat. "No, Janelle, honey, you know we wouldn't ever do that to you."

"No?" Janelle's growl could be heard clearly over the whir of her mixer.

"No, babe, that's straight-up."

"Okay, so why you be tellin' me this?"

"Because when we turned him down, the fool tried to make us change our mind by tryin' to intimidate us."

"He have a death wish?"

They all shrugged this time, and Mr. Manatee said, "We just thought you ought to report this guy to the man, since you tol' us not to get into any fights here."

"Why didn't you all report him, 'stead of botherin' me?" Janelle frowned as she smoothed a concoction into her casserole pan.

"Babe," Mr. Elephant answered, "you know the man don' listen to dudes like us."

Janelle slid the dish into the oven and set the timer, then turned and asked, "So, how am I supposed to report this chump if I didn't see him?"

"They won't have no trouble findin' this cracker," Mr. Manatee blurted out. "He a little guy, 'bout five-seven, five-eight, with tats up and down both arms. He don't weigh no more than a buck twenty, twenty-five, and he bald on top, with a ratty old ponytail down his back."

"That all?"

Skye could hear the sarcasm in Janelle's voice, but obviously her crew couldn't, because Mr. Wildebeest said, "No, he got a stomach on him like a big ol' muskmelon, and he's dressed all in camo."

"I'll take care of it as soon as my casserole is done." Janelle waved toward the door. "Now you all get the hell out of here."

Skye jumped back from the peephole and hastily walked away. The herd had described Earl Doozier, right down to his little pot-belly. What in the world was he thinking, trying to buy votes, and with fake money? Not to mention threatening guys who would find a Hummer a tight fit.

Of course, the simple answer was that Earl didn't think. His impulse control was less than that of a two-year-old with attention deficit disorder. And, while he had a mind like a steel trap, it had long ago been left out in the rain and rusted shut.

Which meant she'd better find him right away. She needed to stop him before he got Glenda kicked out of the competition, or one of Janelle's guys forgot their vow of nonviolence. Because if Earl didn't stop his nefarious activities, either his darling wife or one of the animal pack would end up kicking his poor scrawny butt from here to St. Louis.

But what about her casserole? If she didn't get back to it soon the sprinklers would be going off again. Still, even though Earl deserved whatever Glenda or the herd dished out to him, he had saved Skye's life on more than one occasion, and it seemed wrong to put a cooking contest ahead of their friendship — no matter how odd and twisted that alliance might be.

Sending a silent prayer that Bunny might actually follow her orders and take the dish from the oven when the timer went off, Skye turned around again, this time heading for the audience.

As she emerged from the glare of the bright lights aimed at the cooking areas, it took her eyes a minute or so to adjust. Once they were focused she saw several people she knew, including aunts and cousins who had come out to support May and her children.

She waved at her relatives and friends, then scanned the rest of the seats for any sign of Earl. It didn't take long to spot him. A crowd had formed a half circle at the rear, and everyone was focused on an unfamiliar woman dressed in jeans and a plaid flannel shirt. She was tall and broad, and easily held the errant Doozier off the ground by the scruff of his neck while hitting him on the nose with a rolled-up newspaper as if he were a naughty puppy.

Edging her way through the crowd, Skye tried to come up with something to say, but as she emerged from the mob all she could think of was, "Put the Doozier down."

It sounded familiar. She thought she had issued a similar command during last summer's hundred-mile yard sale when the goat-cheese guy accused Earl of feeding the guy's kids — baby goats, not children — to the Doozier's pet lion.

The order had worked back in August, but this time the woman looked at Skye as if she were a flea, then turned her attention back to Earl. "Bad man, bad man. No cheating. Stop it right now."

Skye hated having her suggestions ignored.

It happened too often in her job as a school psychologist. When parents or administrators disregarded her ideas she could wait them out, as they generally ended up coming back to her for help, but in this situation time was not on her side.

How could she get through to this person? Maybe if Skye blew a dog whistle or offered her a liver treat, the woman would put Earl down. But before Skye could find a muzzle and a leash, Earl wiggled out of the woman's grasp.

Spittle flew from his semitoothless mouth and spattered on the lady's chest as he yelled, "I keep telling you, Miz King, I ain't cheatin'!"

Ms. King bopped Earl again with the newspaper. "What do you call offering people money to assign their points to your wife's recipe?"

Oh, no. Skye tensed, sensing impending doom. Everyone in Scumble River knew you didn't accuse a Doozier of wrongdoing — at least, not to his face and without backup. Clearly this woman was from out of town.

While Skye was trying to figure out what to say or do to defuse the situation, Earl's wife, Glenda, materialized next to her husband, holding a cast-iron frying pan in a threatening grip. Glenda was the epitome of the Red Raggers' ideal woman. She wore a denim miniskirt, the overtaxed material fading to white across her derriere, and a bubble-gum pink halter top that was losing its fight with gravity. She had swept her hair, dyed one shade beyond believability, into a ponytail, and the black roots were an interesting contrast to the rest of the platinum mane.

A movement behind Ms. King dragged Skye's gaze from Glenda. Sneaking up on the group was Hap, Earl's brother. Skye flinched. She hadn't known Hap had been released from prison. He'd been doing a five-year sentence for child abuse and attempted murder — hers. He'd tried to kill Skye when she turned him in for beating his son.

Hap was unarmed, but was scary nonetheless. He was short and skinny like his brother Earl, although not as densely tattooed. While Earl preferred sweatpants and tank tops, Hap liked to dress as if a rodeo might suddenly appear in Scumble River. His tight blue jeans were cinched with a wide leather belt that sported a silver buckle the size of a Frisbee, and his shiny western-style shirt had mother-of-pearl snaps. As he got closer, the stench of his cologne mixed with the alcohol fumes that surrounded him and created an olfactory nightmare.

While Skye had been distracted by Hap's appearance, Earl's twin siblings, Elvis and Elvira, had flanked Ms. King. They both preferred to dress in uninterrupted black, including the switchblades they flicked open and held at the ready. Elvis had dropped out of school, but Elvira was still one of Skye's students. She tried to catch the girl's gaze, but the teen refused to look at her.

Skye knew she had to do something before someone's blood was shed, because without a doubt, no matter who else got hurt, her plasma would be mingled with theirs.

Desperate, she decided to go with the obvious, wishing she had her walkie-talkie and identification card with her. Why hadn't she thought to bring them? This was a crime scene. The only reason she could come up with for her lapse was waking up before the break of dawn two mornings in a row. Skye's mind never did work well when she was sleep-deprived.

Shrugging off the excuses, she said, "Ms. King, I'm the psychological consultant for the Scumble River Police Department. Please put your newspaper down and step away from the Doozier."

Skye wasn't sure if the woman finally noticed that Earl's relatives could have passed for the cast of *The Addams Family* or if she was impressed by Skye's title, but Ms. King stepped back from the little man and turned on Skye. "Are you in charge?" While Skye pondered that question, Ms. King strode over to her and said, "This man is going around offering people money to use their points on his wife's recipe. And if they refuse he intimates that physical harm will befall them."

"Yes, so I've heard." Skye nodded. "I'm here to put a stop to it."

Earl had been backing away from Skye and Ms. King, but when Skye spoke he stopped and bleated, "Now, Miz Skye. You can't do that. There ain't nothin' in the rules that says I can't reward people for doin' a good thing or punish them if they don't."

Skye paused. Why did that sound so familiar?

"After all, ain't you been tellin' me and tellin' me that's what I needs to do with the kids?" Earl answered her unspoken question.

Ms. King glared at Skye and took a step closer. "You told him to do this?"

All eyes swung toward her. The crowd buzzed with comments, all of them malevolent. Skye cringed. With the Dooziers, ignorance was not a barrier to self-expression.

As if to prove Skye's thoughts correct, Glenda pointed her pink acrylic fingernail at Skye. "That's right. She told us it was okay."

Skye gulped. "No. That's not what I meant." They were twisting what she had been trying to show them about positive reinforcement. "Earl, you know that wasn't what I was trying to teach you. Tell them the truth."

Earl squirmed under her stare, but then looked at his wife, who waved her frying pan, and at the large woman, who shook her rolled-up newspaper at him. "I'm sorry, Miz Skye, but you did say it."

Great, she was about to be torn apart by a mob at a cooking contest because she had tried to teach some parenting techniques to two people who should never have been allowed to breed in the first place. There was some irony in this, but she couldn't quite put her finger on it.

She swallowed — her throat had gone dry — then raised her voice and tried to explain one more time. "Look, everyone, I'm a school psychologist. I was trying to teach them parenting skills. I certainly did not tell them they could use those methods to try to cheat in this contest."

Ms. King glared at Skye. "That's all fine and good, except how do we know how many people he's already bribed? My son is entered in this contest, and Butch deserves to win. If he loses to this . . . this . . . tramp, it will be on your shoulders."

Glenda narrowed her rabbitlike brown eyes. "Who you callin' a tramp, you old cow?" She raised the cast-iron skillet, but before she could bring it down on the other woman's head a flash went off.

Skye whirled around. They had been discovered by the media. Reporters were taking notes, photographers were clicking cameras, and the local TV station was zooming in.

Briefly, Skye considered throwing her apron over her face and making a run for it. But since several flashes had already gone off and the TV camera had been rolling for who knew how long, what was the use? Besides, those people who ran from the courthouse to their limos with their coats over their heads always looked guiltier than if they had walked erect, maintaining an innocent expression and saying, "No comment."

Still, someone should try to do something to mitigate the damage. Grandma Sal and her company had been wonderful to the community for years and years, and this type of media exposure couldn't be good for the Fine Foods brand. Where were the business's PR people? Surely they could handle the situation.

Skye's gaze searched the crowd as her mind rummaged around for an idea. On her second sweep of the throng, Skye narrowed her eyes and shaded them with her hand. Was that Brandon and JJ standing just beyond the media?

Yes. JJ, the pudgy one with the blond curls, had just joined Brandon, the slim, dark-haired one. She made her way toward them, and when she could speak without having to shout, she said, "JJ, Brandon, you need to do something. This will look awful on the six-o'clock news."

Brandon asked, "What happened?"

Skye explained the Dooziers as well as she could, then described the situation with Ms. King, ending with, "Then the mob turned on me, but Ms. King insulted Glenda Doozier, and that diverted everyone's attention."

JJ bit his thumbnail. "We'd better get Dad and Grandma."

Both JJ and Brandon had their cell phones out in a flash.

Skye opened her mouth to suggest that

two grown men should be able to handle the situation on their own, but then realized that both these guys were very young for their age, having led protected and pampered lives. Chronologically they may have been in their late twenties, but emotionally they were probably closer to sixteen or seventeen. Frannie and Justin were more mature than these two.

As his fingers flew over the tiny buttons, JJ said, "I'm calling Dad; you get Grandma."

Brandon nodded, pressing a few numbers.

JJ and Brandon were still trying to get a signal on their cell phones when a gunshot rang out through the warehouse. Instinctively Skye went into bodyguard mode and tackled the young men, sending them all to the floor in a gigantic heap.

As Skye worked her way free of tangled arms and legs, having somehow ended up on the bottom of the pile, she heard more screams and shouts. Her first clear view was of running feet and a panicked crowd. Only the thought of her burning casserole motivated her to continue freeing herself rather than pulling JJ and Brandon back over herself like a blanket.

CHAPTER 15
ADD NUTS

It had taken Skye several minutes to persuade JJ and Brandon to get off of her. They had been reluctant to stand up, even after they were reassured that there would be no more shooting.

The situation had disintegrated so quickly, she could hardly blame them for being a bit disinclined to leap into the fray. There had been the gunshot, which caused the audience to charge toward the exit like a tidal wave mowing down anyone and anything in its path. Next there was a dramatic showdown between Hap and the factory security guards, who had appeared just in time to witness Hap twirling his pistol in the air and yelling drunkenly, "Yee-haw! Let's get this here shindig started."

Apparently Skye had been mistaken in her initial assessment — Hap Doozier had been armed after all.

The guards must have been used to dealing with inebriated counterfeit cowboys, because they snuck up behind Hap and had him roped and tied so fast they would have won the first-prize buckle if Hap-busting had been a rodeo event.

As they passed her, Skye heard one of the security men shouting into his walkie-talkie, arranging for the police to pick up the errant Jesse James. She smiled in relief when one of the other guards commented that Hap was on his way back to prison, since possession of a firearm was a violation of his parole.

While the Fines and their PR staff worked on getting the stampeded people back inside and in their seats, Skye finally headed to her workspace. By now her casserole was probably a charcoal briquette, and there wasn't enough time to make another, but at least no one had gotten hurt. She told herself again and again that that was all that mattered, hoping May would buy into that sentiment when she heard about the incident.

Earl had been banned from the premises, and the Fines had announced that his Earl dollars were worthless, but Glenda was allowed to remain and compete. She had somehow convinced Grandma Sal that she was an innocent victim of her husband's stupidity — which was not a far stretch from the truth. It appeared that the only casualty of the Dooziers' antics might be Skye's Chicken Supreme.

Behind the spotlights and inside the cubicles, everything appeared normal. If the contestants had heard the ruckus on the other side of the warehouse, either they had ignored it or taken a look and were already back at their stoves. There were only fifteen minutes left on the clock, and many of the finalists were putting the last-minute touches on their dishes. Those who had finished were cleaning up.

Skye approached her space with trepidation. She sniffed. No smell of smoke. She checked the floor and partitions. Nothing seemed freshly soaked. Could Bunny have actually come through for her?

Stepping around the corner, Skye held her breath, then exhaled it loudly. The stove and counter looked just as she had left them, but Bunny was gone. Skye checked the oven. Her casserole was gone, too.

It looked as if Bunny had actually taken the dish from the oven and brought it to the contest staff. Hope flared in Skye's chest until she remembered that the casserole needed the bread-crumb topping to be complete. Without it she'd be disqualified.

She sank onto the chair and pushed Bunny's abandoned magazine off the seat, watching the shiny pages slither to the ground. *Shit!* If only Bunny had followed instructions and just taken the dish from the oven, Skye could have still gotten it topped and into the contest official's hands in time.

But that was Bunny's curse. She always meant well, but things never turned out right for her. It was hard to understand how she remained such an optimist.

Simon would have said it was because most of the trouble his mother caused was for other people. Nevertheless, no one ended up on the shady side of fifty, managing a bowling alley in a small town, dependent on the goodwill of a son she was estranged from, and with a daughter she had met only a few months ago, without making some really bad choices.

Skye felt drained. There was nothing she could do now. The decision to find Earl rather than save her dish had been made and there was no going back. She only hoped that May wouldn't be too disappointed in her.

Willing herself to get up off the chair, Skye started to rise just as the ending whistle blew. The contest was officially over.

Seconds later Bunny flew into the workspace. She beamed at Skye and threw a pair of pot holders toward the counter, not appearing to notice when they missed by several inches and dropped to the floor.

Skye picked them up, stalling for time while she tried to think of what to say. Bunny had tried her best, and Skye didn't want her to feel unappreciated.

But Bunny beat her to the punch, grabbing her by the shoulders and waltzing her around the little cubicle. "We did it! I got it to the officials with ten minutes to spare, and she said it looked scrumptious."

Skye dug in her heels, forcing the older woman to stop dancing, then squirmed out of her embrace. "I appreciate what you did, Bunny, but you should have waited for me. Without the topping the dish will be disqualified, since it doesn't match the submitted recipe."

Bunny frowned. "But —"

Skye cut her off. "It's okay. I know you were just trying to help, but you need to learn to follow directions."

"No, I —"

"I said it was okay. Just don't tell May. I'll let her think I screwed up. She's prepared for that, but to come so close and have this happen would send her blood pressure into

257

the stratosphere."

"Wait." Bunny stamped her foot. "Listen to me. I put the topping on before I brought it over. You had it all ready, and I saw what you did the other two times. So when you were so late, I just sprinkled on the bread crumbs and browned the whole thing for a few minutes in the oven. You won't be disqualified."

Skye opened her mouth, then closed it, then opened it again. Had she heard Bunny correctly? Had she really saved the day?

Gradually Skye's lips began to twitch. Wait until she told her mother that Bunny, May's archenemy, had salvaged the Chicken Supreme entry.

"That's great!" Giggling, Skye enveloped Bunny in a bear hug. "You're a lifesaver. Thank you."

"You're welcome. Too bad you and Sonny Boy aren't seeing each other anymore. You could tell him his mama finally did something right."

Skye swallowed the lump in her throat and gave Bunny a final squeeze before releasing her. "Don't worry. I'll make sure he knows."

"Good." Bunny picked up her magazine and purse. "You don't need my help cleaning up, do you? Charlie offered me a ride home, and I don't want to keep the darling

258

man waiting." Without pausing for a reply, she trotted out the doorway.

Skye shook her head. With Bunny it was always one hop forward and two hops back. It would have been nice to have help with the cleanup, but considering everything, doing a few dishes and mopping a floor was the least Skye could do for the woman who had saved her casserole.

She was just putting away the last utensil when May bustled into the cubicle. Her critical stare examined every inch of the workspace. She closed a cupboard door that had been slightly ajar, then ran her finger over the stove's cooktop. Impassively she opened the oven door, peered inside, and scraped something off the interior with her fingernail, throwing the debris in the wastebasket before acknowledging her daughter's presence.

When May straightened, she said, "We can go as soon as you bag the trash." She held up a white plastic sack closed with a yellow twist tie. "We can throw mine and yours both in the Dumpster on the way out."

"Don't they have someone to do that?" Skye took off her apron and grabbed her purse from a drawer.

"Yes. Us." May stared at Skye, then looked pointedly at the trash bin. "Didn't you read your rule sheet?"

"Most of it. Why?"

"Because it states that in case of a draw, either in your category or for the grand prize, the cleanliness of your workstation will be the tiebreaking point."

"I saw that, but I didn't see where it said it included garbage duty."

May *tsk*ed. "Better safe than sorry."

Words that had been forming in Skye all during the contest threatened to spill out, but she swallowed them. Maybe her mother was right. It would be awful to lose five thousand dollars because of an unemptied sack of garbage.

From what Skye could tell when she and her mother emerged from the cubicle rows, the other finalists seemed to have all left. The judges and photographer remained, as did a large part of the audience, who were milling around tasting the last few dishes.

As Skye and May headed for the back door, Skye said, "Vince told me you borrowed his cell phone to call Wally, because you remembered something that could help catch the murderer. What was it?"

May lowered her voice. "I remembered that the person who helped me with my box was left-handed."

"How did you notice that?"

"You know how when you reach for something you usually do it with your dominant side? This guy took my tote bag with his left hand; then, when he carried the box, he switched it to his right and had the box in his left hand."

"That's great, Mom." Skye tried to think of anyone involved who was left-handed. She hadn't really paid attention, but she would now. "Did Wally have anything to say? Anything new in the investigations?"

"I left a message with Thea. She said she hadn't heard a thing, and that both Wally and Quirk had been in the field the whole day." May held the door for Skye, then followed her daughter to the Dumpsters.

Skye heaved her bag into the huge black bin, then took her mother's and did the same.

As they walked toward the car, May stopped and picked up a piece of crumpled paper nearly buried in a footprint in the dirt beside the sidewalk. She looked around but there were no trash cans, so she half turned to go back toward the Dumpsters.

"Just give it to me, Mom." Skye held out her hand. "I'll throw it away when I get home."

May handed it over, and Skye thrust it into her jeans pocket.

They got into the car in silence, both exhausted from cooking for nearly eleven straight hours. Skye rested her head on the seat back and closed her eyes, not opening them until she felt the car turn into her driveway.

May pulled the Olds up to the front walkway and asked, "Do you want Dad and me to pick you up for the square dance and pork-chop supper?"

"Are they still having that?" Skye had been certain that the event would have been canceled to show respect for the dead finalist.

"Yes, didn't you get the flyer?" May rummaged in her purse and handed Skye a sheet of paper, but instead of letting her read it, May continued, "It says that they checked with Cherry's husband and he said to go ahead. That Cherry wouldn't want them to call it off."

Skye raised an eyebrow. Kyle must know Cherry better than anyone else, but Skye's impression of the author had been more prima donna and less humanitarian.

"Do I have to go?" Skye knew the answer before the words left her lips.

"Dante went to a lot of work organizing this event, and it would be disrespectful to him, Grandma Sal, and the whole community for you not to show up." May's lips thinned. "Especially since Dante's attending, and he only got out of the hospital this morning."

"I'll take that as a yes." Skye opened her door and slid out.

"You're a grown woman. I certainly can't tell you what to do."

Skye muttered under her breath, "Since when?"

"So, shall we pick you up?"

"No, thanks. I'll drive myself." Skye waved at her mom and started to shut the car door. "Thanks for the ride. See you tonight."

May shouted through the closed window, "It starts at seven. Don't be late." Without waiting for a response, she tooted the horn and drove off.

Bingo met Skye as she walked through the front door. His purr-o-meter was turned to high, making his sides vibrate like a bagpipe playing "Amazing Grace." She scooped him up, rubbing his ears and under his chin.

After thirty-two-point-one seconds of petting, he wiggled out of her arms and trotted toward the kitchen. About halfway down the hall he stopped and looked back to make sure she was following.

Skye had paused to put down her purse and apron, but reassured the feline, "Go ahead. I'll be there in a minute. I doubt you'll starve before I arrive."

Bingo flicked his tail twice — to show he meant business — then continued toward his food dish.

Skye risked the wrath of the feline by poking her head into the parlor as she passed. The indicator light on her answering machine beamed a steady red. No one had tried to contact her.

Darn. She was hoping to hear that some progress had been made on the missing teen, the murder, or even the mysterious disappearing father. In any case, as soon as she fed Bingo she'd call Wally. She knew he was busy, but she needed to update him on all she had heard during the contest.

Bingo was waiting by his food bowls when Skye walked into the kitchen. One bowl held a heaping portion of dry cat food; the other had been licked so clean it looked as if it had just come out of the dishwasher.

According to the vet, Bingo was allowed one small can of wet cat food a day, at the most. He could have as much of the dry as he wished. Unfortunately, what he desired was an unending supply of the canned, and for the dry to disappear in a puff of smoke and never come back.

Most of the time Skye stood firm, parceling out his Fancy Feast a third of a can at a time, once in the morning, once when she got back from work, and the last before bed. But on days like today, when she had no idea what her schedule would be, she gave him the whole can before she left the house, which resulted in a demanding feline when she got home.

She should ignore his plaintive meows, the sad slump of his tail, and the hungry looks — just as she should ignore her own craving for chocolate and cookies. Normally she was about 50 percent successful with either endeavor, but today had been extremely stressful, and she decided both she and Bingo deserved a treat.

After putting half a can of grilled tuna flakes in the cat's bowl, she grabbed a package of Pepperidge Farm chocolate-chunk cookies from the cupboard and headed upstairs. She shed her clothes in the bedroom, then walked into the bathroom and turned on the shower.

While she waited for the water to get hot — it had a long way to come from the water heater in the basement to the second floor — she tore open the cookie package and lifted out the little plastic tub containing four cookies.

The nutrition information on the side of

the bag claimed a serving size was one cookie. Where did these people come from, Planet of the Barbie Dolls? Obviously a real portion should be what the plastic basket held.

Once she had showered, blown her hair dry, and gotten dressed for the square dance, Skye went downstairs to see if any calls had come in. There were still no messages, so she phoned the police department.

After exchanging pleasantries with the afternoon-shift dispatcher, Skye asked for Wally. The woman informed her that he was still working and hadn't taken a break to answer his messages all day.

Skye tried his home number — no one answered, not even a machine — and his cell, which apparently was still broken, since it went immediately to voice mail. Frustrated, she wasn't sure what to do. Trixie needed to get back from her vacation soon because Skye needed a brainstorming partner badly.

It was six o'clock. She had an hour before she had to show up at the pork-chop supper. What should her next move be? Her gaze wandered to the little antique desk in the corner of the parlor, and an idea came to her almost as if someone had whispered in her ear.

She'd write it all down and drop her notes at the PD. Maybe while she was there she could find out what was going on with both the missing girl and the murder.

CHAPTER 16
POUR BATTER INTO PREPARED PANS

The police department parking lot was full, which, at nearly six thirty p.m., was surprising. The PD shared a building with the city hall and library, which meant that from nine to five cars prowled the tiny lot looking for an empty space, but in the evening there were usually only two automobiles occupying slots — the dispatcher's and that of the officer on duty.

Wally must have called everyone in, including the part-timers. What was up? Had there been a break in either one of the cases?

Skye felt a surge of triumph when a young man exited the building and approached a silver Camaro. Skye eased her Bel Air into position and waited for the guy to back out. Instead he rolled down his window and a smoke ring drifted into the night air.

Shoot! This whole not being able to find a parking spot was starting to make Skye feel like she lived in Chicago rather than

Scumble River. Gritting her teeth, she exited the lot and drove down the block until she found a space.

On the walk back she noted that the town was hopping. A steady stream of traffic filled both the road the PD faced and the street it intersected, which was remarkable for a Sunday night, when most of the Scumble River population was usually at home watching *60 Minutes* and preparing for the workweek ahead.

The cooking challenge's change in schedule had probably thrown everyone off, especially with school being closed the next day. Skye had been shocked to get that message. Dante must have pulled a lot of strings and made a lot of promises to get the superintendent to cancel classes so that the contest could use the auditorium/gymnasium for the award ceremony.

Before the country's heightened security, Fine Foods could have used the auditorium and only gym classes would have had to be canceled, but now the school district policy didn't allow that many strangers in the building while students were present.

Maybe the fact that they hadn't taken any of the year's snow days helped. However, snow days were really only a technicality needed because of the way the teacher contracts were written. They still had to be made up, so now they'd have to go an extra day into the summer, a detail everyone conveniently forgot as they were celebrating their impromptu holiday.

When Skye pushed open the glass door of the PD, she immediately noticed the busy hum. She waved to the dispatcher behind the bulletproof glass window that enclosed the counter on her right, and the woman buzzed her through the door leading to the rest of the station. Cubicles that were normally empty were filled with officers who were on either the phone, the computer, or both.

One young man Skye didn't recognize was performing percussive maintenance on his PC. He didn't seem to realize that smacking the crap out of an electronic device rarely improved its working condition. But then, artificial intelligence had never been a match for natural stupidity.

Skye shook her head and moved on. From the snatches of conversation she heard, half the officers were looking for Ashley and half for the murderer. Had something happened to stir up the search for the missing girl?

She was tempted to stop and ask, but the men looked too busy. Not to mention she had only a short time to turn up at the supper before May sent the search-and-rescue dogs after her.

Dashing to the back of the building, she quickly climbed the steps. Wally's office and a couple of small storage areas were the only rooms in the truncated upstairs space. There was no egress between the PD and the portion of the second floor that was located over the city hall, which contained the three-room Scumble River library.

Skye's heart skipped a beat when she saw Wally leaning back in his chair with his eyes closed. He exuded an attraction that enticed her like a golden box of Godiva chocolates. As she got closer she saw that his features were etched with exhaustion and defeat, and a soft gasp of pained empathy escaped her.

He immediately straightened, his eyelids flying open. At first he scowled, but his expression brightened when he saw Skye. In one swift movement he rose to his feet and met her halfway across the office in a fierce embrace.

She buried her face against his throat, enjoying a moment of pure pleasure.

His breath hot against her ear, he whispered, "How did you know I needed to hold you?"

"Bingo told me." She wound her arms inside his jacket and around his back.

His chuckle shed years from his face. "In that case he must be the one hanging up the phone every time I try to call you."

"What?" Skye was distracted by the touch of his thumb stroking her jaw.

"I tried two or three times today and your machine hung up on me every time."

"Guess I need a new answering machine." She struggled to focus, but the tingle where his thigh brushed her hip was hard to ignore. Breathlessly she continued, "And while I'm at it, I might as well get a cell phone, too."

"It's about time," he growled as he nipped at the sensitive cord running from her ear down her neck.

"Did you find out what was wrong with your . . ." Skye tried to concentrate. There was a reason she had stopped by, and something else she had to do tonight, but darned if she could remember. ". . . cell?"

"No. Bingo must have thrown it down the stairs last time I was over." His lips hovered above hers as he spoke.

Suddenly impatient, she pressed her open mouth to his. He needed no further invitation, and his kiss devoured her.

A few seconds, or minutes, or hours later — she had no idea how much time had passed — an apologetic cough from the doorway made her lift her head.

Anthony, one of the part-time patrol officers, stood on the threshold, his face beet red. "Uh, I'm really sorry, Chief, but your phone must be off the hook, and I finally got Mr. Alexander on the line. I know you wanted to talk to him."

After a quick squeeze and kiss on the nose, Wally released Skye. "No problem. What line?"

"Four. He sounded drunk or high or something," Anthony added over his shoulder as he retreated down the hall.

"I'll put it on speakerphone so you can tell me what you think," Wally said to Skye as he turned to his desk. "This jerk has been avoiding me all day."

Skye sat down and took a pad of paper and a pen from her purse.

Wally pressed the button and said, "Mr. Alexander, thank you for calling. I'm sorry for your loss."

"Thanks, dude. It's so bogus. She was so young. Who'd want her dead?" The voice on the speaker broke. "Are you sure it wasn't an accident?"

Wally shot a look at Skye, making sure she heard that, then ignored the man's question. "I'd really like to talk to you in person, Mr. Alexander."

"Uh, actually, man, my last name's not Alexander; it's Hunter. Cherry used her maiden name — you know, professionally."

"I understand." Wally made a note. "Sorry for the confusion. So, Mr. Hunter, would it be possible for you to come into the station now and talk?"

"Sorry, no can do. My son's asleep and I don't have anyone to watch him."

Skye scribbled the words *housekeeper* and *nanny* on her legal pad and held it up for Wally to read.

He nodded and said, "How about your housekeeper or the nanny?"

"I gave Juanita the day off, and we fired the nanny Friday night when we got home from the dinner."

"I see." Wally made another note. "Well, maybe you can come in tomorrow, Mr. Hunter, when your housekeeper is back at work."

"Maybe. There's just so much to do," Kyle whined. "We'll see."

"Okay. Try to get some rest, Mr. Hunter."

After Wally hung up, Skye raised an eyebrow. "Why do I think that Kyle Hunter will have company tonight rather than take a nap?"

Wally gave her a wolfish grin. "Hey, I've been trying to have a face-to-face with that

274

guy since Saturday morning. At least now I know he's home and will be staying there for a while."

"Interesting that the nanny was fired right before Cherry's murder."

"If he's telling the truth."

"Good point." Skye got up from her chair. "Listen, I know you're in a hurry to go see Hunter, and I need to get to the pork-chop supper/square dance before Mom sends out the FBI's missing persons unit, but I wanted to share some info with you."

"How about you come over to my house when the supper and dance are over?" Wally put his hand on the small of her back and walked her out of his office.

Skye studied her watch. "That should be around ten. Is that okay?"

"Great." He locked the door. "If something comes up, leave a message with the dispatcher, and I'll do the same." He frowned. "Tomorrow after the cooking contest is over, we're both going to Joliet to buy us cell phones."

As they descended the stairs Skye said, "Oh, remember that argument I told you about between Hunter and the nanny? I forgot to mention that he said Cherry had an airtight prenup so he couldn't divorce her, but Bunny said he's been a frequent flier in the bar at the bowling alley and is a real hound dog."

"Thanks. I'll keep all that in mind when I question him."

"Also, ask him if Cherry ever hired private investigators to look into the people she wrote about. She seemed to have found out a lot of secrets about the judges and the other contestants. Oh, and ask him who was going to be the subject of her next book."

"Got it." Wally opened the door leading from the PD to the garage. "See you at ten."

It was exactly seven p.m. when Skye arrived at the Brown Bag banquet hall. People stood two deep all the way from the buffet tables to the entrance. Skye spotted her parents near the front and waved. May motioned for her to join them, but Skye shook her head. In Scumble River, cutting into a food line was a crime punishable by social death. May, one of the queen bees, might be able to get away with it, but Skye, a drone, knew she could not.

Instead she walked into the hall's attached bar and ordered a Diet Coke with a slice of lime. The place was empty except for the owner, Jess Larson, who was sitting on a stool reading a book.

As he slid the glass in front of her, he said,

"I hear you all had some excitement at the cooking contest. I told Dante I didn't have a good vibe about having it here."

"Yeah." Skye took a long drink and sighed. "Why doesn't anything ever go smoothly in Scumble River?"

"What would be the fun in that?" Jess was a relative newcomer to town, having bought the Brown Bag a couple of years ago from his cousin when she retired.

"You sound like some of my ADHD kids."

"I probably was, but we moved around a lot, so the school never had a chance to stick a label on me."

"Hey," Skye said sharply. "I do not stick labels on kids. I identify them so they can get the help they need."

"Whoa. Sorry." He held up his hand. "See, it's that poor impulse control coming out."

"Right." Sarcasm dripped from the word. "So, you hear much about the murder?"

"The usual." Jess pushed a dish of snack mix toward Skye, who helped herself to a handful. "Since the victim's from out of town, no one seems to know much."

"Yeah." Skye's voice retained its sarcastic tone. "Laurel is a whole forty-five minutes from here. Might as well be a foreign country."

Jess chuckled. "You sure you don't want some rum in that Diet Coke? You sound less perky than usual."

"Perky!" Skye glared at him. "I am never perky. Perky is for cheerleaders and Miss America."

This time Jess raised both hands in surrender. "I meant . . . uh . . . not in good spirits."

"Well, okay." Skye examined the bar owner. He was only an inch or so taller than she was, with black eyes and brown hair. She didn't know his age, but guessed he was nearing thirty. He seemed friendly enough, but didn't socialize and rarely mentioned his past. She grinned. He needed a girlfriend. Who could she fix him up with?

"I don't like that smile," he said, his gaze wary.

"I don't know what you mean." Skye waited for a beat, then asked, "Do you ever take a night off?"

"I think you're real cute and I like talking to you, but . . ." Jess backed away. "One thing I've learned is never to mess with a cop's girlfriend."

"Not me, silly." Skye giggled. "But I have some single friends."

"No. I do not do blind dates or fix-ups." Then, as if to distract her, he said, "Speaking of cops, the chief's father has been in here a couple of times — though I almost didn't recognize him this time, what with him having shaved his head and all."

"Yeah, that was a surprise," Skye bluffed.

"Is he moving to Scumble River or something?"

"I don't think so." Skye's thoughts started to race. Or was he? Maybe that was why he was visiting. No, that was silly. The head of a multinational company would not live in Scumble River. "Do you remember the last time he was here?"

"He left just a few minutes ago."

Damn! "He have anything interesting to say?"

"Nothing special." Jess shrugged. "Mostly we talked about the stock market and baseball — I was trying to explain to him why the fans stick by the Cubs even though they continue to lose year after year. He had a hard time with that concept. Seemed to think winning is the only thing that matters."

That was certainly consistent with the picture Wally had painted of his father. "Anything else?"

"I mentioned the murder, and he said it was a shame, because the bad publicity would hurt Grandma Sal's business."

279

Jess and Skye chatted for a few minutes more; then Skye paid for her drink and walked back to the banquet hall. The line had disappeared, and Skye stepped across the room to the buffet. She made her selections, then looked over the sea of faces, trying to find a place to sit.

She spotted an arm waving. Not surprisingly it was her mother. She waved back and made her way to the table. When she got near enough to see who else was sitting with May, a sense of déjà vu washed over her once again. This whole weekend seemed to keep repeating itself.

Just like at Friday's dinner, her parents had somehow managed to sit with the people Skye most wanted to avoid.

How in the world had both Simon and Kathryn Steele, the owner of the *Scumble River Star,* ended up at the same table as May and Jed? Simon was clearly escorting his mother, whom May loathed, which should have guaranteed they wouldn't choose to sit together.

And Kathy really had no connection with Skye's family, unless . . . Could Vince have asked her out? He was supposed to be dating Loretta Steiner, Skye's sorority sister. If he was cheating on her, Skye would have to kill him, but if she never found out, she wouldn't have to do anything. Thus it would be better to sit at another table. But she hesitated a second too long before attempting her escape.

Her mother shot her a stern look and said, "Where did you go? We've been saving you a seat, but we're almost ready for dessert."

Skye gave in and sank into the empty chair between her brother and Uncle Charlie. No matter what she did, this conversation would not be pretty.

May pursued an answer to her question. "We saw you come in and then you disappeared. What's going on?"

"I bought a soda at the bar while I waited for the line to go down."

"Iced tea and coffee are free." Skye's father spoke between bites.

Before Skye could respond, Bunny, seated on Uncle Charlie's opposite side, said, "But, Jed, when you were fixing up my car you said you get what you pay for. So, if something's free, wouldn't that mean you get nothing?"

May glared at Bunny, then turned her laser stare on her husband. She hated any reference to the time Jed had spent in the redhead's company, still believing in her heart of hearts that the two had had an affair.

Next to Bunny her son, clearly wanting to stop his mother from continuing on the sore subject, said, "So, Skye, did your contest entry turn out well?"

Skye was grateful for the chance to divert her mother's attention. "Better than any of my practice ones. I doubt I'll win, but at least I didn't embarrass myself." She remembered Bunny's wish that Simon know she had been a help, and added, "Your mom saved my last dish."

"That's great." Simon smiled at his mother, then beamed approval at Skye. "That's really nice of you to share the credit. I know cooking has never been your forte, so you must have worked extremely hard. But then, I know you can do anything you set your mind to."

Skye basked in his admiration. There was something different about him tonight. Except for Friday night's dinner, she hadn't talked to him since the fight they'd had at a diner Thanksgiving weekend, and at that time his harsh words had caused her to finalize their breakup. Now he seemed changed, but how?

Before she could analyze Simon's transformation, Vince said, "You are way too nice, Simon. Skye at a cooking contest is like the pope at a bar mitzvah. Both have heard of the concept, but neither really wants to be involved in the ceremony."

Kathy Steele leaned around Vince and added, "Didn't I hear that Skye set off the sprinklers over her cooking area?"

Skye worried briefly that that would be the headline on this week's *Star,* but Kathy's next words replaced that concern with a worse one. "Of course, a little water is nothing compared to Earl Doozier trying to bribe people for their voting points, then claiming Skye gave him the idea."

Shit! She should have realized the media would pick up on that — at least the local paper. Too bad she couldn't tell Kathy anything about the murder investigation or the missing teen. That might at least move the Doozier story from the front page to the inside, and with any luck the article about the sprinklers would get cut completely to make room for the school cafeteria menu.

May must have been thinking along the same lines, but had no compunction about trading info about the murder or the kidnapping to get what she wanted. "Kathy, I'm surprised you're interested in the fantasies of a fool like Earl when there's been a murder committed and a teenager is still missing."

Kathy laughed. "Don't worry, May; those

283

two crimes are my headline for tomorrow's special edition. But there will be plenty of room in Wednesday's regular newspaper for Skye's sprinklers and the Doozier debacle."

Skye hissed in her brother's ear, "Stop her from running that story."

Vince whispered back, "Me? How?"

"Since you're dating her, figure out a way."

"What are you talking about?" Vince looked confused. "I'm not dating Kathy. You know I'm going with Loretta."

"Then why is she sitting at our table?"

"How should I know?" He shrugged. "She came in with Simon, Bunny, and Charlie. Maybe she's Charlie's date, or Simon's."

Skye flinched. Simon was an attractive, intelligent man. May had warned her that he wouldn't have any trouble finding a new girlfriend.

She swallowed hard. It really wasn't any of her business. She certainly wasn't jealous. She was happy with Wally. She just wanted Simon to find someone wonderful. True, Kathy Steele was beautiful and smart, but she was too cold, too aloof. Simon needed a woman who would love him with all her heart, not just be with him for his money and position. Just as Skye had once tried to explain to him, he needed a soul mate.

Before Skye could continue fretting about Kathy's presence, Charlie said, "I'm surprised you're going to the expense of a special edition tomorrow. Everyone already knows about the murder and the kidnapping. They aren't exactly a scoop."

"Maybe." Kathy's eyes glowed. "But I have an exclusive interview with the girl who supposedly abducted the missing teenager. Her story is definitely breaking news, and not even the *Chicago Tribune* has that."

Xenia! Skye's heart skipped a beat. Why hadn't she thought to talk to Xenia herself? The only reason Skye could come up with was that the girl frustrated her. She did not respond to any of Skye's clinical training, and Xenia's superior IQ put the adults around her at a disadvantage.

Skye hated being made to feel stupid by a sixteen-year-old, which was why she avoided the teen. Had Skye's ego made her miss a chance to rescue Ashley? If Ashley had been harmed because Skye had been protecting her own self-esteem, she would never forgive herself.

CHAPTER 17
BAKE FOR TWENTY-FIVE MINUTES

"And then Kathy Steele said she had an exclusive interview with Xenia, and I realized how stupid I'd been in not talking to the girl myself."

Skye sat with her back against the armrest of the sofa. She and Wally were in his living room, and she had been giving him a rundown of her day.

Wally lifted her feet onto his lap and began to massage her toes. "Quirk talked to Xenia, but she denied everything. He said she was a tough nut, and it would take more than a visit from a police officer to crack her."

"Yeah, she's had too much experience with cops to be intimidated by them." Skye closed her eyes and enjoyed the sensation that Wally's fingers were producing. She'd been on her feet for nearly eleven hours and his massage was heavenly. "But I could take a different tack, try to convince her I'm on her side."

"Would Xenia go for that?" He moved on to Skye's arch and she sighed in pleasure. "Didn't you say she doesn't trust you, and you haven't been able to establish a good relationship with her?"

"True. But I could try again. Maybe approach it as being good for the student newspaper." Skye opened her eyelids a crack. "For some reason she's really fierce in defending the *Scoop*."

"I don't think you ever told me what Xenia wrote that made Ashley's parents so upset that they decided to sue."

"I can't believe she hacked into our files and inserted her story just before we sent it to the printers. Of course, it wasn't too difficult; all she needed was our password, which we foolishly kept in the desk drawer. We're not used to the kids doing stuff like that." Skye added, half to herself, "Or maybe we just never caught on before."

"But what did she write?"

"Oh, she claimed that Ashley was having sex with the basketball team in their locker room the night they won the championship."

"Yep. That would stir up her parents, all right." Wally switched feet and started rubbing her left one. "I'm guessing the school is threatening to have the boys testify if the parents don't drop the suit."

"Right. Unfortunately, the parents don't believe the boys. They say that they're being coerced by the school to lie about Ashley."

"So, they're going ahead with the lawsuit?"

"Uh-huh. I think the only way they'd ever be convinced is if there were pictures." Skye paused. A memory nibbled at the edge of her consciousness. What was it? She concentrated. No. It was gone, but another recollection popped into her head. "Oh, I just remembered something that happened the morning the contest started. When we were finally dismissed from the stage, everyone had to go to the bathroom, so I headed for the teachers' restroom, figuring no one else would think of using that one. I had just gotten down to business when I heard two people talking in the lounge next door. Someone was berating someone else about not getting complete info on one of the finalists."

"Could you tell who they were?" Wally finished with her feet and moved on to her calves.

"No, not even their gender, although I'm pretty sure one was a woman. Oh, wait, the second voice said the woman had paid him to get her into the finals, so I guess that person would have to be on the Grandma Sal's staff. If I had known there would be a murder, I would have tried harder to find out." Skye's expression was sober. "Anyway, I've told you everything I learned today. What about you?"

"I never did find my dad. From what you said, I guess I should have checked the bars, but he's not usually a big drinker." Wally's brow wrinkled. "Other than that, I spent the whole time interviewing the contest people. I've got the entire force either doing background checks or looking for Ashley."

"Anything on either front?"

"Not a thing."

Skye *tsk*ed, then asked, "What did Cherry's husband have to say? I bet he was surprised to see you."

"He wanted to slam the door in my face, but he knew that was the wrong thing to do, so he let me in and tried to make me believe that he didn't know a thing."

"Don't they all?"

"Yeah." Wally leaned forward and picked up his can of beer. "He claims he has no idea who would want to kill Cherry — she had no enemies, and he stayed home when she went to the factory that morning. She went early to check and make sure everything was perfect."

"Did he claim the housekeeper could alibi him?"

"He said she was there, but they weren't in the same part of the house."

"What about the prenup?" Skye took a sip of her wine.

"He says there is no prenup. Told me to check with his lawyer if I didn't believe him."

"Hmm. Why would he lie to his girlfriend about having one?"

"Because he really didn't want a divorce." Wally's grin was devilish.

"What makes you think that?"

"Because he told me. Hunter enjoyed his life as Mr. Cherry Alexander. He didn't have to work; she made enough money for both of them. And she bought him anything he wanted — a motorcycle, a boat, trips to Hawaii to surf."

Skye nodded thoughtfully. "And he really does love his son."

"Right. The prenup line is something he brings out when the current girlfriend gets too serious."

"He used it to get rid of them." Skye finally understood.

"He liked them to break up with him, but if that didn't work he pretended to be noble and said he couldn't keep seeing them, knowing he'd never be able to get free of his marriage." Wally finished his beer and got up to throw away the can. "This time, though, the nanny endangered his child, so the breakup wasn't amicable."

"Did Cherry ever hire a PI?"

"Yes. Hunter gave me the name, and I was able to get hold of the investigator just before you got here. The PI said that Cherry did have him investigate the judges. He found something on all of them. The food editor is being treated for bulimia, the cookbook author was once accused of plagiarizing a recipe, and the radio restaurant critic is under suspicion for taking kickbacks to write good reviews. I'll be talking to each of them again tomorrow, but none of what Cherry had on them seems enough to kill for."

"Especially since it would all be public knowledge if anyone really wanted to dig around for it." Skye tilted her head, thinking. "Did you ask who Cherry's next book was going to be about?"

"Hunter said she never told anyone except her investigator, and he said she hadn't selected a new subject yet."

"Shoot." Skye frowned. "I bet Kyle isn't left-handed either."

"Nope." Wally's voice was flat. "But we

found out a lot of people are. Heck, even my father is a lefty."

"So Kyle's no longer a good suspect, is he?"

"Not if what he said checks out with his attorney. There was no life insurance or savings, and everything was mortgaged to the hilt. They lived beyond Cherry's real means. Her royalties go to the kid's trust, so Hunter will have to go to work to survive. He'll learn real soon that it's not so easy to play the clown when you have to run the circus."

"I bet he finds himself another sugar mama." Skye got up and joined Wally in the kitchen. "Who's our lead suspect now? The nanny? Maybe she thought if Cherry were dead and he didn't have the prenup to stop him, Hunter would marry her."

"I doubt it. According to Hunter, he fired her before Cherry was killed. If the nanny did it, it was revenge, not love." Wally leaned a hip against the counter. "I've got Quirk looking for her. Hunter claimed he has no idea where she would go."

"Which means we're back to square one." Skye rinsed out her wineglass and put it on the drainer. "What's the plan?"

"Tomorrow we reinterview all the contestants and contest people who don't have alibis." Wally stepped behind her and slipped his arms around her waist. "If the murder's not personal, maybe it's professional. Who had the most to gain with Cherry out of the picture?"

"Good question." Skye found it hard to think with his warm breath fanning the sensitive spot below her ear.

Wally's nuzzling was interrupted by his yawn. "Sorry," he murmured.

"I'll bet you're exhausted. Thea said you were at the PD by six this morning and never took a break." Skye turned to face him, tracing a fingertip across his lip. "I should go home and let you get some rest."

Slowly and seductively his gaze slid downward. "I think I'm getting my second wind."

Her heart jolted and her pulse pounded. His appeal was undeniable. His hands burrowed under her sweater and locked against her spine. Skye inhaled sharply at the contact, a shiver rippling through her.

He whispered into her neck, "You're driving me crazy. I can't concentrate. I think about you all the time."

She had thought that once they had made love the first time her craving for him would lessen, but it seemed to grow each time they were together. She buried her hands in his hair and lifted his head, staring into his dark eyes.

It had taken them years to get to this point, and somewhere in the back of her mind she was always afraid that she would lose him. His father's unexpected and unexplained presence intensified those fears and paralyzed her tongue. She wanted to tell him how much he meant to her, but the words refused to come.

Wally gazed at her, waiting for her to respond. After a moment his broad shoulders heaved as he sighed.

She knew she had hurt him, and gathered him close, trying to show him how she felt with her kiss.

His lips devoured her and the room spun.

Skye didn't notice that they had moved into his bedroom until she felt the mattress press against the back of her knees. Gently he eased her down on the comforter, sliding her sweater off over her head, then stood to discard his own clothes.

She watched as his powerful, well-muscled body emerged, and when he lay down and gathered her in his arms, all her doubts and fears drained away.

Skye pressed the accelerator to the floor, increasing the Bel Air's speed until it almost seemed to skim the ground. She had fallen asleep at Wally's and hadn't woken up until his alarm clicked on at seven thirty. Which would have allowed plenty of time to get home, shower, dress, and still be at the awards ceremony on time if he hadn't persuaded her to stay for an encore of the night before.

Now she had less than an hour to get herself together and arrive at the school auditorium by ten. Gravel flew from under her tires as she turned into her driveway, and her brakes squealed as she slammed her foot on the pedal to avoid rear-ending the Ford Escort parked in front of her house.

Who did she know who drove an Escort? Certainly no one in her family; they all drove either pickups or cars the size of parade floats.

As she ran down a mental list of names, a tall, good-looking man in his early sixties emerged from the driver's-side door. He wore crisp khakis and a black polo shirt with a little alligator embroidered on the pocket. His head was shaved and his eyes were hidden behind mirrored sunglasses.

Shoot. What was Wally's father doing at her house at nine o'clock on a Monday morning? No possible answer she could come up with suggested he was the bearer of good news.

Skye considered throwing her car into reverse and getting the heck out of Dodge, but she had a feeling he would follow her — possibly to the ends of the earth. He had that look, like a pit bull that had chomped down on a hand and wasn't letting go until he had reached the bone.

Dang. She did not want to meet Wally's dad for the first time dressed in yesterday's clothes, with no makeup on, her hair skinned back into a ponytail, and smelling of . . . well, a lot of things, none of them a morning shower. Could this be any more awkward?

She glanced in the rearview mirror. Nope, nothing she could do about her appearance. She had approximately five seconds before he reached her car. She clawed through her purse, closing her hand on a small glass vial — a bottle of Chanel. She whipped it out and sprayed. The spicy scent gave her the self-confidence to face what was coming; even if she looked like the Bride of Frankenstein, at least she smelled like Miss America.

Opening her door a second before he reached the Bel Air's front fender, Skye stepped out of the car and said, "Mr. Boyd, I presume?"

"Carson Boyd, at your service, ma'am."

He held out his hand. "And you must be Skye."

She nodded, but narrowed her eyes. He had called her *ma'am.* How old did he think she was? She couldn't say what she wanted to, and couldn't think of anything else to say, so for once she kept her mouth shut.

"I'd like to have a word with you, if you have a moment." His request sounded more like an order.

Skye bristled. "I'm sorry, Mr. Boyd; as a matter of fact I don't. Perhaps we could schedule something later in the day, or tomorrow."

"Would that we could, but I'm leaving Scumble River this afternoon, and I know you'll be tied up with the cooking contest all morning."

How did he know that? Probably Uncle Charlie or Jesse had mentioned that she was a finalist. "Unfortunately, that's the reason I don't have time right now. I need to freshen up and get back to town for the awards ceremony." Skye bit her lip to stop from smirking. Freshen up — that was a good one. What she really needed was to be run through a car wash, complete with the wax option.

"If you could just give me fifteen minutes," he persisted, following her as she walked up the steps. "It's about my son. I need your help to do what's best for him."

Holy crap. How could she say no to that? "Okay. But I really have a limited amount of time."

Skye unlocked her front door and led him into the parlor. At least this room was freshly painted and contained some beautiful antiques. If he would just not notice the worn and stained carpet, she might be able to pull off a good first impression.

She sat on the settee, offering the delicate Queen Anne chair to her guest. She hoped its uncomfortable seat would make him leave that much sooner.

After a few minutes of silence, she prodded, "What can I do for you, Mr. Boyd?"

"Call me Carson."

"Okay, Carson, what is it you wanted to say?"

He took off his sunglasses, and she was struck by his resemblance to Wally.

He cleared his throat. "I understand you and Walter are seeing each other."

"Yes. It's not exactly a secret."

"How serious are you?"

Skye tilted her head. "Are you asking me what my intentions are?"

"Yes, in a way I am."

"Shouldn't my dad be having this conversation with your son, instead of the other way around?"

Carson gave her a serious look. "I'm sixty-four years old. I own a multinational corporation, and instead of preparing to take my place in the business, my only son is off playing Sheriff Andy Taylor in some Northern Mayberry. I'm not playing around here."

"So you've suddenly traveled to Scumble River to persuade Wally to return to Texas with you and run your company." Skye's stomach cramped. It was just as she had feared.

"In part, yes."

"What does Wally's choice of occupation and hometown have to do with me?"

"My dear, don't be so modest." Carson ran his fingers over his head as if he'd forgotten he had no hair. "From what I hear, my son has been infatuated with you since you were a teenager, and now that you two are finally together, I doubt a Texas twister could tear him from your side."

"Interesting." Skye forced herself not to beam. After the last couple of days of self-doubt, it felt wonderful to have Wally's father verbalize his son's devotion. Even if it turned out not to be true, she would bask in the moment. "But I still don't know what you want from me."

"Before I answer that, let me ask you something." Carson stared into her eyes. "Would you be willing to pack up, move to Texas, and live there for the rest of your life?"

His question caught her unprepared. If he had asked it of her when she first graduated from high school or college, or even just a few years ago, she would have jumped at the chance to leave Scumble River, but now . . . she had friends, family, a house. She wanted to know how things would turn out for the kids she was working with at school. She just didn't know if she could leave all that.

"Your silence is enough of an answer." Carson shook his head. "What in the world does this little nowhere town have that makes you and my son want to stay here?"

"It's home." Skye shrugged. That really wasn't a good answer, but it was the only one she could put into words. "Now that we've settled that, I repeat — what do you want from me?"

"I want you to break up with Wally. Tell him you don't love him. You've changed your mind. You really love that funeral director you were going with before dating my son."

Skye couldn't stop her gasp. "Why would

I do that?"

"I had planned to offer you money, but I understand you gave away a painting that was worth hundreds of thousands of dollars, so maybe cash doesn't motivate you." He stared at his sunglasses, almost as if he had forgotten she was there. "Still, it's worth a try." He looked up at her. "I will help you set up an offshore account and transfer a million dollars into it, if you will agree never to speak to my son again."

"You were right. I'm not as motivated by money as I used to be." She smiled to herself. She'd come a long way since she'd been blinded by her ex-fiancé's wealth and position. "How Wally makes me feel is worth ten times that amount."

"Then I'll ask you to do it because it's the right thing for my son. The only way he'll fulfill his destiny and be the great man he was born to be."

"But that's not the life Wally wants." Skye tried to calm her emotions and think straight. "He moved here and became a police officer long before he ever met me."

"He did that as a young man's foolish act of rebellion. He's more mature now."

"So, now that he's older and wiser, what did he say when you asked him to quit his job, move back to Texas, and take over for you?" Skye held her breath.

"He turned me down." Carson continued before Skye could comment. "But not because of his love for this town or his job — because of his love for you. If you were willing to move with him, he would come home."

"Did he say that?"

"Not in so many words. But a father can tell what his son really means."

Skye briefly contemplated turning Wally's dad over to her mother — of course, first she would tell May that Carson was trying to get Skye to move to Texas. She smiled thinly before realizing that her mother would be thrilled with Carson's other suggestion — that she break up with Wally and get back with Simon. *Hmm.* No, her mother would be no use in this situation.

"I'm a firm believer in hearing something from the horse's mouth," Skye said, watching the older man's expression carefully. "If Wally tells me that he wants to move home and take over for you, but doesn't want to leave me, I'll either break up with him or agree to move with him."

"He'd never tell you that, but what if I arranged for you to overhear him say it to me?"

"Fine." Skye stood up.

Carson followed suit and she led him into the foyer.

"I'll let you know where and when."

"You do that."

"I'm not a monster, you know." He paused, one foot over the threshold. "All I want is what's best for my son."

"I know." Skye closed the door after him and leaned against the smooth wood, her emotions at war. "Me, too."

After several minutes, she sighed and started up the stairs to change. Her heart was focused on her feelings concerning Wally, but her brain was telling her she had missed something important in her conversation with his father. But what?

CHAPTER 18
TOOTHPICK INSERTED IN CENTER SHOULD COME OUT CLEAN

Why am I always running late? Skye fumed as she hurriedly bathed, threw on clean clothes, and jumped into her car. *Just once I'd like to get dressed without feeling as if I'm a quick-change artist.*

Cursing Carson Boyd, she roared out of the driveway toward town. His visit was not only extremely upsetting; it had cut her primping time in half.

Skye's bad temper worsened when she arrived at the high school a little before ten and discovered the parking lot was full. By the time she drove around the block to the middle school, found a spot to park there, cut across the stretch of lawn that divided the two buildings, and walked into the auditorium, her irritation had blossomed into a full-fledged huff.

Her mother's glare did not improve her disposition. Skye glared back at May as she crossed the stage and took her position among the other One-Dish Meals contestants.

From what Skye could tell, the ceremony had just begun. Grandma Sal wrapped up her welcome speech, then introduced Dante, who spoke for a few minutes about how pleased Scumble River was to be this year's host for the contest. He also managed to squeeze in a mention of his own self-sacrifice in being wounded for the good of the town before turning the stage back to Grandma Sal.

A serious expression on her face, she said, "As you all know, a terrible tragedy occurred during this year's challenge. We lost one of our wonderful finalists, Ms. Cherry Alexander."

Someone in the crowd yelled out, "She was murdered, not misplaced."

Skye cringed.

Grandma Sal ignored the outburst and went on. "To honor Cherry's valiant spirit, we have created a special award to be given to the finalist who showed the most stick-to-itiveness. And here with us today to present it is her husband, Kyle."

Dressed in a sober black suit, his hair gelled back from his face, he looked ten years older than the man who had been with Cherry backstage three days ago. He stepped up to the microphone and read from an index card, " 'Cherry would be honored to have this award named after her. She was a person who never gave up and demanded the best from everyone, especially herself.' "

A voice from the audience bellowed, "You should be taking Fine Foods to court, not giving out an award for them. Their negligence contributed to your wife's murder."

Skye squinted past the stage lights. The heckler sounded a bit too well educated to be one of the Scumble River regulars. Who was trying to make Grandma Sal's company look bad in front of all the press?

There was no way to tell, and Skye's focus returned to Kyle, who pulled at the neck of his white shirt and darted a glance toward Grandma Sal.

She murmured in his ear, and he straightened and said, "The winner of the Cherry Alexander Award for Perseverance is . . ."

He squinted at the card Grandma Sal handed him, and Skye wondered just how much Fine Foods was paying him to do this, rather than file a lawsuit.

"Glenda Doozier." Kyle waited for the applause to end, then continued, "Not only did this plucky little lady come into the contest late and as an alternate, but she made it through some very difficult family issues, still managing to turn her dish in on time."

Skye would have swallowed her chewing gum if she'd had any. Glenda Doozier, plucky? Little lady? Family issues? Her husband had been trying to bribe people, and her brother-in-law had shot up the place. How did that constitute being worthy to win a prize?

The Red Ragger queen pranced up to the mike in four-inch spike-heeled black plastic sandals and a Dolly Parton wig. Her leather skirt was the size of a Post-it note, and her lipstick-red tube top was no bigger than a rubber band. Every man in the place held his breath and prayed for a wardrobe malfunction.

Kyle seemed to be having trouble forming words. Finally managing to gasp, "Here," he thrust the silver spoon-shaped trophy at Glenda's 38DD chest. When it caught in the elastic of her top, several men in the audience growled like hyenas about to tear into their dinner.

Clearly Grandma Sal had dealt with testosterone-induced stupidity before. She casually reached over, disengaged the utensil's handle from the stretchy material, and gently moved Kyle backward, taking his place. She then grasped Glenda's arm, and as she walked her to the stairs said, "Mrs. Doozier, thank you so much for participating in our little contest. You'll be contacted to come and pick up your check at the factory."

Skye overheard Grandma Sal mutter to herself as she walked back to center stage, "Why in the world would he pick *her* to win the special prize? Is he trying to ruin us?"

The older woman straightened as she approached the microphone, pasted a smile on her face, and addressed the audience again. "Now, for our regular awards. We'll be giving one in each of our four categories; Special-Occasion Baking, Healthy, Snacks, and One-Dish Meals. The grand prize will go to one of those winners."

Skye looked at the little table placed on Grandma Sal's right. Several plaques and one trophy — the size of a small child — were waiting to be passed out.

Jared stood between his mother and the table. He picked up the first plaque and handed it to her.

She peered at the name, then announced, "The winner of the Healthy category is Monika Bradley, our CPA from Brooklyn, for her Gluten-Free, Dairy-Free Sponge Cake and Frosting."

It took several minutes for the attractive blonde to hobble up to the front of the stage, her leg still immobilized by a brace, but when she got there she kept her speech short. "What characterizes a dish as healthy is different for each person. If you have diabetes, it's sugar-free. If you have high cholesterol, it's excluding trans fats. And if you have high blood pressure, it's low sodium.

"While most people are aware of these dietary needs, many are uninformed about life-threatening food allergies. I entered this contest to bring the issue of celiac disease and other life-threatening food allergies to the public's attention. My winning entry has no gluten or dairy and is still delicious. Thank you all for the opportunity."

Next Grandma Sal awarded the Snacks winner. Skye had half believed Charlie would win, but a woman from Laurel took the prize for her Fiesta Italiano Dip.

The Special-Occasion-Baking category was next. Skye looked down the row at her mother. May was holding the hands of the contestants on either side of her as if she were in the Miss America Pageant.

Grandma Sal took the plaque from Jared, checked the nameplate, and said, "The winner of Special-Occasion Baking is . . . Diane

White, our cookie blogger from Clay Center, for her Chocolate Brownie Tiramisu."

The blogger shrieked and ran over to Grandma Sal. Her hug nearly knocked the older woman off her feet. After releasing Grandma Sal, Diane whipped a piece of paper from her pocket. She unfolded it like an accordion, grabbed the microphone, and began to read, "I'm grateful to my wonderful husband, my three lovely children . . ."

The thank-you list was endless, and when Diane expressed her appreciation to the fish in her aquarium for being a calming influence, naming each individually, Skye tuned her out and looked back at May. Her mother's smile was shaky, and Skye could tell that it cost her a great deal not to burst into tears.

Her own throat closed; she knew how much it had meant to May to win. Skye wished she had done a better job on the casserole, so she could have won for her mother. *Darn.* She should have practiced more and kept her mind on the cooking rather than on sleuthing.

Diane showed no sign of coming to an end of her roll call, but Grandma Sal wrestled the mike away from the excited woman by tempting her with the plaque. The blogger was still thanking people as she returned to her place clutching her prize.

Grandma Sal took the fourth award from her son, squinted at the engraving, and frowned. She whispered something to Jared, who answered her. She shrugged and said, "Last but not least, the winner of our One-Dish Meal is . . ."

Skye glanced to her left and smiled at Butch King, the firefighter whose mother had tried to obedience-train Earl Doozier. She hoped Butch would win. He'd been so nice that first day when they'd had lunch together.

". . . Syke Denison."

Had her name — at least, a version of her name — really been called? Skye was rooted to the spot. Even after she heard her mother screaming and saw her jumping up and down, she didn't believe it was possible she had won.

Skye shot Grandma Sal a questioning look, and the older woman nodded. Finally Skye managed to move her feet, and she walked carefully to the front of the stage. She was still more than half afraid that she'd misheard and was about to make a huge fool of herself.

Grandma Sal handed her the plaque and said, "Syke is a school psychologist from right here in Scumble River, and she wins for her Chicken Supreme Casserole." Skye whispered in the older woman's ear and Grandma Sal said, "Sorry, her name is Skye. I thought the other was wrong, but my son insisted. You know these youngsters; they think they know everything."

The crowd laughed politely, and Grandma Sal handed Skye the mike.

Skye took a deep breath and tried to think of something to say. "Uh, well, I just want to thank my mother for teaching me to cook, and Wally Boyd for eating all of my practice attempts, even the burned ones."

As Skye stumbled back to her spot, May met her halfway, hugging and kissing her. "You did it! You really did it! I knew you could."

Grandma Sal waited for May to calm down, then turned to the audience. "Now for what you've all been waiting for. The grand prize of ten thousand dollars goes to . . ."

May's nails dug into Skye's hand.

". . . Diane White for her Chocolate Brownie Tiramisu."

Skye's shoulders sagged. She had no right to be disappointed. It had been a miracle she had won her category, and there was no way she'd had a chance to win the grand prize. Still, for just a second she was let down.

Then May hugged her and whispered, "She was probably sleeping with the judges."

Skye shook her head. "Two of the judges are women."

May raised an eyebrow. "So?"

Skye giggled and May hugged her again. "We did great. Next year we'll get the grand prize."

"There won't be any next year." Skye hugged her mother back and stepped out of her embrace.

"We'll see."

"No next year," Skye insisted.

"Sure. Whatever you say." May nodded toward the front of the stage. "Now be quiet. I want to hear what our winner has to say."

This time the cookie blogger's speech was even longer, and not even being handed the huge trophy shut her up. Twenty minutes later she wound down, after thanking her Kindergarten teacher, her minister, and the manufacturers of the Easy-Bake oven, in which she first learned to cook.

Grandma Sal asked the winners to stay so the media could ask questions, then dismissed the audience and the rest of the contestants. The Grandma Sal's Soup-to-Nuts Cooking Challenge was officially over.

Most of the media wanted them to talk about Cherry's death, but they all professed to have nothing to say. After several "No comments," "I have no ideas," and "What are you talking abouts?" the press gave up, and the winners were free to go.

Before they dispersed, Jared told them all they would be notified when their checks were ready. They would need to pick them up at the factory so they could fill out the paperwork for the IRS.

Waiting for Skye when she was finally released were the four huge guys who had been rooting for Janelle to win the contest. Skye's heart skipped a beat as the largest man, the one she had dubbed Mr. Elephant, stepped forward.

He stared at her without speaking, then turned his head slightly. Skye followed his gaze and saw the prison cook standing a few feet away making a "go on" motion with her hands.

"My posse and me jus' wanted to give you props on your win. Your recipe was killer."

"Thanks." Skye was pretty sure he had given her a compliment. "Your friend Janelle's recipe was, uh, phat, too."

Mr. Elephant smiled at her use of slang.

"We hears that you got juice in this 'hood."

That was a little easier to translate. "Maybe some."

"Little Boy Blue listens to you, and word is you represent for your peeps."

"I try to help when I can."

Janelle cleared her throat loudly, and Mr. Elephant took a deep breath before saying, "I know the poe-leece ain't goin' listen to a dude like me, but I heard that dead chassis say to that biddie that jus' won the contest that she be a bammer. That she be cheating by bringing in brownies from the bakery — not making her own."

"Oh, my." If Skye understood him correctly, he had accused Diane White of cheating and said that Cherry confronted her about it. The cookie blogger now had a motive for murder.

"You tell your man what I heard." Mr. Elephant turned to leave.

"No, you have to tell Chief Boyd yourself." Skye looked the man in the eye. "I promise, he'll listen to you and not disrespect you."

"That be whack."

"No. Chief Boyd is straight-up."

Janelle had moved closer and spoke up. "Jus' do it and get it over with. You gonna go straight, you gotta learn to live with the man. That chief of police be cool." She gave

315

Skye a level look. "Right?"

"Right." Skye looked around and saw Anthony talking to Diane and Monika.

He had each of them by the arm and was leading them down the hallway saying, "I need you to come this way, please. We have a few more questions for you both about Ms. Alexander's death."

Wally had mentioned that he planned to reinterview the contestants and staff who didn't have alibis for the time of Cherry's murder. Skye hadn't realized he would do it right at the school, but it made sense. They were already assembled, and there were plenty of rooms for the interrogations.

As Anthony led Diane and Monika past her, Skye said to him, "Anthony, this gentleman has some information he needs to tell Chief Boyd. Where is he?"

"In the principal's office."

Skye nodded and escorted Mr. Elephant, his herd, and Janelle toward the front of the building. As Skye walked, she tried to decide whether she should tell Wally about his father's visit, or give Carson the chance he had asked for and see if she really was standing in the way of Wally's desire to go back to Texas.

Part of her said that tricking Wally like that would damage their relationship forever. But another part wondered if she would ever know the truth if she didn't go along with Carson's plan.

She still hadn't decided what to do when she reached the main office. She'd just have to wing it and see what popped out of her mouth. Perhaps not the best plan, but the only one she had.

The outer office was empty, and Skye asked the group to wait there. Once they complied, she proceeded down the narrow hall and knocked on the door at the end.

"Yes?" Wally's voice held a slightly annoyed tone.

She inched open the door, poking her head inside. "Could you step out here for a minute?"

"Now?"

"Now."

When he was outside the office with the door closed she explained about Mr. Elephant and what he had heard. Wally immediately went to talk to them, saying to Skye over his shoulder, "After we get done with this guy, do you have time to help me reinterview Jared's wife?"

"Sure."

Mr. Elephant repeated to Wally what he had reported to Skye. Friday night at the dinner he had overheard Cherry tell Diane

White that if she didn't drop out of the competition, Cherry would inform Grandma Sal that Diane had used brownies from a bakery during the practice session that afternoon, and that she had an order for three more pans of brownies from that same bakery the next morning.

Wally asked a few questions, but it was clear Mr. Elephant didn't have any other information, and since he and his crew had alibis for the time of the murder, there was no reason to suspect he was lying. Wally took his address and phone number, then let them go.

When Wally and Skye returned to the principal's office, he said to the woman sitting in one of the visitor's chairs, "Mrs. Fine, this is our psychological consultant, Ms. Denison."

Tammy appeared impatient, and as Skye took a seat next to her, she demanded, "Are you nearly finished? We have a dinner party in Chicago tonight and we need to get on the road. My husband and mother-in-law may have to come back here, but this is the last time I ever have to pretend to want to be in Scumble River."

Wally leaned forward and rested his elbows on the desk. "Sorry, Mrs. Fine; I still need to talk to your husband and mother-in-law. I was able to catch your sons while the awards ceremony was going on, but Mr. and Mrs. Fine were onstage. Where were you, by the way? I'm told you only arrived at the school fifteen minutes ago."

"I was packing and having the car loaded. I can't wait to get out of this town."

"And yet your factory here provides a good living for your family," Wally reminded the woman.

"Things change." The slim brunette stared at Wally.

Skye caught Wally's eye and silently asked if she could jump in. He nodded, and she said, "Rumor has it your family may be selling Fine Foods. Is that what you're referring to?"

"Well, I can't confirm or deny." Tammy's smile was predatorlike. "All I can say is, read tomorrow's newspaper."

Wally took the conversation back. "So, Mrs. Fine, you were alone in your motel cabin sleeping the morning of Ms. Alexander's death?"

"Yes. How many times do I have to tell you?"

"Have you thought of anyone who might be able to corroborate your story?"

"No, Jared left early to go to the factory. I took the phone off the hook and put the

'Do not disturb' sign on the door."

"Did you know Ms. Alexander before the contest?" Wally steepled his fingers.

"No."

"Have you read any of her books?"

"Certainly not. They're all lies. It's clear she has a grudge against anyone rich or famous."

Wally was silent for a few minutes, then said, "Okay, Mrs. Fine, that's all for now. We have your number." He paused, letting the double meaning of what he had said sink in, then continued, "And your address in Chicago. Don't leave the state."

Tammy rose from her chair in one fluid movement and marched out the door, slamming it behind her.

"That was interesting," Skye commented. "Did she have anything of value to say before I got here?"

"No."

"Who all are you talking to today?"

"I've already interviewed Tammy, JJ, and Brandon. Neither Mrs. Fine nor her two sons seems to have any connection to Cherry. There's no evidence that they ever met her before this weekend, and since they aren't contest judges, she wouldn't have had any reason to blackmail or bribe them."

"Do any of them have alibis?" Skye asked,

making sure she understood. "Are any of them left-handed?"

"No alibis. Tammy and Brandon are both lefties, as is the male judge, and two contestants — Monika Bradley and Diane White."

"But they aren't your top suspects," Skye guessed.

"No. Tammy says Jared is ambidextrous, and he's the one who was at the factory, which places him near the scene of the crime. Also, he could probably change the results of the contest if he wanted to, so he's number one on my list. I'm planning on seeing him next. Then I need to talk to his mother again."

"I should get out of your way then." Skye got up. "Is there anything you need me to do?"

Wally peered down at the legal pad on the desktop. "Anthony and Quirk are interviewing Monika Bradley and all three judges, but considering Mrs. Bradley's leg injury, I don't think she would physically be able to get Cherry into the chocolate fountain."

"No," Skye agreed. "Unless she's faking her injury."

"That would mean she came into the contest knowing she was going to kill Cherry." Wally made a note. "I'll have someone look a little deeper into her background, see if she and the vic ever met before."

"Anything else?"

"Quirk located the nanny. Turns out Larissa went home to her parents after she was fired. They live in St. Louis, and she claims to have driven there that night and arrived about five on Saturday morning. A neighbor walking a dog saw her pull into the driveway, which gives her a pretty good alibi."

"How about the others?"

"The others involved in the contest have alibis, too, except Diane White, and now that we know she had a motive, I want *you* to talk to her."

"Sure, but why me?" Skye asked.

"She's my other top suspect, but she resorts to hysteria anytime I've tried to question her. Which means she's a prime candidate for Scumble River PD's finest psychological consultant."

"You mean Scumble River PD's *only* psychological consultant."

"That, too." Wally got up and escorted Skye to the door. "You ready to rock and roll?"

"Always." Skye put her hand on the knob. "Where is she?"

"Waiting for you next door." He kissed

322

her on the cheek. "Go get 'em, tiger."

"Grr." Skye made a clawing motion with her hands, then walked out of the principal's office and into the nurse's.

While she was explaining her role as psychological consultant to Diane, Skye realized she hadn't told Wally about his father's visit. Did that mean she wouldn't, or had it just slipped her mind?

CHAPTER 19
COOL FIFTEEN
MINUTES

"I'm through with Mrs. White." Skye had finished with the cookie blogger and gone to report to Wally, who was ushering Grandma Sal into the principal's office.

He seated the older woman and said he'd be right back. Closing the door behind him, he asked Skye, "Anything?"

"She's a much cooler customer than I'd expected. That slightly daffy cookie-blogger persona of hers is as fake as Bunny's boobs, although not as uplifting. At first she tried the hysterical routine with me, but once she saw that I wasn't buying it, she shifted to her real self."

"What did she say then?"

"I told her we knew about Cherry threatening her and about her cheating. She denied cheating. Said that Cherry had been mistaken; she only used the bakery brownies in her practice recipe to save time, but never intended to use them in the contest.

The bakery must have made a mistake if they thought she had ordered three pans for Saturday." Skye leaned against the wall. "Diane also insisted that she told Cherry that, and thus had nothing to fear from her."

"A logical explanation."

"Right, and, really, she had nothing to fear from Cherry unless she used the bakery brownies during the contest. Nothing in the rules says you even have to participate in the practice session, let alone how you have to prepare your recipe."

Wally crossed his arms. "Not to mention she'd have to be pretty stupid to use the bakery brownies, even if she had originally intended to, once Cherry had discovered her plan."

"True. Diane did admit that she arrived at the warehouse before the official practice time, found the front door locked, and went around back to see if she could get in through the factory, which she did. At that point she spotted Cherry in the chocolate fountain and started to scream."

"Did she say anything else?"

"Nope. Just told me that the police should talk to her attorney if they have any more questions."

"What do you think about her explanation for being at the crime scene?"

"The timing's plausible." Skye drew her brows together. "I wonder how many other people entered the warehouse through the factory entrance."

"Good question. Mr. Fine claims that door should have been locked, too."

"Did Jared have anything else helpful to say?" Skye asked. "I passed him on his way out and he seemed pretty preoccupied."

"He claimed he was doing paperwork in his office in the factory and had no idea what had happened until we called his mother and then she buzzed him on the intercom. Her office is a few doors down from his, so they can't alibi each other." Wally shook his head. "So far we have nothing. After I talk to Mrs. Fine, that's it. We're out of leads. We'll have to wait and hope forensics tells us something. But it could be weeks before we get those results."

Skye made a sympathetic sound and patted his arm, then asked, "Do you need me for anything else?"

"No. Why?"

"Because I'm going to go talk to Xenia about Ashley's disappearance." Skye drew a deep breath. "Which I should have done several days ago."

"Don't be so hard on yourself. I doubt she would have talked to you."

"You're probably right, but I should have tried. Ashley's life may be at stake."

"Or she could have just run away." Wally ran his fingers through his hair. "Listen, we both need a break. Why don't I pick you up around five and we'll go into Joliet for dinner and a movie? And while we're there we can buy a pair of cell phones."

"That sounds wonderful." Skye smiled, thinking that maybe Wally's father would give up if they weren't available, which would mean she wouldn't have to choose between finding out the truth and sticking to the moral high road.

Xenia lived with her mother, Raette, in a newly remodeled house near the river. When Skye pulled into the driveway, she saw that Raette's Sebring convertible was in the garage. Skye felt a small ray of hope. Maybe she'd be lucky and both of the Craughwells would be home.

Raette threw open the front door before Skye could even ring the bell. She was a tiny woman, less than five feet, with platinum hair that hung straight down to the middle of her back. She and Skye had a history, some good and some bad. Skye hoped the favor she had done Raette and her daughter in the fall would gain her access to Xenia.

Raette looked as if she would have liked to close the door, but instead she said, "Oh, what a surprise. You weren't who I was expecting."

"Is it okay if I come in?" Skye put her foot on the threshold.

"Uh, sure, but I'm leaving soon."

"Then I'll try to be quick." Skye stepped into the foyer, forcing Raette to back up. "Is Xenia home?"

"Yes. She's in her room."

"Could I talk to her?"

"Well, uh, I guess so. Is it about school?"

"In a way." Skye smiled noncommittally. "Do you want to get her for me, please?"

"Okay. Why don't you have a seat in the great room and I'll be right back."

Skye walked down the hall Raette had pointed to, and found herself in a large room with a sweep of windows that faced the water. It was a beautiful panorama, and whoever had decorated hadn't tried to compete with the natural beauty by putting any art on the other three walls.

Not wanting to be distracted, Skye chose a chair with her back to the view. As she settled in, she could hear Xenia protesting from the other end of the house.

The girl entered the room alone, a sullen

328

expression on her face. "What do you want?"

"Hi, Xenia. Nice to see you, too." Skye kept her tone cool. The teen loved to cause adults to lose their tempers. "Have a seat."

"Why should I?"

"You're right. Just because my feet are tired doesn't mean yours are. Feel free to stand."

Xenia frowned and sat down in the chair facing Skye. "So, what do you want?"

"I understand that Ashley Yates is missing, and you may have been the last to see her." Skye figured enough people had accused the teen of the kidnapping, so she'd try a different approach.

"Yeah. So what? That doesn't mean I had anything to do with her disappearance."

"That's right. It doesn't. In fact, one of her friends told me that she thinks Ashley is holed up somewhere with a guy."

Xenia raised her chin. "Whatever."

"After all, Ashley is a beautiful girl; she could get any boy she wanted."

"If you like that type." Xenia studied her black Doc Martens. "Or maybe she knew she was a lying whore, and when she found out there was proof of her being a two-faced slut, she ran away."

"Why do you think that?" Skye made sure

not to make eye contact. Xenia was like a wolf — she had to be the alpha in any situation.

Xenia shrugged. "Just a guess."

"You know, it's been more than three days now. At first I wasn't too worried, thinking maybe her friends were right. But now, even if she were with a guy or had run away because she didn't want to face some truth about herself, I'm starting to think she might be hurt or in trouble. Don't you think so?"

"How should I know?" Xenia toyed with a hole in her black T-shirt, making it larger.

"Maybe you could put yourself in her place, which is hard for me to do because I'm too old." Skye hoped she wasn't laying it on too thick. "Maybe we could figure out what happened that way."

"What if I do that and I'm right? Everyone will think I was involved, and I'll get into trouble."

Skye tried to keep the surprise off her face. This was the first time Xenia had ever admitted to caring if she got in trouble. Was the teen actually starting to develop a conscience? Could Skye use it to find out about Ashley?

"I'm here as your school psychologist, and I promise you anything you say to me is confidential, and I can't tell anyone what you told me, unless you say you're going to hurt yourself or someone else." Skye wanted to make it clear she was not here as the police consultant.

"What if I told you I already hurt someone else?"

Skye shook her head. "Unless you tell me you'll do it again or do something else in the future, I can't tell anyone."

Xenia tugged her short skirt down toward her knees. "Yeah, that's what my other shrink says, and she's been cool about stuff."

"So, if you had to guess, what happened with Ashley?" Skye held her breath.

"Maybe someone caught her by herself, with none of her posse around, you know, and sort of forced her into a car?"

Skye nodded.

"Then maybe this person drove her away from school and showed her proof of something that Ashley was claiming was a lie. Something that her parents were suing the school about. Something that would get Ashley in big trouble with her parents, who don't know what a slut their daughter is."

Skye nodded again, afraid anything she said would interrupt Xenia.

"And Ashley got out of the car and ran away crying and hasn't been seen since."

"So, this person who forced Ashley into the car has no idea where she is now?"

"Right." Xenia's attention was focused on peeling the black nail polish from her thumbnail.

"Where do you think this person drove Ashley to?"

"Well, the town's been sort of full of people, especially over by that factory where they're having that stupid cooking contest. So, if it were me, I'd go over there, because who would remember seeing any one car when there are lots and lots of them around?"

"Like in the parking lot?" Skye asked.

"Not the one in front, but there's one around back where the employees park, where people aren't coming and going that much."

"And I suppose once Ashley ran off, maybe whoever was with her might have spent some time looking for her. Then maybe been too scared to come home right away, but after a while figured it was better to be home, because if she was missing, that might make people think she was connected with Ashley being missing?"

"That sounds about right." For the first time that afternoon Xenia looked Skye in the eye. "You know, Ashley's a twit, but I

332

bet whoever snatched her didn't mean for any of the rest of this to happen."

"I'll bet you're right." Skye got up to go. "Thank you for talking to me. If you ever want to talk at school, just put a note under my door and I'll send you a pass."

Skye drove back to the factory, parked in the employee lot, and made notes on what Xenia had said. By the time she was finished her legal pad was full of squiggles and arrows. Staring at the yellow paper, Skye chewed on the end of her pen. What had she learned?

1. *Xenia forces Ashley into her car Friday morning and drives her to the Fine Foods factory's back parking lot.*
2. *Xenia shows Ashley "proof" of what was written in the school newspaper. (Must be a picture — probably taken with one of those cell phones that take pictures.)*
3. *Ashley flees the car and no one has seen her since. Could she have hopped one of the trains that stop there to deliver supplies and pick up finished product?*
4. *Xenia searches for Ashley, but can't find her. Xenia hides out for a while,*

realizes that is suspicious behavior,
comes home, erases her blog, and
claims she has no involvement.
5. So where is Ashley?????

Where hadn't they looked? Skye gazed out of the Bel Air's windshield. The factory sat on several acres of land bordered by a cornfield, which in early April was nothing but chunks of dirt and the occasional weed, certainly no place to hide.

The buildings were set about a quarter mile back on the property. The front was a large expanse of green lawn with a reflecting pool and a fountain. The water was too shallow to drown in, and besides, it was clearly visible from the road. Surely someone would have noticed a teenager lying in it for the past three days.

The back of the factory was taken up by the employee parking lot, where Skye was sitting, and truck bays that the semis used to load and unload the product. If Ashley were in trouble, inside the factory were guards and hundreds of workers she could go to, or there were phones she could use to call for help.

Which meant Skye still had no idea where to look for the missing girl. She might know what had happened, but that knowledge

334

didn't help her find Ashley.

After a quick walk around the grounds, Skye checked her watch. It was already three thirty. The employees worked a seven-to-four shift. Should she wait around and look through the factory after they all left?

No, not unless she was willing to try to get permission for the search. During their tour of the factory the guide had explained that since September 11, because they manufactured food that could easily be poisoned, all of the factory entrances and exits were kept locked except for the employee entrance, which had a guard who checked identification.

During the day, if there was a crisis, workers could get out through doors with alarms wired directly to the fire department. But once the employees left for the day, the emergency exit doors were locked from the inside.

So, unless she had the Fines' consent, even if she were able to sneak in to look for Ashley, Skye wouldn't be able to get back out. She'd just have to wait until Wally came over at five; then she'd tell him what she had figured out from her chat with Xenia — not revealing how she had come to those conclusions — and see if he could get a search warrant.

A few minutes later she was pulling into her own driveway. It was a relief to be home for a little while, and after showering she decided to do some laundry. She gathered up the clothes she had worn over the last few days and took them downstairs. Before she stuffed them into the washing machine, she emptied out the pockets — she had a bad habit of sticking Post-its, used Kleenex, and change in them.

As she stuck her hand into the pocket of the jeans she had been wearing the day before, she pulled out the piece of paper May had found by the factory. Flattening it, Skye drew in a startled breath. It was a March schedule for Scumble River High cheerleading practice. Was this proof that Ashley had been around the factory in the past couple of days? Another thing to discuss with Wally.

After she started the machine, Skye checked her messages. The little light was blinking merrily, and she pushed the PLAY button.

The first voice was Trixie's. "Hi. Sorry I missed you. Owen and I got word that school was canceled, so we stayed another day. I should be home by midnight or so tonight. See you tomorrow morning before the first bell. Can't wait to hear what you've been up to."

The second message was from Carson Boyd. "Wally tells me he's picking you up at five at your house. I'll be there at quarter to, and we can get set up so you can hear the truth for yourself."

Holy shit! Not only was Carson still in town; he still wanted to set Wally up. What should she do?

CHAPTER 20
REMOVE FROM PANS

The doorbell rang at precisely four forty-five. Skye looked through her peephole, but almost didn't recognize the man standing on her front porch. Instead of the khakis and polo shirt he had worn earlier that day, Carson was dressed in a British tan Armani suit with a cream-colored Egyptian-cotton shirt and a chocolate brown Italian silk tie.

On his head was an ivory Stetson, and ostrich-skin cowboy boots had replaced his Wal-Mart tennis shoes. His sunglasses were no longer cheap rip-offs; instead they were expensive Ray-Bans. His current ensemble probably cost more than her annual salary.

For a moment Skye felt her throat tighten. This was what Wally would be giving up if he stayed in Scumble River, which was why it had to be completely his decision with no influence from anyone, including her. Taking a deep breath, she opened the door and let Carson Boyd inside.

He immediately took off his hat and said, "Miss Skye, I'm real grateful you're allowing me this chance to get my boy back."

"Well . . ." Skye noted that he now had a Texas accent. He hadn't had it that morning.

"I know that with your help, Walter will be home with me soon."

"Uh . . ." Skye's heart pounded. She hated this. Why? Why had she been forced into this position, and more important, had she made the right choice?

"Right?"

"Please." She swallowed with difficulty and found her voice. "This is between you and Wally."

"If that's what you want to believe. But you'll keep your word?" His stare drilled into her. "If you hear Wally say he wants to come back to Texas, you'll either agree to go with him or break up with him. And if you break up with him, you'll convince him you love that other fella."

Skye nodded. "If I hear him say he wants to live in Texas, I'll keep my word." She led him into the parlor and sat on the settee. "So, how are you going to do this?"

"When he arrives, I'll answer the door and say you had to run to town for something, but you'll be back in a few minutes. I'll tell him I'm leaving and I know he's only staying here because of you, and I understand and respect his decision, but I would like to hear the truth. Would he come home if you agreed to go with him or if you were no longer in his life?"

"So you'll lie, because you don't really respect his decision?"

"That's a minor detail. A means to an end." He glanced at his Rolex. "He'll be here soon. Where will you be so you can hear?"

"She can have my spot, Dad. You can hear really well what's said in the parlor if you stand in the hallway." Wally strolled through the archway and took a seat next to Skye.

"Walter." Carson's tanned face paled. "I can explain, son." He shot Skye a confused look.

"I'm sorry, Mr. Boyd, but I couldn't set Wally up that way. It just wasn't right," Skye stammered. "It's better all around if the three of us discuss this openly and together."

Carson slumped in the chair. "You've ruined everything."

"No." Skye leaned over and put a hand on his shoulder. "Really, I haven't. Not if what you want is a better relationship with your son. This is the way to get it. Not by deceiving him."

"But he'll never come back to Texas now. He'll never take over for me as CEO of CB International."

"That would never have happened anyway, Dad." Wally shook his head. "I told you more than twenty years ago when I was in college that I didn't want that kind of life. I'm happy here. Yes, a lot of that is due to Skye, but even if she dumped me or agreed to move to Texas with me, I don't want to be a CEO."

"I'm getting old. I want to retire." Carson tried to regain some ground. "Who'll take over for me?"

"I hear my cousin is doing a mighty fine job. He'd be the clear choice to take over."

"You have a nephew who works for you?" Skye demanded, outraged that Carson had let her believe that he was alone, with no one to turn to. "You never mentioned a nephew."

Carson nodded, not meeting her stare. It was clear he was beaten. He stood up and thrust his hand out at Wally. "I hope that we can at least stay in closer touch. I've enjoyed visiting with you the past few months."

Wally shook his dad's hand, then put his other arm around the older man's shoulder and hugged him. "Anytime, Dad. You're always welcome here. And maybe Skye and I can take a vacation to Texas this fall."

"I'd really like that." He put his hat on. "Well, I'd better go. I told my pilot to have the Cessna ready for takeoff by eight."

"Wait one minute." Skye struggled to put together the bits and pieces that had been bothering her. "You were here for another reason, besides to bring Wally back into the fold. What was it?"

"I guess it won't hurt to tell you now." Carson shrugged. "It'll be in the papers by tomorrow."

Where had she just heard that?

She glanced at Wally questioningly and he gave a slight nod and murmured, "Tammy Fine."

"That's right." Carson nodded. "For the past several months CB International has been in talks with Fine Foods. I've been traveling here to negotiate the deal."

Skye wondered if Wally felt betrayed that his father hadn't been coming just to see him.

"Why the disguise this time?" Wally asked.

"Previously I was meeting with the Fines to look over profit-and-loss statements, check out the condition of the factory, and examine their distribution networks, but this time I was interested in their morals and values. I only acquire companies that have a good reputation, which is why I usually only go after businesses that are family-owned."

"That seems a little hypocritical, Dad, considering your own morals aren't exactly squeaky clean."

"Nothing personal." Carson shrugged. "It's just good business."

Skye and Wally exchanged a knowing glance. Evidently Carson's thinking was like that of a lot of the parents she dealt with, who wanted their kids to do as they said, not as they did.

"So, that's why you toned down your appearance and lost your accent — you wanted to fit in to Scumble River, be able to hang out and ask questions during the contest," Wally guessed.

"That, and I didn't want the Fines to recognize me, although I think a couple of them did."

"Quite a coincidence that you decided to buy a factory in Scumble River," Skye commented.

"Not really," Carson corrected her. "I was hoping that if all else failed, maybe Walter would at least agree to run that part of my company. He's the reason I got interested in Fine Foods. I had my people look for something for us to buy that was within thirty miles of Scumble River."

"So, why didn't you offer me that job, Dad?" Wally looked puzzled.

"Because he's decided not to buy the factory after all," Skye blurted out. "Right?"

"Right." Carson grinned at Skye. "Maybe I should offer *you* a job with the company."

"Thanks, but no thanks." Skye smiled back, then explained to Wally, "Fine Foods didn't pass the reputation test. There was dissention among the family — Jared and his mom arguing over the loudspeaker at the dinner, the contest practice being sabotaged, and, of course, the murder."

"There were a few other things, too, but those were the major issues," Carson agreed. "Someone in that company doesn't want it sold, and that's a sure sign that an acquisition is going to bomb."

"The Fines don't know you're backing out. Right?" Skye remembered what Tammy had said.

"No." Carson moved toward the door. "They'll get a notice delivered from my lawyer tonight at eight, and I want to be in the air headed back to Texas when they read it."

"Have a safe flight, Dad." Wally shook Carson's hand.

Skye kissed his cheek. "You be good now,

you hear?"

As Carson made his way down the front steps to his rental car, Skye shut the door and asked Wally, "You okay with what just happened?"

"Yeah. I am." Wally took her hand in both of his. "I feel good about us. I'm glad you told me what my father had planned; otherwise it would have felt like you two had ganged up on me. And strange as it may seem, I think Dad and I are better now than we have been in years. I think he may finally understand me a little more, or at least accept who I am."

"I'd say trying to buy a factory for you proves his love, too."

"So you want me to buy you a factory?" Wally teased.

"You are so not funny." Skye stuck out her tongue. "Hey, speaking of factories, I need to tell you something about Ashley Yates."

"Did Xenia admit to kidnapping her?"

"Because I talked to Xenia as her school psychologist and not as the PD's psych consultant, all I can tell you is that Ashley was last seen alive and well Friday morning at the Fine Foods factory. She got out of a car at that location of her own free will, and hasn't been seen since."

"Let me see if I can extrapolate. Xenia and Ashley were together at the factory for whatever reason, and Ashley got out of Xenia's car." Wally scratched his chin. "At least it wasn't the day of the murder."

"Can we get a search warrant for the factory?"

"I doubt it. There's nothing to suggest she went inside. Is there?"

"Maybe." Skye reached into her pocket and handed him the March schedule for the high school's cheerleading practices. "Mom found this near the sidewalk in back of the factory."

"That's not enough to show she went inside, but tomorrow I will ask the Fines to let us look around." He tilted his head. "I'm surprised you didn't sneak in and take a peek this afternoon."

"I would never do that, now that I'm with the police force." Skye crossed her fingers and didn't mention the factory's elaborate security measures. Then she changed the subject. "Did you find out anything from your interviews after I left?"

"No, Quirk and the others couldn't break anyone's story. I'm still thinking it's Jared. He had opportunity and he's strong enough."

"That's means and opportunity, but what

about motive?"

"Maybe Cherry was blackmailing him," Wally suggested. "Now that we know about my father's interest in buying Fine Foods, and his requirement that the company have a good moral character, that would make sense."

"Any idea how to prove it?"

"No. I'm hoping that when the forensics come through, there'll be something I can use."

"Shoot. Our first unsolved case." Skye frowned.

They were silent for a few minutes; then Wally asked, "Do you still want to go to Joliet for dinner?"

"No. It's too late. By the time we drive back and forth that's at least an hour and a half, say a couple hours for a movie and an hour for dinner and an hour to buy the phones — we wouldn't be home until midnight, and I have school tomorrow."

"Right. Let's do it this weekend instead."

Wally followed Skye into the kitchen.

She looked in the fridge, shook her head, and closed it. "I'm starving, but the cupboard's bare. Unless you want me to whip up my prizewinning casserole."

"Hey, congratulations, I heard you won. That's great, but . . ."

"But you never want to taste that dish again. That's okay; neither do I."

"Phew." Wally mimicked great relief. "I was afraid that since you had won, you'd want to make it all the time."

"Right." Skye snorted. "So, back to the age-old question — what shall we do for dinner?"

"How do Italian beef sandwiches sound?"

"Yummy. From where?"

"That place in Braidwood. Antonia's."

"Sounds good. Just let me put some lipstick on, and I'm ready."

Wally dropped her off back home at ten. They had talked some more about Wally and his dad's relationship. It seemed that Wally really was fine. Skye wished she could be that casual about the twisted branches of her family tree, but that would probably never happen.

She was exhausted, and for a second considered sleeping in the sunroom rather than climbing the stairs to bed, but the thought of trying to stretch out on the short love seat spurred her up the steps. Once she successfully made it to her bedroom, she fell across her mattress fully clothed. The next thing she knew her alarm was buzzing and Bingo was licking her nose. The workweek merry-go-round had begun, and she needed to move her butt, or her carousel horse would gallop away without her.

After more than a week off, school was crazy. She had only a few minutes to say hi to Trixie before Homer swept her into his office. He sat behind his desk and rubbed his beer belly as if he were about to give birth. The kids had several nicknames for him, including Nitpicker, Homie, Crapik, but Skye thought the most appropriate was Hairy.

Homer was the most hirsute man she had ever seen. Hair grew in tufts from his head, ears, and eyebrows, and covered his body like a pelt. The principal's habit of petting himself while he talked made it hard to concentrate during a conversation with him. Even after having worked with him for several years, Skye had to make a concerted effort not to stare as he stroked his furry forearms.

At first Homer drilled Skye about Ashley's disappearance, the lawsuit, and other issues she had little or no control over, but finally he got to the real reason he had snatched her from the hallway — Mrs. Cormorant, the oldest teacher in the district and Homer's archnemesis. "You won't believe what Corny has done this time."

"What?" At this point in her career Skye was ready to believe almost anything.

"She added a box in the comment section of the report cards."

"Oh?" Skye was cautious in her reply. "I was under the impression that teachers were encouraged to write in additional remarks."

"Not anymore. Last time she did it the parents sued us, so we discontinued the policy of allowing teachers to insert unapproved statements." Homer ran his fingers through the clumps of hair sticking up from his scalp. "But that didn't stop old Corny."

"What comment did she add?"

" 'Shallow gene pool.' "

Skye held back a snort of laughter and tried to look serious when she said, "But report cards came out nearly a week ago. Why is this just coming up now?"

"Someone explained what the comment meant to the parents. Before some freaking Good Samaritan enlightened them, they thought the teacher wanted them to have their son swim in deeper water this summer."

Skye bit the inside of her cheek to stop herself from laughing. "I take it once the parents received this little nugget of wisdom, they were not amused."

"They're demanding an apology from the

school and the teacher."

"And my guess is Cormorant refuses to say she's sorry." Homer nodded, and Skye went on, "And my second guess is that you want me to convince her."

Homer nodded again.

"We've been through this before; Pru Cormorant does not like me. I am the wrong person to get her to do anything."

"Hey, we all know her receiver is off the hook, but everyone else is afraid of her."

"What makes you think I'm not?" Skye demanded.

"Anyone who has faced down as many murderers as you have should be able to handle one little old lady."

"Except that she isn't little, and she isn't a lady."

Homer took up another hour of her time whining about various other situations, then glanced at his watch and verbally shoved her out the door with the admonishment, "Remember, talk to Corny and make her see the light."

As Skye walked away, she muttered, "I'd rather make the harridan go into the light than try to make her see it."

Despite her grumbling, Skye had long since realized that it was easier to do what

351

the principal told her to and get it over with, rather than argue. With this in mind she checked the master schedule and saw that Mrs. Cormorant was free for the next seventeen minutes. Perfect. By the time the next bell rang, the distasteful task would be done.

Pru Cormorant had one of the best class-rooms in the building. It had actual walls — instead of folding curtains — windows, and even a door to the outside. Because of this it was a well-known fact that if the weather was nice she usually spent her planning periods on a lawn chair on the grass.

Skye found Pru there reading a spicy romance, which she quickly hid under a copy of *Moby-Dick.* Skye pretended not to notice, not that she cared what the other woman read, and said, "Hi, are you enjoying the sunshine?"

"Yes, it's so nice to be able to pop out here during the day." Pru's watery blue eyes were malicious. "Your office doesn't have a door to the outside, does it, dear?"

"No, but then, I'm usually too busy to notice."

"Yes, I suppose you are." Pru raised an overplucked eyebrow. "The students nowadays aren't like they were when I started at Scumble River High School."

Skye bit her tongue to stop herself from asking what it was like to teach in the Stone Age, and instead said, "Actually, that's what I wanted to talk to you about. Homer asked me to see if you might have changed your mind about apologizing to those parents who were insulted by your comment on their son's report card."

"No."

"No?"

"No, I haven't changed my mind and I won't." Pru patted her stringy, dun-colored hair. "We need to stop coddling these parents. No Child Left Behind, my eye. Anyone with the slightest knowledge of the bell curve knows the largest portion of students are going to be average; then there's going to be a certain number who are gifted, and, sadly, there are going to be an equal number who are dim-witted. The sooner the parents accept that not every child is going to Harvard or even to a community college, the better. Look at the poor Fines."

"The Fines?" Skye had been letting Pru ramble, having heard her opinion on the subject before, but suddenly she tuned in. "You mean the family that owns Fine Foods? What about them?"

"They spent a fortune on tutors and

donations getting those two boys through college." Pru licked her thin lips. "At least they were satisfied when JJ got a BA in business, but they poured even more money into getting Brandon through law school."

"But he got his degree, right?" Skye frowned. "Money is never wasted on an education."

"He got his degree, all right, but it's useless."

"Why?"

"He can't pass the bar exam." Pru smiled meanly. "He's tried and tried, even other states' bar exams, but there's only so much being rich can do for you. And buying you a license to practice law isn't one of them."

After leaving Pru, Skye checked with Frannie and Justin, as well as Ashley's fellow cheerleaders. No one had heard from Ashley, and no one seemed particularly worried. They all claimed the girl was behind her own disappearance, and that she'd show up when she got bored, but Skye suspected the students knew more than they were saying — maybe not about where Ashley was, but about why she had disappeared.

The rest of the day whizzed by as Skye prepared for and attended both the junior high and the high school's bimonthly Pupil

Personal Services meetings. She was kept busy pulling and reading files, taking notes, and getting paperwork ready to start several reevaluations.

Students in special education had to be evaluated by the psychologist triennially, so every three years a third of the kids receiving services had to be tested. These assessments often took up the majority of a school psychologist's time, and Skye was no exception.

When the final bell rang at three, Trixie Frayne burst through Skye's door. Skye hurriedly finished filling in a consent form, tucked it into its folder, and filed it away. She was anxious to talk to her friend, hoping Trixie would provide a fresh take on both the murder and the disappearance.

Trixie was the school librarian, cheerleading coach, and cosponsor of the student newspaper. She reminded Skye of a brownie — not the Girl Scout, the forest imp. She had short nut brown hair and cocoa-colored eyes, a size-four body, and high spirits.

Her first words were, "Why does everything exciting happen when I'm gone?"

Skye ignored Trixie's question — Trixie had been involved in lots of Skye's past adventures — and asked, "Did you have a romantic getaway?"

"Yes." Trixie's grin was lascivious. "Times like this weekend remind me why I married Owen. Woo, that man has stamina."

"My number one criteria for a good husband," Skye said dryly.

"Yeah, right." Trixie sneered. "That's why you dumped Mr. Nice for Mr. Hot."

"We are so not going there."

"You brought it up." Trixie snatched a piece of Easter candy from the jar on Skye's desk.

"Can we talk about something else, like our missing student and the murder?" Skye filled Trixie in on what she could about what Xenia had told her about Ashley, avoiding breaking confidentiality by a hair.

"Boy." Trixie crossed her legs and dangled her pink high-heeled sandal from her toe. "That girl is a pepperoni short of a pizza."

"True," Skye agreed, then gave Trixie the lowdown on the murder and Wally's dad, concluding with, "It all seems to coalesce around the Fine Foods factory."

"It does, doesn't it?"

Skye got up and went over to a portable blackboard someone had stored in her office. She'd asked the custodian to remove it, but hadn't bugged him enough yet to stir him to action. For now she'd put it to good use.

She picked up a piece of chalk and began to outline. "The first thing that happened is that Wally's dad decides to look into acquiring Fine Foods. He'll buy it only if the company has a good reputation, so he comes to town in disguise during the cooking contest — their biggest PR event — to check that out."

Trixie nodded. "Number one: The sale of the factory hinges on its good name."

"Second, the Friday morning before the contestants get to the factory, Ashley runs away from her abductor in the Fine Foods parking lot and has not been seen again."

Trixie grabbed a foil-wrapped candy egg. "Number two: Does Ashley get inside despite the security measures you mentioned, and if so, is she still there?"

"Third, the contest has an unusual number of problems this year. The practice round is sabotaged. Jared and Grandma Sal's private argument is broadcast on the PA, doors that were supposed to be locked aren't, and to top it off, a woman is murdered." Skye paused, thinking. "Not to mention, who in his or her right mind would think Glenda Doozier's cooking is worthy of finaling?"

"Number three: Someone knew Carson Boyd was here watching the contest. Knew he wouldn't go through with the deal if Fine Foods ended up looking bad, and so this person made sure that it did."

"That's it!" Skye jerked as if she'd been zapped by a cattle prod. "Wally and I have been thinking that Cherry was murdered because she had something on the company that would ruin its reputation, but it's the opposite. I'll bet she caught someone sabotaging the contest, and that person killed her to keep her quiet."

Trixie licked the chocolate from her fingers. "So who wouldn't want the company sold?"

Skye wrote a list of names on the board. "Jared and Tammy can't wait for it to sell. If I remember my brief conversation with Brandon and JJ, both of them don't like it here at Scumble River either, so that only leaves Grandma Sal and maybe all the factory workers, if they're afraid for their jobs."

"Isn't Grandma Sal a little old to be lifting bodies into chocolate fountains?"

"She may be in her late seventies, but she's a big, strong woman who could probably outrun me in a race, maybe even you if it was an endurance event." Skye bit her lip. "The big question is, would she be willing to make her own company look bad in order to keep it? And since she owns the majority percentage, why would she have to?"

"Yeah. As Nancy Reagan used to urge, she could just say no." Trixie pursed her mouth. "On the other hand, would anyone outside the family know about the terms of the sale? The employees might know CB International is interested in buying Fine Foods, but would they know the one thing that would stop the sale?"

"Good question."

Trixie and Skye sat in silence as they tried to think of another suspect.

Finally, when neither of them could come up with anything new, Trixie jumped up from her seat. "I'd better get home. There's a pile of laundry with my name on it. And I need to stop at the grocery store. Owen will be looking for his supper at five on the dot, and I don't have a thing to cook."

Skye waved good-bye to her friend, then closed her eyes and thought about what she and Trixie had discovered. *Hmm.* If Grandma Sal was not a suspect — and since she could stop the deal simply by refusing to sign the papers, she didn't look likely — that meant maybe she'd agree to answer a few questions. It was only three thirty, and she might still be at the factory.

A quick phone call verified that Skye was in luck. Mrs. Fine wasn't officially there, but she had stopped by to sign some papers. However, she was leaving in an hour, and although she was willing to talk to Skye, Skye needed to arrive within fifteen minutes.

While dialing the police station, Skye hurriedly packed up her tote bag. The dispatcher said that Wally was out, but had left a message that he hadn't been able to secure permission to search the factory and would stop by her house when he got off work at five. Skye left him a message saying she was going to talk to Grandma Sal, and would try to change the older woman's mind about giving them permission to look for Ashley.

Wishing she and Wally had stuck to their plan and gone to buy cell phones yesterday, Skye got into her car and headed toward the factory. As she drove, she fingered the container of pepper spray in her blazer pocket, wondering if she was making a bad move. If she was wrong, and Grandma Sal was the killer, Skye could end up looking very stupid . . . and possibly very dead.

CHAPTER 21
COOL COMPLETELY

Entering Grandma Sal's office, Skye was taken aback at both the decor and Grandma Sal herself. Instead of the sweet old lady she had met at the cooking contest, whose image was on all the products, a well-dressed, attractive woman sat behind a sleek chrome-and-glass desk.

Gone were the gray curls, the wire-rimmed glasses, the flowered dress, and the old-fashioned hat. Instead Grandma Sal's hair was now ash blond and styled in a smooth French twist. She wore a stylish pink Chanel suit with matching high-heeled pumps.

Skye stood staring while the secretary announced her.

Even after Grandma Sal looked up and said, "What can I do for you, dear?" Skye was speechless.

The older woman prodded, "A lot of people are surprised when they see the real Sally Fine, after meeting 'Grandma Sal.' I only dress like a little old lady for public appearances."

"Oh, of course." Skye's cheeks flamed. "I understand completely."

"I'm so sorry we had your name wrong throughout the contest. I assure you we'll get the spelling fixed on your plaque, and it will be correct on your check."

"Thank you. It's an unusual name. I completely understand the mix-up."

"Then I take it you're here for another reason. Have a seat."

"Thanks." Skye sat in one of the leather-and-chrome visitor's chairs, put her tote bag by her feet, and craned her neck to look around a huge rolling pin–shaped trophy that was directly in front of her.

"Go ahead and move that thing over." Mrs. Fine blew out an exasperated breath. "I can't quite figure out what to do with it. Fine Foods won it for having the most homemade-tasting packaged foods."

Skye reached out her right hand to shove the prize to the side, and was surprised by the weight of the marble award. Grunting a little as she pushed, she said, "I'm here as the police department's psychological consultant."

"Is there news about Ms. Alexander's unfortunate death?"

"Well, we have put some pieces of the puzzle together, but still haven't quite found that final part — the name of the murderer. Which is why I wanted to talk to you."

"You think there's something I can do to help?"

"I hope so." Skye wrinkled her brow, choosing her words carefully. "Once we learned about CB International's interest in Fine Foods, and the fact that they would buy the company only if it had an exemplary reputation, we figured that whoever killed Cherry did so to stop the sale of the business."

"No." Mrs. Fine toyed with her Montblanc pen. "I don't believe that for one minute."

As Skye tried to decide the best way to respond to the older woman's denial, she was startled by a loud whistle. "What was that?"

Mrs. Fine put down the pen and smiled, seemingly relieved at the interruption. "It's just quitting time."

"Right." Skye nodded to herself. "You don't run an evening shift anymore."

"Not for quite some time. That's one of the reasons it would have been good for us to sell to CB International. They would have expanded our sales by three or four times, and we could have gone back to running around the clock."

Skye filed that piece of info away, then asked, "Who was familiar with the conditions of the transaction with CB?"

"The only ones who knew about their stipulations were the family." Mrs. Fine paled under her artfully applied makeup. "The only ones with anything to gain or lose are Fines."

"Would any of the workers not want the factory sold?"

"They were all assured that no one would lose their jobs, and, in fact, it was highly likely that more positions would be created."

"In that case, *who* didn't want the transaction to be completed?"

"No one." Mrs. Fine's voice cracked. "I was the only one who was the least bit against the sale, and Jared and JJ convinced me it was for the best."

"What about Brandon and Tammy?"

"They don't have a say in the matter. Tammy has nothing to do with the company, and Brandon is only Jared's stepson. Although we allow him to use the Fine name, Tammy had Brandon before she married Jared. He was already six months old at the time of their wedding."

"Jared never adopted Brandon?"

"No, not officially. Brandon and Tammy aren't really Fines. My husband left fifty-five percent of the company to me, thirty percent to Jared, and fifteen percent to JJ. He felt strongly that only blood relations should own Fine Foods." Mrs. Fine closed her eyes, lines of pain etched in her forehead. "Which is why I didn't want to sell it to CB International."

Skye refrained from pointing out that Mrs. Fine wasn't a Fine by blood either, and instead asked, "If the company is sold, would Tammy and Brandon get a share then?"

"Well, Tammy would have access to Jared's money, but I doubt Jared or JJ would give any significant amount to Brandon. They just aren't that close. And I'm leaving all my money to the Fine Foundation for the Arts."

Interesting family dynamics, not that Skye was surprised. After several years as a school psychologist, she'd seen a lot worse. "So, you can't think of anyone who had anything to gain or lose if the company was sold?" She knew she was on the right track and was frustrated that she couldn't figure out what she was missing.

"No, but I'll think about it and give you a

call if something comes to me."

"Thank you." Skye pushed back her chair and grabbed her tote bag; then as she got up she remembered Ashley, and asked, "I know you've already said no, but is there anything I can say that will convince you to reconsider, and allow us to search the factory for the missing girl?"

"What missing girl?"

Skye explained, ending with, "So the last time she was seen was outside your factory."

"No one told me about this. Of course you can search for her." Mrs. Fine rubbed her temples as if she had a headache. "I can't imagine how she'd get in here or why she'd stay, but feel free to look around."

"That's wonderful. Can I do it right now?"

"Certainly." Mrs. Fine reached into a black lacquer box on the desk and took out a key. "I have to leave for an appointment in the city, so you'll need this master to look around and to get out — the guards lock up when everyone goes home for the night."

"Everyone's already gone?" Skye looked at her watch. It was only four thirty.

"The building empties out fast once the whistle blows. Even the guards are gone by this time."

"You don't have twenty-four-hour security?"

"Not inside the building. They have a booth near the gate and patrol the perimeter of the property."

"Oh." Skye nodded. "What should I do with the key once I let myself out?"

"You can drop it off tomorrow."

Mrs. Fine walked with Skye as far as the lobby. "If you need to use the phone, the only one that works after hours is the one in my office. Help yourself." She waved, unlocked the front door, and left.

Skye paused to figure out what to do next, then decided the best course of action was to return to Mrs. Fine's office and call the PD for help with the search. The factory was just too big, with too many nooks and crannies to look through all by herself.

As she walked back, she read the name-plates on the doors she passed. Jared's office was closest to the front, then the business office, then the legal department, then . . .

She stopped and stared at the door. Suddenly the memory of what Pru Cormorant had said, added to what Mrs. Fine had just revealed, and what she and Trixie had figured out about the killer coalesced and she blurted out, "That's it! Brandon killed Cherry because —"

Before she could finish her thought,

someone grabbed her arm and she shrieked. Brandon Fine loomed at her side, a scowl on his face. Had he heard her? She had to quit talking out loud to herself — a habit she had picked up since adopting Bingo.

She quickly ran through various mental scenarios and decided that if he hadn't heard her, maybe she could distract him. "Uh, hi, Brandon. I, um, was just getting permission from your grandmother to search for a missing teenager."

"Shut up!" His fingers dug into the flesh of her upper arm, and her tote bag thumped against her hip. "I thought you were supposed to be so smart. Who do you think turned down the cops in the first place?"

"Oh." Great, he wasn't just the murderer; he had something to do with Ashley's disappearance as well. "Anyway, your grandma said yes, and the cops will be here any minute, so I'd better get to the door to let them in before they break it down." Skye's laugh was forced.

"Drop the act. I was standing at my grandmother's secretary's desk when you called earlier this afternoon. I'd heard how nosy you are and that you 'help' the police, so I hung around and found out you were coming here to talk to Grandma. I've been following you and eavesdropping on you since you got here."

Skye fought to keep her face expressionless. If she played dumb, maybe she could convince him she thought his brother was the killer. "But why would you do that? Are you protecting JJ?" She slipped her free hand into her jacket pocket and grasped the small can of pepper spray.

She read the hesitation in his dark eyes as he considered what she had said, and whether he could put the blame on his half brother. Taking advantage of his momentary distraction, she jerked her left arm free and used her right hand to empty the pepper spray directly into his eyes.

He howled, clawing at his face.

Now what should she do? He stood between her and the exit, and she was afraid he would recover before she could get around him and unlock the dead bolt. She had only one choice: She dashed into the factory and was frantically looking for a door when she heard Brandon's footsteps thundering toward her. She quickly hid behind the giant mixer — ironically the same one he had demonstrated during last Friday's tour.

A second later Brandon came into sight. He paused, looked around, then approached the huge machine. As he leaned over the rim and peered down into the enormous bowl, Skye darted from behind the control panel and shoved him with all her strength. At first he teetered, then nearly regained his balance, but one more thrust from her and he fell inside. She whirled around, flipped the switch to the ON position, and ran.

Skye came to a dead end in the area Brandon had called the Boneyard. Here ancient machinery was piled against the rear wall, and there was a feeling of longtime disuse and abandonment. She anxiously scanned the equipment for a hiding place. Draping the straps of her tote bag across her chest, she wiggled behind an apparatus bristling with rusting steel hooks. As she stood holding her breath, she examined the spot she had wedged herself into.

The walls were puke green, and there were no windows or doors. Her gaze dropped to the wooden floor and stuttered to a stop on a section to her right where the seams didn't seem to meet evenly. It probably didn't mean anything, but just as she always had to check the coin tray when she passed a vending machine, knowing it would be empty, she scooted over and nudged the wood with her toe. Had it wobbled just a tad?

It was a tight squeeze, but Skye managed

to get down on her hands and knees. She found a nail file in her tote bag and slipped it into the irregular area. She could feel a definite wiggle this time as she used the file as a lever.

For a heart-stopping moment nothing happened; then a square of the wooden floor swung upward . . . and stuck halfway open. It had caught on a piece of equipment shoved against it. Skye braced herself against the hook machine and pushed.

The door moved only a few inches, but Skye thought she could fit — maybe. She peered over the edge and saw a ladder nailed to the wall. Slithering into the small space like a dancer going under a limbo bar backward, she managed to get her foot on the first rung.

She was still half in and half out when she heard the mixer stop. Had Brandon escaped or had the motor burned out?

Ignoring the painful scraping of the skin on her back, Skye jerked herself through the opening, blindly stepping down until she could shut the door. She'd been prepared for total darkness, but once her eyes adjusted she could see a light coming from somewhere beneath her.

As she descended, she prayed for help. She was afraid to take her eyes from the ladder, so she was surprised when her foot encountered solid ground. Stepping away from the wall, she saw that she was in some sort of storage basement.

Now what? Her only hope was that if Brandon had escaped from the mixer he wouldn't find the trapdoor, which he wouldn't see unless he stood in the exact place Skye had been standing. If he only gave the area behind the old machinery a cursory look, he wouldn't notice it.

At first all she could see were old file cabinets, desks, some boxes, and bookcases, but as she took a few steps farther into the area, she swallowed a scream. Lying on a worn leather sofa, eyes closed, perfectly still, was Ashley Yates.

A tear slipped down Skye's cheek. Ashley was dead. She was too late to save her.

But a husky voice penetrated her grief. "Is that you, Ms. Denison? How'd you find me?"

Skye's head jerked up, and she ran to the sofa. "It's me, all right." She knelt beside Ashley. "Are you okay?"

"No." The teen started sobbing. "I think my leg's broken, and I'm hungry and thirsty."

Skye lifted the strap of her tote bag over her head and plunged her hand inside.

Grabbing the bottle of water she always kept there, she opened it and handed it to Ashley, cautioning, "Drink this slowly, or it will make you sick."

In between sips, Ashley said, "I ran out of water and food yesterday."

Skye found her emergency candy bar and handed over the Kit Kat. Ashley tore off the wrapper and stuffed a piece of chocolate into her mouth.

Skye had met the girl's basic needs for food and liquid, but there was nothing she could do for Ashley's leg.

After giving the teen a few seconds to compose herself, and remembering to keep her voice low, Skye asked, "What happened? How did you get here? I mean in this basement. I know how you got to the factory."

"Xenia told you?" Ashley followed Skye's lead, keeping her voice barely above a whisper. "When Xenia showed me the pictures Friday morning, I knew my parents would kill me, so I decided to run away. I thought I could hide in the factory while I figured out where to go, but all the doors were locked. I was about to give up when a semi pulled away and I noticed that the big door it had been backed up to was still open. I climbed up onto this kind of wooden deck thing and suddenly I was inside. I spent most of the rest of the day hiding in a storage closet, and then I spent the night in the employee lounge."

Skye examined the area they were in as Ashley talked. She was listening to the teen, but also searching for a way out. So far there was no sign of Brandon. Had she killed him by shoving him in the mixer and turning it on?

When Ashley paused, Skye asked, "Then what happened?"

"I figured I'd have the place to myself on Saturday, since the factory would be closed, but way early I started hearing noises. First an old lady came in with a middle-aged guy. They went to the front part of the plant and into separate offices. Then I saw this younger guy unlock the back door where the workers come in and put on one of those white jumpsuits they wear. He went into the warehouse, and I could hear all kinds of rattling and clunking."

Skye nodded to herself. That must have been when Brandon sabotaged the cooking contest. No doubt he arrived early on Friday, too, and substituted ingredients, messed with timers, and switched the dials on the ovens.

Ashley had paused to lick chocolate from her fingers, but continued, "Next this

374

redheaded woman slips in and it's quiet for a while, but suddenly it sounds like a battle of the bands. So I sneak in and that's when I saw it."

"Saw what?" Skye glanced nervously upward. Had she heard footsteps?

"The guy in the jumpsuit hit the red-headed lady over the head with this ham-merlike thing my mom uses to flatten meat. After he hits her, he dumps her in this fountain and holds her under."

"What did you do?"

"I ducked into one of the little kitchens." Ashley took a swig of water. "I could still see what was happening through the gap where the partitions went together."

"What happened next?"

"I heard a noise in one of the other little kitchens; then Mayor Leofanti came around the corner. When he spotted the woman in the fountain he ran up and bent down to help her; then Jumpsuit Guy threw a table-cloth over his head, spun him around, and stabbed him in the stomach with this little knife he had in his pocket. Blood gushed out like a geyser." Ashley took another drink. "That's when I screamed."

"And?"

"And Jumpsuit Guy must have followed the sound, because he found me and tried to kill me." Tears welled up in her eyes. "He really tried to kill me."

Skye patted the girl's hand. Most teenagers had no concept of their own mortality, but Ashley had looked the Grim Reaper in the face and seen her own death in his expression. "Is that how you broke your leg?"

"No." Ashley took a deep breath and went on. "He came after me with that hammer thingy, and just as he swung downward with it to hit me I fainted, and it must have just grazed my forehead. He obviously thought I was dead, because when I came to I was wrapped in a sheet and lying in the back of one of the Fine Food vans. As I was getting out I spotted Jumpsuit Guy coming toward me, so I ran the other way around the van and circled over to the side of the factory."

Skye patted her again and made an encouraging sound.

"My head hurt and I was dizzy, but I knew he'd kill me if he found me. I was looking for someplace to hide when I saw these windows." Ashley pointed up.

Skye looked at the row of windows near the ceiling of the basement. Weren't basements supposed to have low ceilings? This one had to be twelve or fourteen feet high.

"The locks were all old and rusted, and I

was able to push one open. Just as I was climbing inside I heard the guy coming, and I miscalculated, so instead of stepping in and hopping down, I crashed to the floor. Luckily the window must have snapped closed behind me, because Jumpsuit Guy walked right by and never found me. I think I passed out again, because when I came to it was dark and I couldn't move my leg."

Skye sucked in her breath, feeling the pain and terror that Ashley must have experienced. "And you've been trapped here ever since?"

"Yes. I was able to drag myself around using that." She pointed to a wheeled stenographer's chair. "But I couldn't climb the ladder you came down, and I couldn't get back up to the windows, and my cell battery died before I could get a signal in here." She took a teary breath before going on. "At first I tried screaming. Then I realized: What if Jumpsuit Guy was the one who heard me yelling? There's a bathroom over in the back there, but after the second day the faucet stopped working. I had a bottle of water and some energy bars in my backpack, but I ran out yesterday. I thought I was going to die here."

Skye opened her mouth to reassure Ashley, but before she could come up with any comforting words, the teen asked, "So, how did you get here, and how do we get out?"

CHAPTER 22
FROST THE CAKE

After Skye explained to Ashley how she had found her, Skye tried to come up with an answer to the girl's second question. How could they get out?

Pacing the length of the basement, Skye searched for an exit. She found evidence of a door that had long since been bricked over, but there was no way to remove the concrete blocks.

Her next objective was a weapon, but there was nothing except abandoned office furniture and box after box of tightly packed paper files dating back to the first year the company was in business. Clearly Fine Foods' philosophy was the same as the school system's: Never keep just one copy of a document when you can keep twelve instead.

After several circuits Skye was forced to accept that the only way out was via the windows that Ashley had entered through.

Unfortunately there were a couple of problems with that solution. First and foremost, with her broken leg, there was no way the teen could climb up that far, and second, even if Skye could make the climb — which was iffy — that would mean leaving Ashley behind.

Skye went over to the girl, knelt back down, and took her hand. "It looks like I'll have to go out the window you came through."

"No." Ashley's fingers clutched Skye's. "Please don't leave me. I'm sorry for everything. For having sex with all those boys, for lying about it, for getting the paper in trouble. I'll be good if you get me out of here; I promise."

"Ashley." Skye put her other arm around the girl. "I'm not leaving you because I'm mad at you or because you were bad. I'm going because it's the only way out, and I need to get help. We can't wait to be rescued. The guy chasing us is Brandon Fine, and eventually he's going to find us."

"But what if he finds me before you get back?"

"Once I'm out the window, I promise I'll have help back here in ten minutes, fifteen at the most."

"Don't go," Ashley sobbed. "I just know

he'll get me while you're gone."

Skye hesitated. What if the girl was right? No. She had to play the odds. If Brandon hadn't found Ashley before now, that meant he didn't know about this basement. Judging from the dates on the files, the room hadn't been used since before he was born.

"I'm sorry, honey, but I have to. I just can't figure out any other way to save us both."

Before starting to build her ladder to freedom, Skye climbed back up the wooden one and listened at the trapdoor. She couldn't hear anything. Either the floor was extremely thick, which would explain why no one had heard Ashley's screams for help, or Skye had killed Brandon when she pushed him in the mixer. Better yet, he might have simply given up — but she kind of doubted that. He was probably lying in wait like a shark at a shipwreck, poised to pounce once Skye jumped overboard.

Skye pushed a double filing cabinet under the window bank. Next to it she shoved a desk and a chair; then she went to work piling boxes full of paper on the desktop. Once she figured she had enough, she got onto the desk and transferred the cartons onto the file cabinet. She followed this system

381

until she had steps that reached nearly to the sill.

She took her car keys and the factory key from her tote and stuffed them both down her bra, then stripped off her blazer. When she was down to slacks and a cami, she considered her shoes. They were loafers with an inch-and-a-half heel; was she better off with or without them?

Deciding to try the ascent with the shoes and discard them if they got in the way, she started up the shaky box staircase. With each step she felt as if the whole structure were about to come tumbling down, but she reached the top unscathed.

Taking a deep breath, she grasped the handle of the window and pulled. Cool, fresh air poured into the dank basement. Skye took a greedy breath before placing her foot on the ledge and heaving herself upward.

She teetered — caught halfway between the top box and the windowsill. *Crap.* If she made it out of here alive, she really had to work on her upper-body strength. Steeling her arms and praying to the gym gods, Skye pulled.

Suddenly she was on the sill, then through the window. Stunned, she stood there for a moment. A few seconds later she was running toward the parking lot, keys in hand. She skidded to a stop by the Bel Air and suppressed a scream of frustration. Someone had slashed all four tires — probably Brandon.

Okay, plan B. The guards Mrs. Fine had mentioned earlier that afternoon. She had said they had a booth near the road. Skye jogged the quarter mile down the lane, gasping for breath. She really needed to get more exercise if she was going to keep running away from killers. Now she knew why Charlie's Angels were so skinny.

Skye arrived at the security booth, only to find it empty. Now what? Plan C was to wave down a car, but who would drive by on a road that dead-ended at the gate? That left plan D, otherwise known as Dumb Move — go back to the building and try to use Grandma Sal's phone. But she couldn't think of a plan E — it would take her at least half an hour to walk into town, which was just too long to leave Ashley alone with Brandon on the prowl. If only she knew whether she had incapacitated him in the mixer.

Maybe she could find a guard patrolling the factory's perimeter. Summoning up the last of her energy, Skye ran back down the lane and around the building, but there was nothing stirring, not even a mouse. Where were the fricking guards? If she got out of this alive, she would make Mrs. Fine fire them all.

Finally she faced the fact that there was no one to help her; if she wanted to save Ashley, she would have to do it herself. Having come to that conclusion, Skye knew she had to go back inside and get to the telephone. Too bad Ashley had used up her cell phone's battery trying to get a signal.

With no other choice, hoping she wasn't being as stupid as she felt, Skye used the key Mrs. Fine had given her and slipped back inside. She stopped briefly to wedge the door open with a flattened soda can she had found in the parking lot.

She kept to the wall, edging around the lobby and down the hall to the offices. She eased into Mrs. Fine's office, closed and locked the door, then grabbed the phone and dialed.

The dispatcher answered on the first ring. "Scumble River police, fire, and emergency. How may I help you?"

"Thea, this is Skye. I'm in the Fine Foods factory and need backup right away. I've found Ashley Yates, who is injured. Cherry Alexander's killer is in the building trying to find and kill both of us."

Thea gasped and dropped the receiver. Before she came back on the line, Skye heard the sound of splintering wood. The office door crashed down and Brandon rushed in. His maniacal grin reminded her of Jack Nicholson in *The Shining*, except that instead of brandishing an ax, he was wielding a wooden mixing paddle, and instead of his being covered in blood, batter dripped off him like alien sweat.

Skye grabbed one of the chrome-and-leather chairs and backed toward the window, wondering if she could break the glass and escape before Brandon reached her.

He advanced, yanking the phone cord from the wall, then swung the paddle at Skye. She leapt to the side and he missed, cracking the windowpane.

Backing away, she kept poking the chair at him as if he were a lion and she his tamer. Her goal the door, she moved around the desk, trying to keep it between her and her attacker.

Unfortunately Brandon had not read the same self-defense book that Skye had, because instead of chasing her around the desk, as he was supposed to, he employed a flying tackle that would earn him a place on the Chicago Bears football team, if they ever decided to recruit homicidal maniacs. Landing on top of her, he wrapped his hands around her neck and squeezed.

Skye tried to pry his fingers from her throat, but he tightened his grip. She knew she had only a few minutes before she lost consciousness, and she groped blindly behind her in search of a weapon.

Just as she was starting to black out, her hand encountered the rolling pin trophy. With her last bit of strength she grasped the handle, dragged it off the desktop, and brought it down on Brandon's skull.

His hands relaxed a fraction, but he didn't remove them from around her neck. She didn't have the strength to lift the heavy trophy and hit him again. This was it. She would die. She would die at the hands of a wannabe lawyer who couldn't even pass the bar exam, and was willing to kill in order to ensure the huge salary he couldn't earn anywhere but in his family-owned business.

Suddenly he stiffened, then collapsed on top of her. When his fingers fell away from her throat and she was able to draw in desperate breaths, she shoved him off of her and got unsteadily to her feet.

He lay limp, unmoving. Had her blow killed him? Skye wasn't taking any chances. She had to get away from him. She limped toward the exit, and had just put a foot on the downed door when the thunder of pounding footsteps was followed by a blur of navy blue uniforms rushing through.

Wally was in the lead, and he swept her up in his arms and out of the way of the column of officers swarming the room. He helped her out into the hallway.

"Are you okay?" His dark gaze searched her face.

She nodded, gulped in more air, and managed to get out, "Now I am."

Wally's arms tightened around her. "Forget about me buying you a cell phone. I'm having a GPS chip implanted in your butt."

EPILOGUE
MAKES TWELVE
SERVINGS

As per tradition, May and Jed entertained his side of the family for Easter. Also, as per tradition, May invited anyone she thought might be alone for the holiday. Which meant that in addition to the Denison clan, Frannie, Xavier, and Uncle Charlie were also present. Mr. and Mrs. Boward had declined, but allowed Justin to attend without them.

Vince was absent, as well. He and Loretta had opted for her family's celebration. It was clear to Skye that her mother was torn regarding that situation. On the one hand, this was a first for Vince and showed that he was serious about his relationship with Loretta. On the other hand, Vince was not at May's table — nor under her control.

Knowing her mother as she did, Skye had wondered briefly if May would invite Simon and Bunny. After all, she had included them in the past. But thank goodness, there was no sign of either Skye's ex or his mother.

Dinner was over, and the men who had followed Jed to the living room were sprawled in various stages of digestive stupor, watching — or at least snoozing in front of — the television set, which was tuned to a baseball game.

Skye had stayed in the kitchen with her mother and most of the other women, having long since given up on the notion of ever achieving equality between the sexes in her family. As she helped clear the table, she thought of the hope and renewal she'd felt while attending Easter Sunday Mass.

After she'd spent the past week enmeshed in the greed and despair that had ultimately resulted in the murder of Cherry Alexander and the attacks on Ashley Yates and Dante Leofanti, the service had been exactly what she needed.

As usual, Father Burns had ended with a bit of gentle wisdom. "If you're having trouble sleeping at night, don't count the sheep; talk to the shepherd."

Skye smiled, thinking of the priest's advice. May asked, "What are you so happy about?"

"I was just thinking about Father Burns's comment at the end of Mass."

"Yeah, that was one of his better ones." May nodded. "At least he didn't try to be funny." She took a breath and changed the subject. "I'm glad I took this week off from work. Thea tells me it's been crazy around the station."

"That's for sure. Even though Brandon is still in the hospital under guard, his lawyers have been all over us." Skye delivered another pile of dirty dishes to the sink. "Thank goodness that at least Ashley is okay, her parents have dropped their lawsuit, and the school newspaper is up and running."

"Why are Brandon's lawyers all over you?" Uncle Charlie marched in and pulled out a kitchen chair. "They caught the little bastard red-handed."

"Not exactly." Skye wiped the table with a dishrag. "I had already hit him over the head with the trophy by the time the police arrived — though, luckily, I had the bruises around my throat to prove he had tried to strangle me."

"Yeah." May snorted. "That was real fortunate."

"Ms. D." Frannie walked into the kitchen and sat next to Charlie. "I know at first you said you didn't want to talk about it, but can you tell us now how you figured out who the murderer was and why he did it?"

Justin had followed Frannie, and now sat on her other side. "Yeah. We're dying to hear what happened."

"Okay." Skye wasn't really ready to discuss the subject, but there was no escaping some things in life. "Since you and Justin have been so good about visiting Ashley while she recovered this week, and have promised to help her get around once she comes back to school, I'll tell you the whole story.

"Let's see, it all started when the Fines decided to sell their company to CB International. All the 'real' Fines would make a lot of money from the deal, but Brandon, being only a stepson and not owning any of Fine Foods, would get nothing. Worse than that, he would lose his position as head of the legal department. Where else could an attorney who couldn't pass the bar be put in charge and earn such a huge salary from the very start?"

"So, his motive was to stop the sale?" Uncle Charlie spooned sugar into the mug of coffee May had put in front of him.

"Right, and being family and head of the legal department, he was aware that the sale would go through only if Fine Foods' reputation was squeaky clean. So he set out to sabotage the contest." Skye took a seat on Charlie's other side. "Then, when Cherry caught him switching the temperature-control knob on the oven in my cubicle so I would burn my dish, he lashed out with a meat mallet and knocked her out, then held her down in the fountain."

"How do you know that?" Justin demanded.

"Before Brandon's mother stepped in and got him a team of criminal lawyers to defend him, he claimed he was going to defend himself, and he told Wally everything to 'explain' his actions. His attorneys are now claiming that he wasn't thinking straight due to his head injury and are trying to get the confession suppressed."

Charlie harrumphed. "You'd think a lawyer would know enough to keep his mouth shut."

"Yeah." Justin shook his head. "That guy has to be really stupid to think he could justify murder."

"Well, that would explain why he couldn't pass the bar exam," Frannie pointed out.

From the sink May said, "He could have just bribed Cherry with winning the contest."

"He didn't know she'd be receptive to that, and besides, he wasn't thinking at that point, just reacting to what he perceived as a threat. The problem was, Brandon had counted on the warehouse being empty, not realizing that in Scumble River 'on time' is actually fifteen minutes early."

Frannie snickered.

"So, Dante was nosing around before the official start time and discovered Cherry's body in the fountain. Brandon saw him and threw a tablecloth over Dante's head so he couldn't identify him. Then Brandon stabbed Dante in order to distract him while Brandon made his getaway. Incidentally, they found the pocketknife on Brandon. He'd tried to clean it up, but it contained traces of Dante's blood type. A sample has gone for DNA analysis."

"That's got to be one for the good guys." Charlie sipped his coffee.

"Anyway, as he stabbed Dante, Brandon heard a scream and realized there was another witness — Ashley Yates, who had spent the night in the factory because she couldn't face her parents' knowing there was proof of her sexual escapades. He hit Ashley with the meat mallet, stowed what he thought was her body in a company van, and went to get the keys to the vehicle. While he was gone, she came to and climbed out of the van. Unfortunately he returned at that precise moment. She ran away from him, and he chased her back toward the factory."

May waved her soapy hand in the air. "That must have been when I stopped him to help me carry my cooking supplies."

"Right. He was the person in the jumpsuit and hairnet." Skye shook her head. "Only you, Mom, could get someone in the middle of committing multiple murders to stop and do what you wanted."

May's smile was smug. "Why didn't he find Ashley? He ran away as soon as Dante came barreling out of the warehouse."

"First she got lucky in that the window closed behind her as she fell, so from the outside it still looked locked. Second, Brandon wasn't aware of the storage basement. The factory had stopped using it before he was born, and the only real door had been bricked over years ago. And third, he never had a lot of time to search."

"It is busy around there." May nodded.

"Yep, and just as he rounded the corner of the building, he caught a glimpse of his brother coming around the opposite side. He barely had time to take off the jumpsuit and hide it behind some boxes before JJ spotted him. Then, once his brother saw him, JJ grabbed Brandon and hustled him back inside the plant because Grandma Sal was looking for him."

"Didn't Brandon go back later to look for Ashley?" Frannie asked.

"He couldn't do much while people were working in the factory. Then he had to be available for the contest, and he was rooming with his brother, who would have wondered where he was if he left in the middle of the night."

"What I don't understand is why he didn't at least dispose of the jumpsuit." Uncle Charlie frowned. "It was one of the few pieces of physical evidence that tied him to the murder."

"Remember how windy it was that day?" Skye asked. "It had blown away by the time he was able to get back to pick it up. When I found it later, there were too many people around and he couldn't do anything about it, except hope it would never be linked to him. But the lab found traces of Dante's blood type and chocolate similar to the fountain. They're testing to see if the blood really is Dante's and if the other DNA on it is Brandon's, but we know it is."

May finished the dishes and opened the drain. "What else did he do to interfere with the contest?"

"Three things I know about." Skye got up

and poured herself a glass of Diet Coke. "One, he arranged for Glenda Doozier to take Cherry's place. He'd heard stories about the Dooziers his whole life, so when he saw she had entered, he figured her family would stir things up during the contest. Second, he made sure she won the special Cherry Alexander Award, counting on her doing something during the ceremony to make the contest look bad."

"You said there was a third thing?" Justin reminded Skye.

"After the press conference the first day, I overheard two people talking in the teachers' lounge, and I finally figured out Brandon might be one of those people, so I had Wally ask him about it. Turns out one of the contestants, Imogene Ingersoll, bribed Brandon to give her all the background info that Fine Foods had gathered on one of the other contestants. He was glad to do it, figuring that if she got caught it would be another black mark for the contest, and the company."

"Wasn't Brandon afraid Imogene would take him down with her?" asked Justin.

"I guess he didn't think his family would believe Imogene over him." Skye shrugged.

"Imogene Ingersoll was the woman I said looked so familiar." May wiped her hands on a dishtowel and came over to the table. "I wish I could place her."

"Hey, I almost forgot." Skye grabbed her tote from the utility room, where she had left it on top of the dryer. "Here's a picture of the finalists that was taken during the awards ceremony, and there's Imogene." She pointed to a woman standing next to Vince. "Does anyone know her?"

While everyone around the table examined the print, Wally came in from the living room and joined them. "Maybe I do, but I'm not sure."

"Who do you think it is?" Skye prodded.

"If you visualize her without the glasses and wig, and a little thinner, she's that woman who impersonated a state police officer when we were investigating the murder of that model last November." Wally leaned closer to the picture. "Only then she was going by the name Veronica Vale."

Skye reexamined the photo. "You could be right." She turned to him, frowning. "How come you recognized her when Mom and I didn't?"

"I spent a lot more time with her than either of you did," Wally explained. "You both saw her for at most thirty to forty-five minutes while you were stressed out, while I spent several hours with her."

"If you're right, and Imogene is Veronica, that's pretty creepy." May made a face. "Why would she turn up again, and with a new name?"

Skye suddenly felt a little light-headed and abruptly sat down. Wally turned to her in concern. "Are you all right?"

"Yes. It's just that Brandon said that the person whom Imogene/Veronica was asking him about was me. Why would she want to know about me and my family?"

Everyone was silent as they considered Skye's question. Finally Wally said, "Maybe she had you confused with May. Everyone thought she had the best odds to win, so maybe this woman was trying to get a leg up on the competition."

"But why pretend to be a police officer and change her name?" Skye shook her head. "I don't like it. She's after something. I just wish I knew what it was."

They all spent the rest of the afternoon and evening trying to figure out who the mysterious woman was and what she wanted. Everyone had a guess, but no one had an answer.

By the time she and Wally left, Skye had a headache and wanted nothing more than to go to bed, even if it was only eight o'clock at night. She said good-night to him without inviting him in, then fed Bingo and went upstairs.

After changing into her nightshirt, she crawled into the big four-poster and lay staring at the ceiling. Tired as she was, she couldn't shut off her whirling thoughts. Was Imogene Veronica? Why would she change identities? Why would she want to know about Skye and her family?

A half hour went by, and Skye still couldn't think of a reason. Another half hour went by and Skye stared at the clock. Something else was bugging her, but what?

Was it that Wally hadn't had her meet his father when Carson Boyd first came to town? He had explained his reasoning, but did she believe him? Not being introduced to the potential in-laws was a red flag that a guy wasn't that into you. Was that the case with Wally?

Skye pulled the blanket up over her head. She couldn't answer either question tonight. She needed to sleep. Everything would look better in the morning.

■ ■ ■ ■

WINNING RECIPES FROM GRANDMA SAL'S SOUP-TO-NUTS COOKING CHALLENGE

■ ■ ■ ■

Try these four "winning" recipes, personally created by Denise Swanson, her friends and family. Denise likes to cook a lot more than Skye does. . . .

WINNER OF THE HEALTHY CATEGORY
MONIKA'S GLUTEN-FREE AND DAIRY-FREE
SPONGE CAKE

6 eggs
1 cup white sugar
5 tablespoons white rice flour
5 tablespoons cornstarch
2 teaspoon baking powder
1/2 teaspoon xanthan gum*
Optional: 1/2 cup Hershey's cocoa powder

Preheat oven to 350 degrees. Break eggs into a warm mixing bowl and beat with an electric mixer on medium-high speed until thick (several minutes). Gradually add half the sugar and continue beating until the mixture holds together. Sift together flour, cornstarch, remaining sugar, baking powder, xanthan gum, and cocoa, if using. Fold dry

* Xanthan gum is used in gluten-free baking to give the dough or batter a "stickiness" that would otherwise be achieved with the gluten. It is available in health food stores and specialty grocery stores.

mixture into egg mixture. Beat on low speed for one minute.

Spray two 8-inch round cake pans with PAM, then pour in batter.

Bake in preheated oven for 15 minutes or until toothpick inserted into center comes out clean.

Immediately remove cakes from their pans. Cool on a cake rack. **Warning:** Be gentle — cakes break apart easily. When cakes are completely cooled, frost and assemble layers.

GLUTEN-FREE AND DAIRY-FREE FROSTING

Blend together in a mixer on medium speed: One stick Nucoa Margarine* and one stick Crisco until fluffy.

Gradually mix in one box (or 1 lb.) confectioners' sugar — more as needed to make a fluffy frosting.

Beat in one teaspoon vanilla extract.

Add a few drops of soy milk until frosting is easy to spread.

* Nucoa is the brand name of a margarine that does not contain any milk solids and is thus dairy-free, as well as free of protein and phenylalanine. It is a lactose-free, cholesterol-free margarine that is distributed by GFA Brands, Inc., Cresskill, NJ, and is available at most large grocery stores.

WINNER OF THE SNACKS CATEGORY
FIESTA ITALIANO DIP

1/4 cup sour cream
1/2 cup mayonnaise
10-oz. package frozen finely chopped spinach, thawed and drained
14-oz. can artichoke hearts, finely chopped
1 teaspoon garlic salt
1/4 teaspoon basil
1/4 teaspoon oregano
1/4 teaspoon red pepper
4 oz. mozzarella, shredded
4 oz. provolone, shredded
8-oz. can of Italian-seasoned chopped tomatoes
Thinly sliced rounds of Italian bread

Preheat oven to 350 degrees.

Mix together the sour cream and mayonnaise. Add spinach, artichokes, and seasonings. Mix well. Stir in cheeses. Pour into a medium-sized casserole dish and bake at 350 degrees for thirty minutes, or until cheese is melted. Sprinkle with room-temperature tomatoes and serve on bread rounds.

WINNER OF THE ONE-DISH MEALS CATEGORY MAY'S CHICKEN SUPREME CASSEROLE

Note: You'll notice that for purposes of the plot, Skye's version of this recipe differs slightly from mine, which comes from Grandma Swanson.

2 cups cooked chicken, diced
7 oz. elbow macaroni, uncooked
2 cups milk
1 can cream of mushroom soup
1 can cream of celery soup
1/2 pound Velveeta cheese, cubed
1 4-oz. jar pimentos, drained
1/4 cup chopped green pepper
1 small onion, chopped
1 teaspoon salt
1/2 teaspoon pepper
1 cup bread crumbs
1/4 cup butter, melted

Preheat oven to 350 degrees.

Combine all ingredients except for the

bread crumbs and butter in a large bowl. Pour into a greased casserole dish and refrigerate overnight. Bring back to room temperature before baking. Bake at 350 degrees for 50 minutes.

Combine 1 cup bread crumbs and 1/4 cup melted butter. Sprinkle on top of hot casserole and return to oven for 5 to 10 minutes, until bread crumbs are browned.

WINNER OF THE SPECIAL-OCCASION BAKING CATEGORY AND THE GRAND PRIZE
CHOCOLATE BROWNIE TIRAMISU

For the brownies:

1 cup shortening
4 1-oz. squares unsweetened chocolate
4 eggs
2 cups sugar
2 teaspoons vanilla
1 1/2 cups flour
1 tcaspoon baking powder
1 teaspoon salt

Preheat oven to 350 degrees.

Melt shortening and chocolate together in double boiler. Cool to room temperature. In a separate bowl, beat eggs with a mixer on high speed until light. Stir in sugar, then add chocolate mixture and vanilla. Sift together dry ingredients, then add to batter and mix well. Pour into a greased 9-by-13 pan and bake at 350 degrees for 30 minutes. Set aside to cool.

For the topping:
8 egg yolks
1/2 cup sugar
1/4 cup milk
2 cups whipping cream
16 oz. mascarpone cheese
1/2 cup sugar
2 cups brewed and cooled Godiva
   raspberry-flavored coffee
1/4 cup Godiva liqueur
2 1/2 oz. semisweet chocolate, grated
Cocoa powder
Chocolate shavings

Whisk together egg yolks, sugar, and milk
in a 2-quart saucepan until smooth and
blended. Bring to a boil over medium heat,
stirring constantly. As soon as mixture
reaches a boil, remove from heat. Immediately refrigerate until cool.

With an electric mixer, beat whipping cream
at high speed until it forms very stiff peaks.
Set aside in the refrigerator.

Mix the mascarpone cheese and sugar. Stir
in the yolk mixture. Fold in the whipped
cream.

Combine the coffee and Godiva liqueur in
a large mixing bowl.

To assemble:

Cut brownies into 2-by-1/2-inch strips. Quickly dip each strip in the coffee mixture and place on the bottom of a 9-by-13 baking dish. Sprinkle with half the semisweet chocolate. Cover with half of the cheese mixture. Add another layer of dipped brownies. Sprinkle with remaining semisweet chocolate and finish with the cheese mixture.

Sift cocoa powder over the top and garnish with chocolate shavings.

Refrigerate overnight for best flavor. Serve in chilled dessert bowls.

ABOUT THE AUTHOR

Denise Swanson worked as a school psychologist for more than twenty-two years. She lives in Illinois with her husband, Dave, who is a classical music composer, and their cool black cat, Boomerang. For more information, visit her Web site at www.denise swanson.com.